Menopause Essentials

Renuka Malik • Kiran Aggarwal
Anuradha Singh • Vandana Agarwal
Editors

Menopause Essentials

Clinical Insights and Management

Springer

Editors
Renuka Malik
Professor and Principal Consultant,
Department of Obstetrics and Gynaecology
Atal Bihari Vajpayee Institute of Medical Sciences and Dr. Ram Manohar Lohia Hospital
New Delhi, India

Anuradha Singh
Professor, Department of Obstetrics and Gynaecology
Lady Hardinge Medical College
New Delhi, India

Kiran Aggarwal
Director Professor, Department of Obstetrics and Gynaecology
Lady Hardinge Medical College
New Delhi, India

Vandana Agarwal
Assistant Professor, Department of Obstetrics and Gynaecology
Atal Bihari Vajpayee Institute of Medical Sciences and Dr. Ram Manohar Lohia Hospital
New Delhi, India

ISBN 978-981-95-7497-1 ISBN 978-981-95-7498-8 (eBook)
https://doi.org/10.1007/978-981-95-7498-8

This Springer imprint is published by the registered company Springer Nature Singapore Pte Ltd.
The registered company address is: 152 Beach Road, #21-01/04 Gateway East, Singapore 189721, Singapore

Foreword

It gives me immense pleasure to pen the Foreword for this book, *Menopause Essentials-Clinical Insights and Management.* At the outset, I would like to congratulate Professor Renuka Malik and her team for bringing out a comprehensive book on an extremely pertinent, yet not completely understood, phase of every woman's life, i.e., the menopause.

Menopause and midlife management have become an entire sub-specialty in the field of Obstetrics and Gynecology, in today's era. With increasing life expectancy, women worldwide now spend about one-third of their lives in this phase. The peri- and post-menopausal phase comes with its own set of unique challenges, which needs to be thoroughly understood in order to render personalized care. Numerous interventions ranging from lifestyle modifications, nutritional adjustments, pharmacological interventions, and alternative remedies make it possible for women to overcome these challenges successfully and have a good quality of life. This one-of-a-kind textbook is designed beautifully with chapters covering all important aspects of the menopause, ranging from the pathophysiology, clinical spectrum, management as well as preventive aspects of the various symptoms which a menopausal woman may encounter.

I congratulate all the eminent authors from across the nation who have drafted each chapter so comprehensively using their vast knowledge and expertise. The 27 chapters have been systematically designed and presented in a very reader friendly, lucid format. I am sure this book will indeed serve as a ready reckoner not only for postgraduate students but also for clinical practitioners and equip them with up-to-date knowledge in the rapidly advancing field of menopause, empowering them to serve with clarity and confidence.

I wish Professor Renuka Malik and the entire team my heartiest congratulations and best wishes for future endeavors.

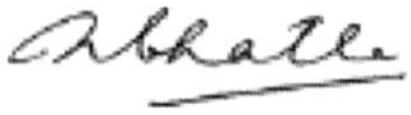

Professor Neerja Bhatla

Preface

Life is a journey, and menopause is just another step on the path. Keep moving forward.
—Anonymous

Menopause is a natural, inevitable phase of life that every woman is going to encounter. This phase of life represents an "*opportunity*" that should be fully seized. The period of transition from perimenopause to menopause comes with its own unique set of challenges. However, in countries like India, majority of women suffer in silence owing to cultural and societal stigma. There are many unspoken aspects of this integral phase of life which needs to be correctly addressed.

There is paucity of standard textbooks, covering the entire gamut of "*Menopause*" which has become a sub-speciality in itself, in today's era. There is dearth of up-to-date, evidence-based information on this pertinent aspect of women's health. It is not covered in depth in the postgraduate curriculum as well. However, it is extremely imperative that every gynecologist is well versed with the ailments that a menopausal woman may present with and provide her quality care.

This textbook was conceptualized to fill this gap in knowledge. It comprises of 27 chapters designed meticulously, covering all the aspects of menopause ranging from the pathophysiology to the various symptoms, their assessment and management. The authors have been carefully chosen as experts in their field and their efforts are well appreciated by the editors. Awareness, preventive measures, and medical intervention at this crucial stage of life offer women years of benefit—with respect to bone health, mental health, sleep, cognition as well as cardiovascular health. Stalwarts in their specific field of expertise have comprehensively drafted each chapter, providing up-to-date, evidence-based information in a lucid, reader-friendly format. Questions in the form of short and long questions along with multiple choice questions have been included at the end of each chapter to facilitate better comprehension.

We hope this textbook serves as a handy, comprehensive, ready reckoner, a source of up-to-date information for the postgraduate aspirants, the practicing gynecologists, and all interested in this topic. Clinicians who interact with women in this phase of their life have a wonderful opportunity along with a significant obligation to provide individualized, quality care and also empower them to live this potentially challenging, yet beautiful phase of life with grace and confidence.

Happy learning!

Renuka Malik
Kiran Aggarwal
Anuradha Singh
Vandana Agarwal

Contents

Contributors

Vandana Agarwal Assistant Professor, Department of Obstetrics & Gynaecology, Atal Bihari Vajpayee Institute of Medical Sciences & Dr. Ram Manohar Lohia Hospital, New Delhi, India

Anshita Aggarwal Associate Professor, Department of Endocrinology, Atal Bihari Vajpayee Institute of Medical Sciences & Dr. Ram Manohar Lohia Hospital, New Delhi, India

Kiran Aggarwal Director Professor, Department of Obstetrics and Gynaecology, Lady Hardinge Medical College & Smt Sucheta Kriplani Hospital, New Delhi, India

Ragini Agrawal Director, A.A. Dermascience, Complete Clinic for Women Health, Gurugram, Haryana, India

Sana Ahmed Senior Resident, Department of Obstetrics and Gynaecology, UCMS & GTB Hospital, Delhi, India

Meenakshi Ahuja Senior Director, Fortis la femme, New Delhi, India

Mrinalini Ahuja Santosh Dental College, Ghaziabad, Uttar Pradesh, India

Asna Beg Ashraf Consultant & Director, Ujala Medical Center, Lucknow, India
Ex-Officio Secretary, Lucknow Menopause Society, Lucknow, India
Founder Member & Joint Secretary, Stillbirth Society of India, Lucknow, India

Jyoti Bhaskar Additional Director, Cloudnine Noida and Delhi, New Delhi, India
Secretary, Delhi Menopause Society, Delhi, India

Monal Garg Fellow, Gynaecological Oncology, National Cancer Center, Goyang, South Korea

Sharmistha Garg Consultant, Department of Obstetrics and Gynaecology, Sir Ganga Ram Hospital, New Delhi, India

Deepti Goswami Director Professor, Obstetrics & Gynaecology, Maulana Azad Medical College, New Delhi, India

Shobha N. Gudi Professor & Head of Department, St. Philomenas Hospital & Consultant, Manipal Sagar and Excel Care Hospitals, Bengaluru, India

Ananta Khurana Professor, Department of Dermatology, Venereology and Leprosy, Atal Bihari Vajpayee Institute of Medical Sciences and Dr Ram Manohar Lohia Hospital, New Delhi, Delhi, India

Jaismine Kaur Kohli Senior Resident, Department of Dermatology, Venereology and Leprosy, Atal Bihari Vajpayee Institute of Medical Sciences and Dr Ram Manohar Lohia Hospital, New Delhi, Delhi, India

Kavita Kumari CMO (NFSG), Department of Obstetrics & Gynecology, Atal Bihari Vajpayee Institute of Medical Sciences & Dr. Ram Manohar Lohia Hospital, New Delhi, India

Akanshi Madan Lead Medical Gynaecology, Obstetrician, Tanvir Hospital, Hyderabad, Telangana, India

Renuka Malik Professor and Principal Consultant, Department of Obstetrics and Gynaecology, Atal Bihari Vajpayee Institute of Medical Sciences and Dr. Ram Manohar Lohia Hospital, New Delhi, India

Geeta Mediratta Senior Consultant, Department of Obstetrics and Gynaecology, Sir Ganga Ram Hospital, New Delhi, India

Meeta Meeta Consultant, Head Obgyn and Co-director, Tanvir Hospital, Hyderabad, Telangana, India

Dr. Rajat Mohan Senior Consultant, Department of Cardiology, Sir Ganga Ram Hospital, New Delhi, Delhi, India

Vandana Parti Consultant, Department of Men's Health, Women's Health & Gerontology, Baba Farid University, Faridkot, Punjab, India
Consultant & Visiting Faculty & Advisor for Children & Adolescent Health, Scottish High International School, Gurgaon, India

Padmini Prasad Consultant Obstetrician & Gynaecologist and Sexologist & Marriage Counsellor, Institute of Sexual Medicine, Ramamani Nursing and Maternity Home, Bangalore, India

A. G. Radhika Senior Consultant, Department of Obstetrics and Gynaecology, UCMS & GTB Hospital, Delhi, India

Deepshikha Rajput Senior Resident, Department of Gynaecological Oncology, King George's Medical University, Lucknow, India

Brijesh Saran Associate Professor, Department of Psychiatry, Santosh Deemed to be University, Delhi NCR, India

Bipasa Sen Senior Consultant, Department of Obstetrics & Gynecology, Sterling Hospital, Kolkata, India
Vice President, Indian Menopause Society, IMS, Sterling Hospital, Kolkata, India

Nalini Sharma Professor, Department of Obstetrics and Gynaecology, Geetanjali Medical College and Hospital, Udaipur, Rajasthan, India
President, Indian Menopause Society (IMS), Mumbai, India

Sudhaa Sharma Former Professor, Department of Obstetrics and Gynaecology, GMC Jammu, Jammu, India

Aarshika Singh Associate Consultant, Fortis la femme, New Delhi, India

Pranav Mohan Singhal Fellow, Thoracic Surgical Oncology, National Cancer Center, Goyang, South Korea

Anuradha Singh Professor, Department of Obstetrics and Gynaecology, Lady Hardinge Medical College, New Delhi, India

Nisha Singh Professor, Department of Gynaecological Oncology, King George's Medical University, Lucknow, India

Anshul Solanki Junior Resident, Obstetrics & Gynaecology, Maulana Azad Medical College, New Delhi, India

Jyotsna Suri Professor and Senior Consultant, Department of Obstetrics & Gynaecology, Vardhman Mahavir Medical College & Safdarjung Hospital, New Delhi, India

Tejas Menon Suri Assistant Professor, Department of Pulmonary, Critical Care & Sleep Medicine, All India Institute of Medical Sciences, New Delhi, India

Neha Pruthi Tandon Associate Professor, Department of Obstetrics & Gynecology, Atal Bihari Vajpayee Institute of Medical Sciences & Dr. Ram Manohar Lohia Hospital, New Delhi, India

Tanvir Tanvir Lead Gynaecological Surgeon, Urogynecology, Tanvir Hospital, Hyderabad, Telangana, India

Jyothi Unni Director, Department of Obstetrics and Gynecology, Jehangir Hospital, Pune, Maharashtra, India

Yukti Wadhawan Director & Fertility Specialist, Yukti IVF & Gynaecology, New Delhi, India

Menopause—An Overview

1

Vandana Agarwal and Renuka Malik

And the beauty of a woman, with passing years only grows!

Audrey Hepburn

Abstract

This chapter is an introduction to a topic which often gets swept under the rug in the world of health and wellness—*Menopause*. This chapter provides an overview about the topic, attempting to debunk the myths about menopause, explaining the science behind the body's hormonal shift. It sheds light on the epidemiology, genetic basis, and the often-overlooked challenges and symptoms of menopause. This chapter is an introduction to the various practical solutions for meeting these challenges, from lifestyle changes, stress management to hormonal therapy and community support. This aims to lay the foundation for the subsequent chapters in the textbook, as we embark on this journey of empowering ourselves with knowledge. Menopause is not the end; it is a new beginning, a time for women to "tune in" to their bodies and embrace this new chapter of life with zeal and confidence.

Keywords

Menopause · Pathophysiology of menopause · Epidemiology of menopause · Barriers to menopause care

V. Agarwal (✉) · R. Malik
Department of Obstetrics & Gynaecology, Atal Bihari Vajpayee Institute of Medical Sciences & Dr. Ram Manohar Lohia Hospital, New Delhi, India

R. Malik et al. (eds.), *Menopause Essentials*,
https://doi.org/10.1007/978-981-95-7498-8_1

1.1 Introduction

Menopause is defined as the natural, permanent cessation of menstruation due to estrogen deficiency, which is not associated with a pathological process. The word "menopause" is derived from Greek words "*pausis*", meaning pause, and "men", meaning month. The period of amenorrhea lasting for 12 months marks the end of a woman's reproductive and childbearing age [1]. It may be natural or iatrogenic. The cause of natural menopause is aging-related loss of ovarian function, while iatrogenic menopause results from medical interventions like the removal of the ovaries. It is a retrospective diagnosis, starting 1 year after the last menstrual period.

The majority of menopausal women experience vasomotor symptoms; however, a myriad of other symptoms, including sleep and cognitive impairment, may also occur. Menopause can affect various organ systems, such as the urogenital, psychogenic, and cardiovascular systems. This increases the risk of certain diseases like osteoporosis, cardiovascular disease, metabolic disorders, etc. In the modern world and changing times, women are living longer. About one-third of one's life is spent in the menopausal period, which is about 30 years on average. Therefore, it is crucial to ensure that these golden years are as healthy and productive as possible [2].

1.2 Epidemiology

Menopause occurs between the ages of 45 and 56 years in the majority of women. The average age of reaching menopause in Indian women is 46.6 years, which is earlier than the global average of 51 years [3]. However, the symptoms of perimenopause may begin as early as the 40s. Women who attain menopause at an age of less than 40 years are termed to have "premature menopause." The women who enter menopause between 40 and 45 years are classified as "early menopause," while the ones who attain it after 55 years are classified as having "late menopause."

Perimenopause and menopause seem to occur earlier in women who have undergone oophorectomy, primary ovarian insufficiency (POI), hysterectomy, pelvic radiation therapy, and who practice active tobacco consumption. Race and ethnicity also affect the variations in the transition to menopause.

According to a longitudinal cohort study of 3302 women in the US (Study of Women's Health Across the Nation, SWAN study), Japanese and Chinese women had longer menstrual cycle lengths as compared to the Non-Hispanic White women [4]. Black women experienced more severe vasomotor symptoms (VMS) and had a longer menopause transition phase. As per an extensive online survey of 68,864 US women, Black, Hispanic, Indigenous, and Middle Eastern women were noted to have more bothersome menopausal symptoms than the Non-Hispanic White women, even after accounting for socioeconomic factors [5].

The average life expectancy of women in India is 72 years, as compared to 80 years in the United States, as per the latest census [6, 7]. Despite its prevalence, perimenopausal as well as menopausal symptoms are often under-reported, underscreened, and under-treated. This results in a significant decrease in one's quality of life and loss of productivity [8]. They have a negative impact on the economy as well. It is estimated that the cost associated with the loss of work productivity due to untreated menopausal symptoms is $1.8 billion in the US annually [9]. Menopausal women face unique challenges in their work life, leading to absenteeism and loss of productivity.

1.3 Barriers to Accessing Menopause-Related Care

Barriers to accessing care related to menopause exist at the patient, provider, as well as at the system level. Patient factors range from a lack of knowledge to stigma and concerns surrounding the discussion of symptoms and adverse effects of therapy. According to an online study of more than 800 postmenopausal women (mostly from the UK), 94% of them said they had never been educated about menopause, and 60% of them first started looking for information about menopause after they began to experience symptoms associated to the menopause [10]. 25% of women did not talk about their symptoms because they believed they were a normal part of menopause, according to another online study that sampled the experiences of 196 US women with menopause and their pursuit of treatment [11]. A survey analysis of women in the SWAN study indicated that 61% did not report urinary incontinence symptoms, citing a perception of mild severity and viewing urinary incontinence as a natural aspect of aging [12].

Patients consider symptoms like dyspareunia, hypoactive sexual drive, and other genitourinary ailments as a social taboo. They do not feel comfortable in discussing them in a clinical setting. Furthermore, a woman's decision to seek menopause-related treatment is influenced by her anxiety and worry about the negative effects of hormone therapy. According to a sub-analysis of 500 US women who took part in the Vaginal Health: Insights, Views & Attitudes (VIVA) survey, majority expressed negative associations with hormone therapy with concerns about the risk of breast cancer and stroke. Enhancing patients' understanding of menopause and available treatments prior to the onset of symptoms may empower them to discuss these concerns. In a study that used a telephone, nurse educator-based intervention with a menopause booklet to educate women about menopausal symptoms and treatment options, participants' knowledge of menopause increased, there was less conflict over treatment options, and 94% of participants said they felt more prepared to talk to their healthcare provider about their symptoms [13].

From the perspective of a provider, time constraints, communication problems, personal beliefs about menopause, and a lack of expertise and confidence in prescribing menopausal hormone therapy can all be major obstacles to providing menopause-related care. Menopause as a subject is not dealt in depth in the medical curriculum as well. It is important that menopause as a topic is incorporated in the curriculum of undergraduate as well as postgraduate medical education. This will improve the trainee's understanding and self-assurance when delivering care linked to menopause. It is a pity that society at large and even many health-care professionals tell women to simply accept the misery of this transition and the related illnesses such as cardiovascular disease, osteoporosis, diabetes, and cognitive decline. The primary reason behind this is the lack of awareness regarding this integral part of a woman's life and the various pharmacological as well as non-pharmacological tools available to face the challenges which might come up in this pivotal phase of a woman's life.

The outlook towards menopause has fortunately started to change and there is renewed interest in menopause since past couple of years. After decades of neglect, research and public awareness have increased regarding this crucial, unavoidable part of a woman's life. It is undoubtedly a therapeutic space with enormous potential payoff. Menopause affects half of the population and disrupts a period when women are in their prime professionally, especially in the urban areas.

1.4 Pathophysiology of Menopause

Menopause's pathophysiology can be complex. Ovarian follicle depletion begins before birth and lasts the entirety of a woman's life. Granulosa cells of preantral and antral ovarian follicles generate large levels of anti-mullerian hormone (AMH) and inhibin B before menopause. To maintain the follicular pool throughout a woman's "reproductive" years, they limit the number of follicles available for ovulation every month. The quantity and size of follicles eventually reach a point where inhibin B and AMH, which limit follicle growth, start to decline. This results in an exponential depletion of ovarian follicles and the beginning of menopause transition [5].

Initially, this causes longer luteal phases and irregular menstrual bleeding patterns. Menstrual irregularity lasting more than or equal to 7 days is a specific indicator of the menopause transition period. Significant hormonal fluctuations, such as variations in estradiol levels, are common during the menopause transition, when menopausal symptoms frequently start to manifest. Over the course of the menopausal transition, the maturation of the ovarian follicle, known as folliculogenesis and estradiol production, gradually decreases, leading to a rise in irregular menstruation and symptoms of estrogen deficiency. In the end, folliculogenesis is no longer possible, and the generation of progesterone and estradiol ceases, resulting in persistent amenorrhea.

Menopause, then, is a physiological process in which the quantity of primary ovarian follicles rapidly decreases to the point where there are inadequate amounts to respond to the effects of FSH. Because there is no LH surge, ovulation does not take place, which results in a decrease in estrogen and the end of menstruation. Years after the onset of menopause, FSH and LH continue to remain at high levels. In certain people, symptoms other than the cessation of menstruation may be insignificant since the adrenal gland can still create small levels of estrogen through the conversion of testosterone [14]. More than 80% of women experience menopausal symptoms. However, a woman's individual experience of menopause changes, varies greatly. The physiological process of menopause is influenced by a number of factors. Body mass index, socioeconomic status, diet, exercise, smoking, ethnicity, pre-existing medical conditions, and overall gynecological health are some of the important determinants which influence menopausal symptoms [14].

1.5 Genetic Regulation of Menopause

Myriad biological and genetic factors influence the timing of menopause. Gaining knowledge about these factors that influence ovarian aging can help one better understand reproductive biology and related medical disorders. Both the onset of menopause and the control of fertility are significantly influenced by the DNA damage response (DDR). The timing of menopause was connected to FSHB (follicle-stimulating hormone subunit beta), one of 37 important genes linked to reproductive outcomes found in a large-scale genome-wide association study (GWAS) [15].

Polygenic risk scores (PRSs) were computed after data from individuals with extremes of age at natural menopause (ANM) (beyond the 40–60-year range) were added in order to examine the genetic drivers of ANM across the entire age range. Premature ovarian insufficiency (POI), or early menopause at less than 40 years of age, can be identified by the PRSs. The findings showed that POI may have a polygenic etiology, despite the fact that it is often thought to be a Mendelian (monogenic) disorder. Premutations in FMR1, a recognized monogenic cause of POI, were equivalent to the risk of POI for women with the top 1% Polygenic risk score for early menopause.

Since the *FMR1* premutation is carried by 1:250 of the population, it is rarer than individuals with the top 1% of PRSs. Therefore, compared to certain specifically recognized monogenic causes, polygenic causes of POI may be more common.

1.6 Stages of Reproductive Aging

The nomenclature for the menopausal transition stages was standardized in 2001 by the Stages of Reproductive Aging Workshop (STRAW). There was no recognized method for identifying the phases of reproductive aging that precede menopause, prior to this workshop. The criterion was revised in 2010 at a follow-up workshop ("STRAW +10") to take into account advancements in changes in hypothalamic-pituitary function that occur throughout reproductive age (Table 1.1) [16]. The STRAW staging system divides female life span into three broad phases: reproductive phase, menopausal transition phase, and postmenopause phase. Based on data from clinical (menstrual cycle pattern, symptoms) and investigative (serum levels of follicle-stimulating hormone (FSH), antimüllerian hormone (AMH), and ultrasound-based ovarian antral) methods, each of the three phases is divided into stages.

1.7 Clinical Presentation of Menopause

Menopause is a physiological period, which coincides with the end of the reproductive period, and is characterized by high variability in symptomatology. It is preceded by a period of about 4–5 years, termed as *Perimenopause.* It is characterized by fluctuations in the hormonal levels which can launch a rollercoaster of symptoms. These symptoms can continue into the postmenopausal years.

Table 1.1 The Stages of Reproductive Aging Workshop 10 staging system for reproductive aging in women [16].

Menarche (at stage −5); FMP (0) (between stages −1 and +1a)

Stage	-5	-4	-3b	-3a	-2	-1	+1a	+1b	+1c	+2
TERMINOLOGY	REPRODUCTIVE				MENOPAUSAL TRANSITION		POSTMENOPAUSE			
	EARLY	PEAK	LATE		EARLY	LATE	EARLY			LATE
					Perimenopause					
Duration	variable				variable	1-3 years	2 years (1+1)	3-6 years		*Remaining lifespan*
PRINICIPAL CRITERIA										
Menstrual cycle	Variable to regular	Regular	Regular	Subtle changes in flow/length	Variable Length Persistent >=7 days difference in length of consecutive cycles	Interval of amenorrhea of >=60 days				
SUPPORTIVE CRITERIA										
ENDOCRINE										
FSH			Low	Variable	$\uparrow$ Variable	$\uparrow$ >25 IU/L	$\uparrow$ Variable	Stabilizes		
AMH			Low	Low	Low	Low	Low	Very Low		
Inhibin B			-	Low	Low	Low	Low	Very Low		
Antral Follicle Count			Low	Low	Low	Low	Very Low	Very Low		
DESCRIPTIVE CHARACTERISTICS										
Symptoms						Vasomotor Symptoms *Likely*	Vasomotor Symptoms *Most Likely*			Increasing symptoms of urogenital atrophy

FMP: Final menstrual period

FMP Final menstrual period

Menopausal symptoms, which include both physical and psychological symptoms, vary greatly in frequency and intensity from person to person. Perimenopause and menopause symptoms can range from vasomotor symptoms (VMS), irregular menstruation, skin changes, genitourinary symptoms, diminished libido, sleep disturbances, mood swings as well as cognitive decline (Table 1.2). Cardiovascular disease, dyslipidemia, type 2 diabetes, metabolic syndrome, osteoporosis, and sarcopenia are among the chronic illnesses that are made more likely by the decrease in estrogen levels during menopause. Approximately 80% of postmenopausal women experience VMS, such as hot flashes and night sweats, while up to 50% report genitourinary symptoms, including vulvovaginal atrophy, vaginal dryness, dyspareunia, incontinence, and urinary urgency. Furthermore, approximately 40% of women experience depression during menopause [4].

Table 1.2 Clinical symptoms of menopause

❖	**VASOMOTOR HOT FLASHES**
❖	**UROGENITAL SYMPTOMS** ▪ Dyspareunia ▪ Urinary incontinence ▪ Vulvovaginal atrophy ▪ Vaginal dryness ▪ Urinary urgency
❖	**COGNITIVE CHANGES**
❖	**MOOD DISTURBANCES**
❖	**SEXUAL DYSFUNCTION**
❖	**SLEEP DISTURBANCES**

1.8 Management of Menopausal Symptoms

Menopausal hormone therapy was the gold standard for treating menopausal symptoms for decades. However, its popularity plummeted in 2002 after the initial report of the US-based study, Women's Health Initiative (WHI) [17]. It stated that women treated with estrogen and progestin had slightly increased risk of breast cancer, cardiovascular accident as well as stroke. Since then, a number of studies have challenged these initial conclusions, emphasizing the advantages and disadvantages of the strategy as well as the significance of taking into account variables including the patient's age, previous diseases, and the route of administration of the therapy.

A review of the WHI trial in May 2024 revealed the study's many subtleties and limitations [18]. They reiterated that the WHI trial's hormone composition, dose, and mode of delivery were different from modern practices. For instance, the transdermal route of medication is better than the oral route in terms of avoiding first pass metabolism, which reduces side effects. Furthermore, the majority of the women who participated in the WHI experiment were at least 10 years postmenopausal. According to research, a sudden increase in estrogen levels may lead to health issues; therefore, the timing of starting hormone therapy is crucial.

MHT is regarded as the cornerstone of treatment for VMS. By avoiding first-pass hepatic metabolism, transdermal MHT provides a clear safety advantage over oral preparations, lowering the risk of venous thromboembolism and other cardiovascular problems. Transdermal MHT is a better choice for women at higher risk; however, oral MHT is still appropriate for those without risk factors for CVD or venous thromboembolism [19].

Neurokinin-1 receptor (NK1R) and neurokinin-3 receptor (NK3R) antagonists, such as fezolinetant and elinzanetant, are non-hormonal therapies for VMS. These emerging drugs affect the thermoregulatory pathways, providing women who are unable or unwilling to take hormonal therapy with a viable option [20]. Furthermore, a useful alternative treatment for vasomotor symptoms and enhancing quality of life is cognitive behavior therapy. During the menopausal transition and the years that follow, lifestyle therapies that promote long-term health and quality of life include weight-bearing exercise, balanced nutrition, and cardiovascular monitoring. It is highly imperative that health care providers are abreast with the latest, evidence-based guidelines inorder to appropriately counsel and treat women, thereby helping them embrace this new phase of life with confidence (Fig. 1.1).

1.9 Menopause as an Opportunity

Menopause is a normal phase of life, much like puberty; it should not be viewed as abnormal. For many women, it is a welcome change—no further menses or premenstrual syndrome (PMS) and no need for contraception/concern for conceiving. Clinicians who interact with women at the time of the menopause have a great opportunity and, consequently, a significant responsibility. Women who receive medical intervention at this stage of life can benefit from preventive health care for years to come. This stage of life represents an opportunity that should be fully seized. While not underrating the importance of good health habits among the young, we would contend that the impact of teaching preventive care is more observable and more tangible at middle age. The prospects of morbidity of chronic diseases and mortality are viewed with understanding and appreciation during these twilight years. The chance of illness is higher, but the impact of changes in lifestyle is greater.

1.10 Scope for Research

Can menopause be reversed? This is a question which has harnessed great interest. Scientific studies have been looking at prospects like Stem cell therapy, Bioidentical hormones derived from plant source, as a better substitute to the traditional Hormone replacement therapy, Ovarian Rejuvenation with Platelet-rich plasma and Epigenetic modifications for prolonging the lifespan of ovaries. However, these are highly debatable issues associated with a lot of ethical dilemmas [21].

1.11 Conclusion

Navigating menopause is a personal journey. A person's quality of life and general health can be greatly impacted by the symptoms of perimenopause and menopause, which can last for an average of 4–10 years. Educating health care providers as well as patients on the various symptoms and treatment options is essential to reduce barriers, improve access to menopause related care, and improve her overall well-being in midlife. Standardized care can be facilitated by debunking previous data and discussing the advantages and disadvantages of MHT. The management of

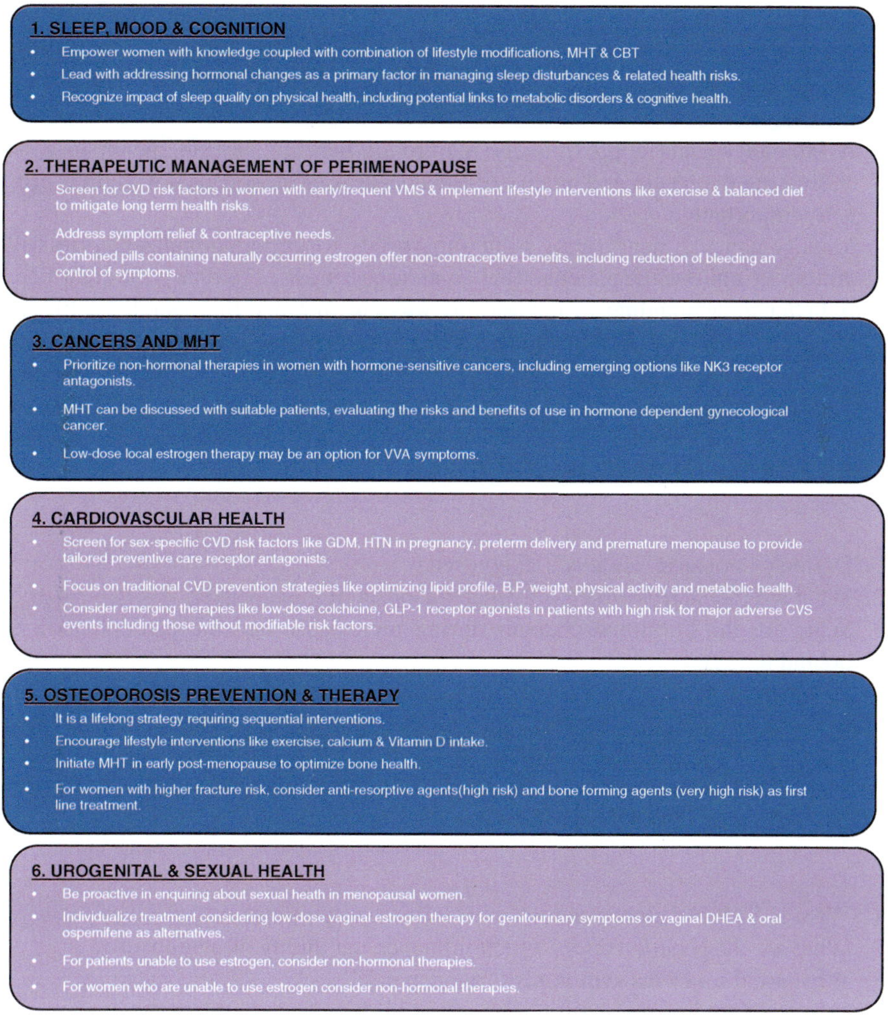

Fig. 1.1 Implementing recommendations from the 19th World Congress on Menopause into standard clinical practice. CBT Cognitive behavioral therapy, DHEA dehydroepiandrosterone, GLP-1 glucagon-like peptide-1, MHT menopausal hormone therapy, NK3 neurokinin 3, VMS vasomotor symptoms, and VVA vulvovaginal atrophy

menopause symptoms has seen a revolution of treatment. There is a shift towards non-hormonal treatment and lifestyle medicine.

Developing specialized skills, putting strategic practices into place, sharing accountability, and promoting interprofessional communication are all important components of a successful menopausal care strategy. Patient-centered treatment for menopausal women can be optimized by pooling the strengths of various healthcare providers, which will improve overall quality of life and lead to better outcomes.

Key Points

- Menopause is a natural stage of life caused by decreased estrogen production in the ovaries.
- A woman spends approximately a third of her life beyond menopause, so addressing the health and quality of life concerns of menopausal women is critically important.
- Management of menopausal symptoms needs to be individualized, primarily aiming to improve the patients' QoL, and respecting her preference for treatment.
- A better understanding of the various ways to improve the overall health and quality of life through menopause transition and beyond is the need of the hour.

Long Answer Questions (LAQs)

1. Define menopause. How is it diagnosed?
2. What are the factors which influence the onset of menopause?
3. What are the hormonal changes during menopause and the pathophysiology behind it?
4. How can menopause be approached as an opportunity?

Short Answer Questions (SAQs)

1. What is STRAW classification?
2. What are the genetic factors which influence the timing of menopause?
3. What are the various symptoms of menopause?
4. Which lifestyle interventions are advised to navigate the natural phase of menopause?
5. What are the various treatment options available for menopausal symptoms?

Multiple Choice Questions (MCQs)

1. Menopause is defined as the natural and permanent cessation of menstruation resulting from deficiency of which hormone?

   A. Progesterone
   B. Estrogen and progesterone

C. Estrogen
D. Estrogen, progesterone, prolactin

2. Menopause is a retrospective diagnosis, starting how many months after the last menstrual period?

A. 6 months
B. 9 months
C. 12 months
D. 18 months

3. Most common symptom experienced during menopause is:

A. Genitourinary symptoms
B. Vasomotor symptoms
C. Sleep disturbance
D. Cognitive dysfunction

4. The average age of menopause in Indian women with respect to the global average is:

A. Same
B. Early onset in Indian women
C. Late onset in Indian women
D. None of the above

5. Menopause occurs earlier in women with the following condition except:

A. History of oophorectomy
B. History of hysterectomy
C. History of mastectomy
D. Pelvic radiation therapy

6. Following are the studies related to menopause except:

A. SWAN study
B. GWAS study
C. GRIT study
D. VIVA study

7. Which key gene is associated with the timing of menopause?

A. Follicle stimulating hormone subunit beta
B. Luteinizing hormone subunit
C. Growth hormone subunit
D. Insulin like factor subunit

8. Which statement is false?

A. MHT is considered the mainstay of treatment for vasomotor symptoms.
B. Transdermal MHT is a preferable option for women at risk of venous thromboembolism

   C. Oral MHT is a preferable option for women at risk of venous thromboembolism
   D. Transdermal MHT bypasses first-pass hepatic metabolism

9. MHT is contraindicated in the following except:
   A. Recent deep vein thrombosis
   B. Acute liver disease
   C. High serum triglyceride
   D. Diabetes mellitus

10. Drugs used in the treatment of menopausal symptoms are all except:
   A. Neurokinin-1 receptor antagonist
   B. Orexin agonist
   C. Orexin antagonist
   D. Neurokinin-3 receptor antagonist

Answers

1. C
2. C
3. B
4. B
5. C
6. C
7. A
8. C
9. D
10. B

References

1. McNeil MA, Merriam SB. Menopause. Ann Intern Med. 2021;174(7):ITC97-ITC112.
2. Simon JA, Davis SR, Lindén Hirschberg A, Kiesel L, et al. State of the art in menopause: current best practice approaches from the IMS World Congress 2024, Melbourne. Climacteric. 2025;28:1–6.
3. Prasad JB, Tyagi NK, Verma P. Age at menopause in India: a systematic review. Diabetes Metab Syndr Clin Res Rev. 2021;15(1):373–7.
4. El Khoudary SR, Greendale G, Crawford SL, et al. The menopause transition and women's health at midlife: a progress report from the study of women's health across the nation (SWAN). Menopause. 2019;26(10):1213–27.

5. Kochersberger A, Coakley A, Millheiser L, et al. The association of race, ethnicity, and socioeconomic status on the severity of menopause symptoms: a study of 68,864 women. Menopause. 2024;31(6):476–83.
6. World Health Organization. India Data | World Health Organization [Internet]. data.who.int. 2023.
7. Statistics CNCfH. Life expectancy. US Department of Health & Human Services 2024. Accessed 16 Nov 2024.
8. Larroy C, Marin Martin C, Lopez-Picado A, Fernandez AI. The impact of perimenopausal symptomatology, sociodemographic status and knowledge of menopause on women's quality of life. Arch Gynecol Obstet. 2020;301(4):1061–8.
9. Faubion SS, Enders F, Hedges MS, et al. Impact of menopause symptoms on women in the workplace. Mayo Clin Proc. 2023;98(6):833–45.
10. Aljumah R, Phillips S, Harper JC. An online survey of postmenopausal women to determine their attitudes and knowledge of the menopause. Post Reprod Health. 2023;29(2):67–84.
11. Shepherd JA, Shiozawa A, Schild AL, Singh D, Mancuso SA. Survey of patient experience and management of vasomotor symptoms due to menopause from the PatientsLikeMe community. Menopause. 2024;31(11):979–86.
12. Waetjen LE, Xing G, Johnson WO, Melnikow J, Gold EB, Study of Women's Health Across the Nation. Factors associated with reasons incontinent midlife women report for not seeking urinary incontinence treatment over 9 years across the menopausal transition. Menopause. 2018;25(1):29–37.
13. Dayaratna S, Sifri R, Jackson R, et al. Preparing women experiencing symptoms of menopause for shared decision making about treatment. Menopause. 2021;28(9):1060–6.
14. Peacock K, Carlson K, Ketvertis KM. Menopause. In: StatPearls Treasure Island (FL): StatPearls Publishing; 2025 Jan-. Available from: https://www.ncbi.nlm.nih.gov/books/NBK507826.
15. Burgess DJ. Dissecting the genetics of ovarian ageing. Nat Rev Genet. 2021;22(10):623.
16. Harlow SD, Gass M, Hall JE, et al. Executive summary of the stages of reproductive aging workshop +10: addressing the unfinished agenda of staging reproductive aging. J Clin Endocrinol Metab. 2012;97(4):1159–68.
17. Writing Group for the Women's Health Initiative Investigators. Risks and benefits of estrogen plus progestin in healthy postmenopausal women: principal results from the women's health initiative randomized controlled trial. JAMA. 2002;288(3):321–33.
18. Manson JE, Crandall CJ, Rossouw JE, et al. The women's health initiative randomized trials and clinical practice: a review. JAMA. 2024;331(20):1748–60.
19. Johansson T, Karlsson T, Bliuc D, et al. Contemporary menopausal hormone therapy and risk of cardiovascular disease: Swedish nationwide register based emulated target trial. BMJ. 2024;387:e078784.
20. Menegaz de Almeida A, Oliveira P, Lopes L, et al. Fezolinetant and Elinzanetant therapy for menopausal women experiencing vasomotor symptoms. Obstet Gynecol. 2025;145:253.
21. Peeples L. The new science of menopause: these emerging therapies could change women's health. Nature. 2025;637(8047):782–4.

Endocrine Changes in Menopause

2

Anshita Aggarwal

Abstract

Menopause is the permanent cessation of menstruation following ovarian follicular depletion, diagnosed retrospectively after 12 months of amenorrhea. It represents a pivotal biological transition with far-reaching endocrine and systemic consequences. The menopausal transition, typically spanning several years, is marked by progressive depletion of ovarian follicles, diminished inhibin B, and compensatory elevations in follicle-stimulating hormone (FSH) and luteinizing hormone (LH). Estradiol concentrations fluctuate initially but ultimately decline sharply around the final menstrual period, accompanied by falling progesterone levels due to anovulation. Anti-Müllerian hormone, reflecting ovarian reserve, also declines and may assist in predicting menopausal timing. These hormonal perturbations underlie the clinical manifestations of menopause. Vasomotor symptoms, notably hot flashes and night sweats, result from hypothalamic thermoregulatory instability secondary to estrogen withdrawal. Estrogen deficiency further contributes to accelerated bone resorption, increasing the risk of postmenopausal osteoporosis and fragility fractures. Urogenital atrophy manifests as vaginal dryness, dyspareunia, urinary symptoms, and heightened infection risk, while adverse metabolic changes—including dyslipidemia, central adiposity, and endothelial dysfunction—contribute to the heightened cardiovascular risk observed after menopause. Understanding the endocrinological basis of menopause is essential to guide evidence-based strategies for optimizing midlife and long-term women's health.

A. Aggarwal (✉)
Department of Endocrinology, Atal Bihari Vajpayee Institute of Medical Sciences & Dr. Ram Manohar Lohia Hospital, New Delhi, India

R. Malik et al. (eds.), *Menopause Essentials*,
https://doi.org/10.1007/978-981-95-7498-8_2

Keywords

Menopause · Ovarian reserve · Vasomotor symptoms · Osteoporosis · Cardiovascular risk

2.1 Introduction

Menopause is the permanent cessation of menstrual cycles following the loss of ovarian follicular activity. It is a retrospective diagnosis made 1 year after the final menstrual period (FMP) i.e. after 1 year of amenorrhea. It may be spontaneous (natural menopause) or iatrogenic (secondary menopause). The latter includes the removal of both ovaries (surgical menopause), as well as ovarian failure resulting from chemotherapy or radiotherapy. Menopause is one of the most significant physiological transitions in a woman's lifespan. Its impact on a woman's physical, mental, and emotional health is remarkable. The experience of menopause varies from woman to woman. While some women have smooth sailing, others may face many challenges that can disrupt their lifestyle to a great extent and require medical intervention.

A drastic and abrupt decline in the levels of various hormones brings about the menopausal transition. Thus, needless to say, there is an intricate and pivotal link between the endocrine system and menopause, and menopause is characterized by a myriad of endocrine-related changes. This chapter delves into the depth of these changes and their clinical relevance.

2.2 The Physiology of Menopause

To understand the physiology of menopause, it is essential to understand the physiology of normal menstrual cycles.

The menstrual cycle is a natural, recurring process that prepares the female body for potential pregnancy. Typically lasting between 21 and 35 days, with 28 days being common, the cycle is divided into distinct phases, each characterized by specific hormonal fluctuations and physiological changes.

2.3 Phases of the Menstrual Cycle

1. *Menstrual Phase* (Days 1–5): This phase begins with the first day of menstruation, where the uterine lining sheds, resulting in menstrual bleeding. Estrogen and progesterone levels are low, which prompts the shedding of the endometrial lining.
2. *Follicular Phase* (Days 1–13): Overlapping with the menstrual phase, this phase involves the maturation of follicles in the ovaries. The pituitary gland releases follicle-stimulating hormone (FSH), which stimulates the growth of ovarian follicles.

3. *Ovulation Phase* (Day 14): Typically occurring around the 14th day of a 28-day cycle, ovulation is the release of a mature egg from the ovary. A surge in luteinizing hormone (LH) triggers ovulation. This LH surge, in turn, is caused due to the "positive feedback" on the hypothalamus and the pituitary by the rising estrogen levels produced by the maturing follicles. The LH surge is critical for ovulation. It stimulates the final maturation of the egg and causes the follicle to rupture, releasing the egg. It also initiates the transformation of the ruptured follicle into the corpus luteum.
4. *Luteal Phase* (Days 15–28): After ovulation, the ruptured follicle transforms into the corpus luteum, which secretes progesterone to maintain the uterine lining. Progesterone levels rise, preparing the endometrium for a potential pregnancy.

Women are born with a fixed, limited supply of ovarian follicles, and this number gradually decreases throughout their lives, unable to be replenished. When the number is depleted, menopause sets in, characterized by several hormonal changes.

2.4 The Endocrinology of the Menopausal Transition

On average, the menopausal transition lasts 4 years in duration and is divided into early and late phases. It begins when menstrual irregularity first appears, classically defined as either a "skipped" period or an increase in variability of cycle length by more than 7 days. The early menopausal transition is characterized by a shortened follicular phase and an associated increase in FSH levels.1 However, early in the transition period, FSH levels are not consistently elevated, and may often vary considerably from month to month as the growing follicle cohort itself varies month to month.

This accounts for the shorter cycle intervals that are experienced by many women in this period of life. Studies have shown that shortened follicular phases are associated with accelerated ovulation, which occurs at a smaller follicle size. The most commonly accepted explanation for this phenomenon is the loss of inhibin B production. Inhibin B is a dimeric glycoprotein hormone, composed of an alpha subunit and a beta subunit, that plays a crucial role in regulating follicle-stimulating hormone (FSH) secretion. It is primarily produced by the granulosa cells from growing antral follicles.

The aforementioned loss of inhibin B leads to increased FSH release and, therefore, to an "overshoot" of estrogen production. This facilitates and accelerates the achievement of the LH surge. Many studies have concluded that a major fall in inhibin-B is one of the earliest changes marking entry into the menopausal transition.2 In contrast to inhibin B, inhibin A is a product of the dominant follicle and levels do not change appreciably until dominant follicles are no longer being generated in the ovary. As time ensues, the age-related hypothalamic modifications lead to a decrease in estrogen sensitivity, and the LH surge becomes more erratic. Follicles also become less sensitive to gonadotropins, which lead to luteal-phase defects and anovulatory cycles, and accordingly, to the first menstrual irregularities.

It is interesting to note that despite estrogen levels being rather high at this stage, symptoms of estrogen deficiency such as hot flashes and night sweats begin to emerge, which can be explained due to the aforementioned hypothalamic resistance to estrogen.

As women approach menopause, one of the earliest and most clinically significant changes observed is the increasing irregularity of the menstrual cycle. This transition is characterized not only by alterations in cycle length but also by a progressive increase in the frequency of anovulatory cycles. Ovulatory dysfunction becomes more common as ovarian follicular reserve declines, reflecting the underlying changes in hypothalamic-pituitary-ovarian (HPO) axis function.

Empirical data suggest that anovulation becomes a predominant feature in the late menopausal transition. In a longitudinal assessment of menstrual cyclicity during this phase, it was observed that 62% of the last ten menstrual cycles before the final menstrual period (FMP) were anovulatory, while only 38% retained normal ovulatory function. It is important to interpret these figures cautiously, as some cycles categorized as anovulatory may have, in fact, represented prolonged cycles with delayed ovulation, potentially escaping detection within the monitoring window. Nevertheless, these findings underscore the fundamental shift in ovarian physiology occurring in the premenopausal years.

The timing of increased anovulation is also notable. Studies have found that anovulatory cycles predominantly emerge within the last 30 cycles leading up to the FMP, with their occurrence being relatively infrequent prior to this period. This temporal association reinforces the concept of a "late reproductive stage", as defined in the STRAW (Stages of Reproductive Aging Workshop) criteria, during which endocrine and ovulatory changes become clinically evident.

From a hormonal perspective, anovulatory cycles are marked by distinctive endocrine profiles. In contrast to ovulatory cycles, which may show relatively stable levels of circulating reproductive hormones, anovulatory cycles are often accompanied by reduced estradiol (E2) concentrations and elevated follicle-stimulating hormone (FSH) levels, particularly during the early follicular phase of the cycle. These findings reflect the loss of negative feedback from estradiol and inhibins on the hypothalamus and pituitary, leading to compensatory increases in gonadotropin secretion.

The rise in FSH levels is a key endocrine marker of the menopausal transition. It typically begins approximately 2 years before the FMP, accelerates most steeply about 10 months prior to the FMP, and then plateaus within 2 years after menopause. The pattern of E2 change mirrors this but in the opposite direction. Estradiol concentrations begin to decline around 2 years before the FMP, with the most rapid decrease occurring near the time of the FMP, followed by a plateau postmenopause. This inverse relationship between FSH and E2 is consistent with the diminishing ovarian follicular activity and the associated decline in estrogen biosynthesis.

Evidence from large-scale cohort studies, such as the Melbourne Women's Midlife Health Project (Burger et al. 1999), has provided valuable insights into these dynamics. This project demonstrated that the most significant hormonal changes occur within 1–2 years before and after the FMP, a critical window in the reproductive aging continuum. The researchers also confirmed that the fall in serum inhibin A and B concentrations, secreted by granulosa cells of developing follicles, is a primary contributor to the elevation in FSH levels, reinforcing the concept of ovarian failure as the principal driver of these hormonal shifts.

Notably, despite these general trends, the search for a single, reliable hormonal biomarker of menopausal status in individual women has proven elusive. While serial measurements of FSH and E2 can provide a general indication of menopausal status at a population level, hormonal fluctuations during the perimenopausal period are substantial and interindividually variable, complicating the clinical utility of these parameters for precise staging in individual cases.

Therefore, while patterns of FSH rise and E2 decline offer valuable epidemiological insights and inform staging criteria for reproductive aging, clinical diagnosis of menopause remains retrospective, defined by the absence of menstruation for 12 consecutive months, in the absence of other pathological or physiological causes.

To put things into perspective, the combined concentration of estrogen, including estrone, estradiol, and estriol typically ranges from 100 to 250 picograms per milliliter in menstruating women, declines to <20 pg/ml a few years before menopause, and is <10 pg/ml after menopause.

Apart from the changes in the FSH levels, there is also a change in the anti-Müllerian hormone (AMH) levels. AMH is produced by granulosa cells of growing follicles (predominantly from follicles <8 mm in diameter) and thus a woman's circulating AMH concentration reflects the number of follicles remaining in the ovary. As expected, it declines towards the menopause. Serum AMH may be of value in the early diagnosis and prediction of age at menopause.

Table 2.1 summarizes the key endocrinological changes occurring during menopause and Fig. 2.1 provides a gist of the key hormonal perturbations in menopause.

By the late transition, prolonged amenorrhea (defined as >60 days) occurs and is associated with a persistently reduced follicle pool and failure of folliculogenesis. At this point in the transition, estrogen deficiency begins to dominate, bone mineral density loss begins, and menopausal symptoms including hot flashes and vaginal dryness increase sharply in prevalence.

2.5 Symptoms of Menopause Due to Endocrine Changes

Many of the symptoms of menopause can be explained due to the hormonal changes that occur.

1. *Hot flashes*

Hot flashes are considered a "sine qua non" of menopause, and are seen in >75% of post-menopausal women. These are episodic sensations of heat, intense sweating, and flushing affecting the face and chest, which are often accompanied by palpitations and anxiety and can last from 3 to 10 min. They can cause immense discomfort and distress to the patient. The frequency of these episodes varies from

Table 2.1 Key endocrinological changes occurring during menopause

Menopause related change	Description
Declining ovarian reserve	With age, the number and quality of ovarian follicles decline This leads to a decrease in the production of *E2, progesterone, and inhibin B*, a hormone that regulates FSH secretion
Increased FSH and LH	Responding to reduced estrogen levels, the hypothalamus increases the release of GnRH This stimulates the pituitary to release more FSH and LH However, despite elevated levels of FSH and LH, the ovaries are less responsive to these hormones, leading to a reduction in E2 production
Decreased estrogen	E2 levels progressively decrease during perimenopause, eventually reaching very low levels after menopause The primary source of estrogen shifts from the ovaries to peripheral tissues, such as adipose tissue, which can produce a small amount of estrogen through the aromatization of androgens
Decline in progesterone	Progesterone levels fall because ovulation becomes irregular and less frequent Without ovulation, there is no corpus luteum to produce progesterone
Increased androgens	In the absence of the negative feedback mechanism provided by E2, there may be a relative increase in androgen levels, such as testosterone This can lead to symptoms such as increased facial hair and changes in libido Free androgen index (FAI) increases by 80% from 4 years before FMP to 2 years after because of a concomitant decrease in sex hormone-binding globulin (SHBG) levels across this time period DHEAS levels are not related to FMP but decline slowly with age Thus, SHBG and FAI levels change at the time of menopause, at least partially due to the decline in E2 Testosterone remained unchanged through the menopausal transition and the early postmenopause

woman to woman. The majority of women have hot flashes for 1–2 years, but 15% may have persistent hot flashes for up to 30 years.

The pathophysiological mechanism involves the narrowing of the thermoneutral zone, such that subtle changes in core temperature elicit thermoregulatory mechanisms such as vasodilation, sweating, or shivering.3 Changes in brain neurotransmitters and peripheral vascular reactivity are involved and can be explained partly due to the declining levels of estrogens and inhibin B, as well as increasing FSH levels. The dramatic response to estrogen therapy also underscores the role of these hormonal changes.

The hot flashes might also be accompanied by frequent night-time awakenings and mood disturbances, and all of these symptoms together encompass the "vasomotor symptoms" of menopause.

However, other factors such as race, weight, lifestyle, etc. also impact the onset and severity of these vasomotor symptoms.

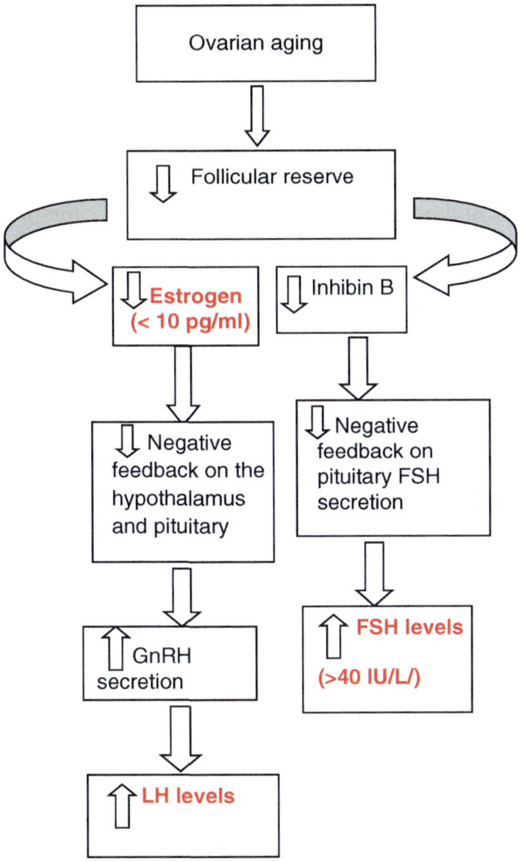

Fig. 2.1 Gist of the key hormonal perturbations in menopause

Management Though estrogen therapy is known to be very effective in the treatment of hot flashes, it is generally not used for this indication because of the associated side-effect profile. Nonhormonal therapies such as paroxetine, fluoxetine, and venlafaxine are effective.4

Isoflavones or phytoestrogens have estrogenic properties and are found in soy products, but these have largely been seen to be ineffective in the treatment of hot flashes. Gabapentin, which is an anti-convulsant has also shown benefits in amelioration of hot flashes.

Apart from these, behavioral therapy and relaxation techniques have also shown good results.

2. *Hirsutism*

Though hirsutism/ other clinical features of hyperandrogenemia after menopause are usually mild, they might be concerning for a few patients. The mechanisms behind this have been discussed earlier in this chapter. Hair growth is generally observed over the face, chin, and upper lip. Hirsutism can be objectively assessed using the modified Ferriman-Galleway score. If the degree of hirsutism is severe or is associated with significant hair fall, clitoromegaly, rapid progression of abnormal hair growth, or other features of virilization, then causes other than post-menopause should be sought.

Management Lifestyle measures to maintain optimum weight are helpful, and in some cases, antiandrogens, such as spironolactone or flutamide can be used for amelioration of hirsutism.

3. *Osteoporosis*

Estrogen is essential for maintaining skeletal homeostasis and regulates bone remodeling, primarily by inhibiting the expression of RANKL (receptor activator of nuclear factor-κB ligand), an essential cytokine for bone resorption by osteoclasts. This results in decreased differentiation and increased apoptosis of the osteoclast, thus favoring bone formation. Hence, estrogen plays a pivotal role in achieving peak bone mass in women. After menopause, due to estrogen deficiency, there is an increase in bone resorption and a precipitous fall in bone mineral density, leading to postmenopausal osteoporosis (PMO).5

Also, estrogen deficiency is associated with decreased production of OPG (Osteoprotegerin). OPG is a cytokine secreted by osteoblasts following estrogen stimulation and is a natural inhibitor of RANKL. Thus, estrogen deficiency further augments RANKL activity.

Based on DXA-derived T-score, PMO has been defined as a T-score ≤ -2.5 and low bone mass (osteopenia) as T-score $< -1 > -2.5$.6

Osteoporosis significantly increases the risk of low-trauma fractures in post-menopausal women and is associated with increased morbidity, mortality, and financial burden. The earlier the age at menopause, the higher the risk of osteoporosis later in life. Since PMO is essentially asymptomatic (until the patient sustains a fracture), active screening for the disease in apparently healthy post-menopausal women is warranted. The candidates for screening are women aged 60 and older, postmenopausal women younger than 60 years, and women in the menopausal transition if there is a specific risk factor associated with increased fracture risk, such as low body weight, prior low-trauma fracture, or high-risk medication.

Management Treatment includes employing fall-prevention strategies, exercising to maintain normal weight and build muscle strength, and regular intake of calcium and vitamin D supplements as indicated. Medications such as bisphosphonates, teriparatide, and denosumab are used in the management of PMO with good results.

Though the pathophysiology of PMO suggests that estrogen should be the first-line treatment, it is seldom, if ever, used for treating it. In a study conducted by the Women's Health Initiative in 2002, it was revealed that using estrogen had many harmful effects, which outweighed its benefits.7

It found that using estrogen hormone replacement for 5 years or more multiplied the risks of congestive heart disease (CHD), venous thromboembolism, stroke, and carcinoma breast, and it could even cause cholecystitis.

4. *Urogenital symptoms*

Estrogen is a vasoactive compound; it promotes the vascularity of the external genitalia, and lower urinary tract, by transduction of fluid and lubrication.8 It also promotes epithelial cell proliferation, mucin production, and collagen turnover. After menopause, due to estrogen deficiency, there is thinning of the labia and vulva, a decrease in collagen, elasticity, decreased vascularity, vaginal atrophy, and reduced vaginal discharge. All of these contribute to vaginal dryness and dyspareunia, and sometimes even postcoital bleeding. There is also atrophy of the bladder and urethra, leading to urinary symptoms like urinary incontinence and increased frequency. It is noteworthy that, unlike vasomotor symptoms, these symptoms tend to persist throughout life.

Also, the pH of the vagina increases, due to the loss of vaginal flora which usually maintains a slightly acidic pH, mediated by estrogen. The increased pH leads to a heightened risk of urogenital infections.9

Management Treatment includes nonhormonal vaginal lubricant during intercourse and the regular use of a long-acting vaginal moisturizer. In women with persistent symptoms, local vaginal estrogen creams can be used. Giving local therapy allows one to use lower doses as compared to systemic therapy, thus minimizing adverse effects while getting more benefits. An initial loading dose of daily applications followed by a maintenance regimen for as long as it is needed to manage symptoms, usually indefinitely, is given.

5. *Cardiovascular disease*

The risk of cardiovascular disease increases significantly after menopause. There is a transformation from a gynoid body shape to an android body shape, along with increasing subcutaneous and abdominal fat deposition after menopause. This abdominal fat is known to be particularly detrimental to cardiovascular health as it is resistant to the lipolytic action of insulin, overexpresses the enzyme 11-beta HSD1, leading to excess production of cortisol, and hence contributes more towards metabolic syndrome.

In women, total and low-density lipoprotein (LDL) cholesterol increases with age, and this increase is accelerated by menopause, whereas cardioprotective, high-density lipoprotein (HDL) decreases.10 Moreover, the protective effect of HDL cholesterol appears to be diminished as women progress through menopause—possibly related to denser subparticle size. A rise in LDL has specifically been associated with the latter part of the menopausal transition and appears to be related to the loss of estrogen at this time of life. Apart from this, estrogen has multiple effects increasing Nitric Oxide synthesis and antioxidant and anti-inflammatory properties;

which are essential for maintaining endothelial function hence its deficiency in menopause causes endothelial dysfunction.

2.6 Conclusion

Menopause is a complex biological process marked by significant endocrine changes stemming from ovarian senescence. The consequent hormonal alterations—most notably the decline in estrogen and inhibins—have profound systemic effects. These changes not only define the menopausal transition but also contribute to a variety of clinical conditions, including vasomotor symptoms, osteoporosis, cardiovascular disease, and urogenital atrophy.

Understanding these endocrinological mechanisms is essential for clinicians to anticipate, diagnose, and manage menopausal symptoms effectively. While hormone therapy remains a potent intervention for some manifestations, it must be employed judiciously given its risk-benefit profile. Nonhormonal strategies and lifestyle modifications are critical adjuncts in optimizing the quality of life in menopausal and postmenopausal women.

Continued research into the hormonal dynamics of menopause will further refine our approach to this vital stage of women's health, ensuring tailored and effective interventions grounded in physiological understanding.

Key Points

- Menopause is confirmed after 12 months of amenorrhea due to ovarian follicular depletion.
- Declining estrogen, inhibin B, and AMH with rising FSH characterize the hormonal shift of menopause.
- Hot flashes are the most common vasomotor symptom, affecting over 75% of postmenopausal women.
- Estrogen deficiency postmenopause increases the risk of osteoporosis and cardiovascular disease.
- Management of menopause involves individualized hormonal and nonhormonal treatment strategies.

Long Answer Questions (LAQs)

1. What are the key hormonal changes during the menopausal transition, and how do they lead to menstrual irregularities and eventual cessation of menstruation?
2. What causes vasomotor symptoms like hot flashes in menopause, and what are the main hormonal and nonhormonal treatment options?

3. How does estrogen deficiency contribute to postmenopausal osteoporosis, and what are the underlying mechanisms?
4. What are the effects of estrogen deficiency on the urogenital tract in menopause, and how are these symptoms managed?

Short Answer Questions (SAQs)

1. What is the average duration of the menopausal transition?
2. Which hormone's early decline marks the onset of the menopausal transition?
3. What is the primary cause of postmenopausal osteoporosis?
4. Which hormone is responsible for the LH surge during ovulation?
5. Why does hirsutism sometimes increase after menopause?

Multiple Choice Questions (MCQs)

1. When is menopause diagnosed?

   A. After 3 months of amenorrhea
   B. After 6 months of irregular cycles
   C. After 1 year of amenorrhea
   D. At the onset of hot flashes

2. Which of the following hormones declines earliest during the menopausal transition?

   A. Estrogen
   B. Inhibin B
   C. LH
   D. Progesterone

3. What causes the LH surge during the normal menstrual cycle?

   A. High levels of progesterone
   B. Inhibition by AMH
   C. Rising estrogen causing positive feedback
   D. Decrease in FSH

4. What is the primary source of estrogen in postmenopausal women?

   A. Ovaries
   B. Pituitary gland
   C. Peripheral adipose tissue
   D. Adrenal glands

5. Which hormone reflects the remaining ovarian follicle pool?

   A. FSH
   B. LH
   C. AMH
   D. Estrogen

6. What is the most common vasomotor symptom of menopause?

   A. Insomnia
   B. Hot flashes
   C. Vaginal dryness
   D. Urinary incontinence

7. What is a key mechanism by which estrogen prevents bone loss?

   A. Increases osteoclast activity
   B. Stimulates RANKL expression
   C. Inhibits RANKL and increases OPG
   D. Enhances calcium excretion

8. Which of the following is *not* typically associated with postmenopausal urogenital changes?

   A. Vaginal dryness
   B. Vaginal atrophy
   C. Increased vaginal discharge
   D. Increased vaginal pH

9. Why does hirsutism sometimes increase after menopause?

   A. Increased androgen secretion from the ovaries
   B. Decrease in SHBG leading to higher free testosterone
   C. Elevated estrogen levels
   D. Increased progesterone levels

10. Which therapy is most effective for hot flashes but is used cautiously due to risks?

    A. SSRIs
    B. Estrogen therapy
    C. Gabapentin
    D. Isoflavones

Answers

1. C
2. B
3. C
4. C
5. C
6. B
7. C
8. C
9. B
10. B

References

1. Talaulikar V. Menopause transition: physiology and symptoms. Best Pract Res Clin Obstet Gynaecol. 2022;81:3–7.
2. Wen J, Huang K, Du X, Zhang H, Ding T, Zhang C, et al. Can Inhibin B reflect ovarian reserve of healthy reproductive age women effectively? Front Endocrinol. 2021;12.
3. Gombert-Labedens M, Vesterdorf, Kristine, Fuller, Andrea, Maloney, Shane K, Baker FC. Effects of menopause on temperature regulation. Temperature. 2025;12(2):92–132.
4. Sahni S, Lobo-Romero A, Smith T. Contemporary non-hormonal therapies for the management of vasomotor symptoms associated with menopause: a literature review. Eur Endocrinol. 2021;17(2):133.
5. Cheng CH, Chen LR, Chen KH. Osteoporosis due to hormone imbalance: an overview of the effects of estrogen deficiency and glucocorticoid overuse on bone turnover. Int J Mol Sci. 2022;23(3):1376.
6. Meeta M, Harinarayan C, Marwah R, Sahay R, Kalra S, Babhulkar S. Clinical practice guidelines on postmenopausal osteoporosis: *an executive summary and recommendations – update 2019–2020. J Mid Life Health. 2020;11(2):96.
7. Stute P, Marsden J, Salih N, Cagnacci A. Reappraising 21 years of the WHI study: putting the findings in context for clinical practice. Maturitas. 2023;174:8–13.
8. Wasnik VB, Acharya N, Mohammad S. Genitourinary syndrome of menopause: a narrative review focusing on its effects on the sexual health and quality of life of women. Cureus. 15(11):e48143.
9. Kalia N, Singh J, Kaur M. Microbiota in vaginal health and pathogenesis of recurrent vulvovaginal infections: a critical review. Ann Clin Microbiol Antimicrob. 2020;19(1).
10. Inaraja V, Thuissard I, Andreu-Vazquez C, Jodar E. Lipid profile changes during the menopausal transition. Menopause. 2020;27(7):780.

Menopause Transition

3

Bipasa Sen

Abstract

Menopause Transition marks the period of changes from normal ovulatory function to cessation of menses and some immediate period thereafter. It falls in −2 and −1 Straw Staging. It is subdivided into Early and Late Menopause Transition. Menopause Transition itself is proinflammatory and disrupts estrogen-regulated neurological system. It prompts an innate immune inflammatory response in female reproductive organs that propagate to the brain. Low estrogen leads to upregulation of neurokinin B in the preoptic area, which acts on hypothalamic neurokinin 3 receptor, precipitating inappropriate hot and cold sensation. There are higher levels of circulating interleukins also. Symptoms of Menopause Transition include menstrual problems, cardiac, vasomotor, genitourinary, sleep problems, cognitive and mood symptoms, sexual, somatic, musculoskeletal, and skin problems. There is increased FSH, LH, and decreased estradiol, AMH, inhibin, DHEA, testosterone. Management involves Lifestyle changes including exercise, avoiding smoking, balanced diet, proper sleep, nutritional supplements, Lycopenes, and Isoflavones. Medications include MHT, Ospemifene, Vaginal Lubricants, moisturizer, SSRI, SNRI, and Gabapentine. An overall positive attitude, mindset, and strong resilience help to sail well through Menopause Transition.

Keywords

Menopause transition · Innate immune response · Inhibin · Neurokinin · Interleukin · MHT

B. Sen (✉)
Department of Obstetrics & Gynecology, Sterling Hospital, Kolkata, India

Indian Menopause Society, IMS, Mumbai, India

R. Malik et al. (eds.), *Menopause Essentials*,
https://doi.org/10.1007/978-981-95-7498-8_3

The World Health Organization (WHO) defines menopause as "the permanent cessation of menstruation resulting from the loss of ovarian follicular activity."

It is the most notable event for women at midlife. The average number of ovarian follicles at birth are 3–4 lakhs—thereafter gradual decline. The count reaches an average of 25,000 at around 37–38 years of age. Menopause occurs when the number of ovarian follicles fall below a critical threshold of 1000, regardless of age. The fall is usually not abrupt. The years prior to menopause and immediately thereafter that encompasses the change from normal ovulatory cycles to cessation of menses and some immediate period thereafter is known as Menopause Transition. Merely 10% of women experienced a sudden cessation of menstruation without a prolonged period of irregularity.

There are 2 standard staging symptoms of Menopause to be followed—Straw & Modified Anklesaria's IMS consensus group staging (Tables 3.1 and 3.2 respectively).

Table 3.1 Straw staging (stages of reproductive aging workshop)

					Final menstrual period (FMP) 0			
Stages	−5	−4	−3	−2	−1	+1		+2
Terminology	*Reproductive*			*Menopausal transition*		*Postmenopause*		
	Early	Peak	Late	Early	Late	Early		Late
				Perimenopause				
Duration of stage	Variable			Variable		(a) 1 year	(b) 4 years	Until demise
Menstrual cycles	Variable to regular	Regular		Variable cycle length (>7 days different from normal)	>2 skipped cycle and an interval of amenorrhea (>60 days)		None	
Endocrine:	Normal FSH		↑FSH	↑FSH		↑FSH		

As per Straw Staging, Menopause Transition Falls in Stage −2 and −1

Table 3.2 Modified Anklesaria's staging

Modified Anklesaria's Indian Menopause Society (IMS) consensus group staging			
Stage I	Stage IIA	Stage IIB	Stage III
About 2 years prior to menopause Early (premenopausal symptoms): IA Vasomotor instability IB Early psychosomatic symptoms menstrual problems	1 year after last period Atrophic changes Genitourinary Vasomotor Weight gain Osteopenia	Up to 5 years after menopause intermediate (postmenopausal symptoms): Late psychosomatic and genital symptoms Sexual disorders Residual changes from stage IIA osteopenia or osteoporosis	From 5 years postmenopause till late (postmenopausal) Complications. Residual changes from stage II Ischemic heart changes Other late complications, e.g. Alzheimer's disease. Osteoporosis
Prevent and treat	*Treat*	*Treat*	*Treat and palliate*

Source: Indian menopause society consensus statement 2008

As per Modified Anklesaria's staging, Menopause Transition falls in stage I and IIA

3.1 Common Symptoms of Menopause Transition

A. *Menstrual problems*—Irregular periods (shorter, longer, heavier, or lighter). Most commonly there is lengthening of cycles (40–50 days in contrast to normal 25–35 days). Amenorrhea episodes and an increase in the frequency of anovulatory cycles may occur later. However, some women do experience significant or persistent bleeding, which is typically caused due to relative estrogen excess.
B. *Cardiac and vasomotor symptoms* (palpitations, nocturnal sweats, and hot flushes).
   The phrase "hot flush" or "hot flash" describes an abrupt onset of skin reddening across the head, neck, and chest that is accompanied by an elevated heart rate and a sensation of body heat. Sometimes the flush is followed by a lot of sweating. It can last anywhere from a few seconds to several minutes, and very infrequently up to an hour. The frequency may be rare to recurrent, occurring once per several minutes. At night, flushes occur more frequently and are more severe.
C. *Genitourinary*—Vaginal dryness, burning, dyspareunia, urinary frequency, urgency, incontinence.
D. *Sleep Problems*—Sleep disturbances [1]—insomnia, frequent waking, difficulty in falling asleep.
E. *Mood Changes*—Anxiety, depression, irritability.
F. Cognitive impairment—Brain fog or memory issues like impaired memory, forgetfulness—which has been suggested to be a prodromal phase of Alzheimer's disease [2].
G. *Sexual*—Decreased Libido.
H. *Somatic*—Weight gain, obesity, metabolic syndrome, skin and hair changes like dry skin, wrinkles, alopecia, frontal balding.
I. *Muscular skeletal*—Joint pain, myalgia, decreased bone and muscle strength.
J. Breast pain in early menopause transition—due to fluctuations in serum estradiol level [3].

According to slight symptom variability, menopause transition can be described as Early and Late.

3.1.1 Early Menopause Transition (Straw Stage—2)

- Menstrual cycle remains regular, but may start to vary slightly in length.
- Hot flashes—mild sensation of warmth, often affecting face and neck.
- Sleep disturbance—occasional insomnia or disrupted sleep pattern.
- Mood swing—increased irritability or mild depressive symptom. This phase can last several years. There is declining level of serum estradiol and progesterone.

3.1.2 Late Menopause Transition (Straw Stage—1)

- Marked by more pronounced hormonal shift.
- Noticeable change in menstrual pattern—skipped cycle or significant variation in flow and duration. Cycles greater than 42 days are frequent and this symptom

predicts menopause in next 1–2 years. The primary factor influencing cycle length is the length of the follicular phase.

- Intensified vasomotor symptoms—more frequent and severe hot flushes and night sweats.
- Genito urinary symptoms—vaginal dryness, discomfort at intercourse, urinary frequency, and urgency.
- Cognitive change—Episodes of forgetfulness or difficulty in concentrating.

3.2 Pathophysiology

In the average women, continuing follicle depletion and irregular cycle length starts almost 12–13 years prior to actual menopause. The length of the follicular phase of the cycle varies depending on the rate of follicular growth, while the luteal phase stays mostly unchanged.

As noted, anovulation often occurs 2–8 years before menopause. During this time, ovarian follicles continue their rate of loss until eventually the supply of follicles is finally depleted. In a study of human ovaries, follicle loss typically begins at age 37 or 38, when the total number of follicles reached to about 25,000. About 8–10 years before menopause, the follicular phase and total cycle length reach their lowest point. Over the following several years, the variability gradually rises as ovulation becomes less frequent and predictable. The number of antral follicles and ovarian volume progressively decline. Inappropriate sensations of heat and cold are caused by the overexpression of neurokinin B in the preoptic area, which acts on hypothalamic neurokinin 3 receptors due to low estrogen [4].

There is growing evidence that the menopause transition affects estrogen-regulated neurological symptoms and is proinflammatory. Through a network of estrogen receptor subtypes alpha (E R—α) and beta (E R—β), estrogen acts as a master regulator. It has been demonstrated that E R-β controls the inflammasome [5], a crucial part of the innate immune response, as well as the mitochondrial activity of neurons. Menopause transition is therefore seen as an inflammatory process, accompanied by inflammation of the central nervous system and the body as well as control of the innate immune response through E R-β-driven mechanisms. Ovarian failure is accelerated by the ongoing low-grade inflammation [6].

It has been proposed that the transition to menopause triggers an inherent immunological inflammatory response in the female reproductive organs, which spreads to the brain and increases the risk of ischemic brain injury [7]. Disturbances in the circulating estrogen cycle pattern during the menopause transition trigger the systemic innate and adaptive immune response because one of estrogen's primary roles is to behave as a powerful inflammatory factor [8, 9]. The multiprotein complex known as the inflammasome is in charge of digesting proinflammatory cytokines including IL-1β and IL-18 and activating caspase-1 [10]. When innate responses start, the adaptive immune response is triggered, which leads to peripheral immune cell infiltration, especially T cell invasion of the brain [11].

The persistent low-grade inflammation associated with aging can ultimately be caused by repetitive or prolonged stimulation of the innate and adaptive immune response. The lack of ovarian steroidal hormones during menopause increases inflammation, making women more susceptible to immunological diseases such rheumatoid arthritis [12]. Higher levels of circulating interleukins IL-6, sIL-6, IL-4, IL-2, and TNF are associated with declining ovarian steroidal hormones during the menopausal transition.

3.3 Hormonal Levels at Menopause Transition

The menopausal cycle change prior to menopause is initially marked by elevated level of Follicle stimulating hormone (FSH) and decreased level of inhibin, but normal level of Luteinizing hormone (LH) and slightly elevated level of Estradiol.

- The FSH level progressively rises to >40 IU/L. the FSH growing rate is modest until 7 years before menopause, then accelerated and larger in 2 years before menopause.
- LH levels first stay within the normal range before rising to >30 IU/L. Therefore, corpus luteum production and function can occasionally occur in the early years of menopause transition, and perimenopausal women are still at risk of becoming pregnant until both FSH and LH reach >20 IU/L and >30 IU/L, respectively.
- Before follicular growth and development stop, the level of estradiol stays slightly increased for around a year. Two years before menopause, there is a significant drop in estradiol levels (10–20 pg/ml). The majority of the estradiol produced during this period comes from the peripheral conversion of estrone, which is mostly produced by the peripheral conversion of androstenedione. The circulating level of estrone is higher than that of estradiol (30–70 pg/ml).
- Both luteal phase of inhibin A and follicular phase inhibin B decrease with aging, but more marked decrease in inhibin B is due to reduced quantity and aging of inhibin secreting follicles. Decreasing level of inhibin reflect either a shrinking number of follicles or reduced functional capacity of older follicles.
- Antimüllerian Hormone (AMH) level is decreased. AMH is a measure of the ovarian follicular reserve. About 5 years prior to menopause, declining levels of AMH and inhibin B approach a low to undetectable level.
- Testosterone production decreased by approximately 25%.
- The levels of DHEA and DHEA sulfate decrease.

3.3.1 Mean Circulating Hormone Levels at Menopause Transition [13]

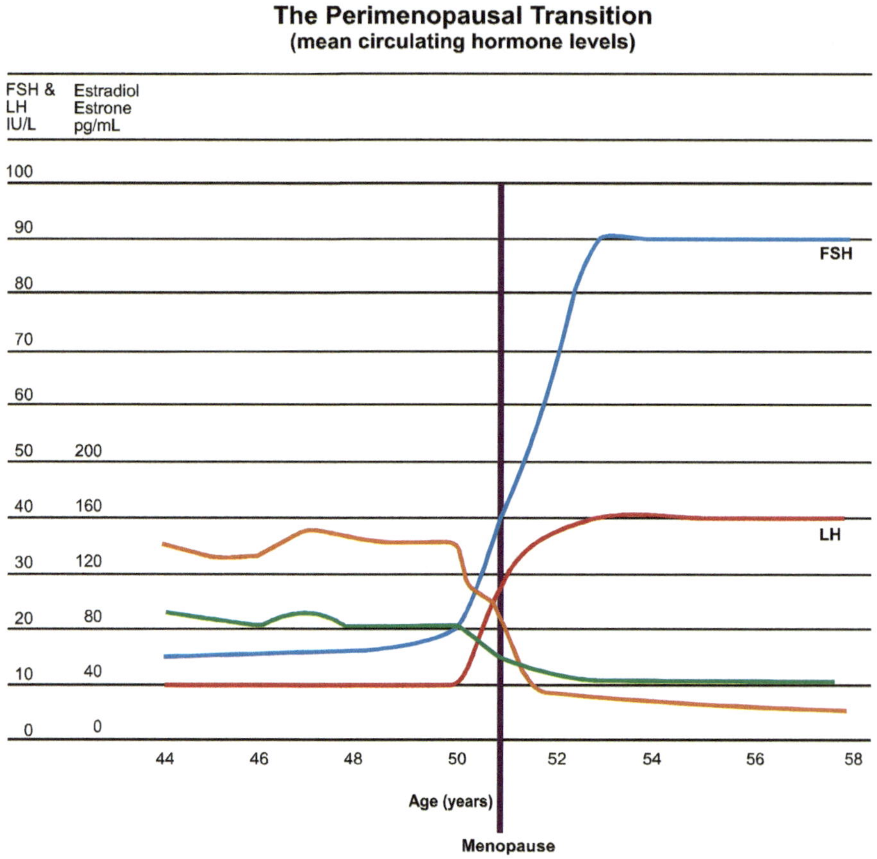

The main symptoms at menopause transition can broadly be described as attributed to 2 categories of hormonal problems [13].

A. Those associated with relative estrogen excess—such as heavy menstrual bleeding, endometrial hyperplasia, endometrial neoplasia.

   The following mechanisms could lead to a rise in endogenous estrogen levels:

   (i) A decrease in sex hormone binding globulin (SHBG), which would raise the amount of free estrogen.
   (ii) Increased aromatization (obesity, thyroid disorder, liver disease).
   (iii) Elevated precursor androgen (stress, functional endocrine tumors).
   (iv) Elevated direct estrogen secretion (ovarian tumors).

   [Although the greater concern provoked by these symptoms are neoplasia, the usual finding is mostly non-neoplastic tissue displaying estrogen effects unopposed by progesterone]

B. Those associated with estrogen deficiency—such as hot flush, atrophic vaginitis, urethritis, cognitive decline, cardiovascular events, metabolic syndrome, and osteoporosis.

3.3.1.1 Menopause Transition and Genitourinary Atrophy

Atrophy of the vaginal mucosal surface due to very low estrogen occurs. Vagina loses collagen, adipose tissue, and the ability to retain water. The surface epithelium thins to a few layers of cells and loses its outer fibrous layer. The ratio of superficial cells to basal cells significantly decreases as the vaginal maturation index changes. Vaginal wall shrinks, rugae flatten or disappear. As a result, the vaginal surface becomes friable and prone to bleeding with minimal trauma. Vaginal wall blood vessels become narrow and the secretion from sebaceous gland diminish. Vagina itself contracts and loses flexibility, labia minora become paler and smaller, vaginal pH becomes alkaline. The vaginal environment becomes less favorable to lactobacilli and more vulnerable to infection by urogenital and fecal bacteria. Different levels of prolapse are caused by vaginal relaxation. Dysuria, urgency, frequency, incontinence, and recurrent UTIs are caused by mucosal thinning of the bladder and urethra. The result of an atrophied vagina and inadequate lubrication is dyspareunia, which can occasionally accompany postcoital bleeding.

3.3.1.2 Menopause Transition and Sexuality [13]

Vaginal lubricating fluid production and volume decrease during the menopausal transition, and there is also some loss of vaginal suppleness and epithelial thickness. Sexually active women have less vaginal atrophy than inactive women; this is likely due to the activity's maintenance of vaginal circulation and vasculature. Dryness, tightness, vaginal irritation, and burning during coitus are symptoms of dyspareunia, which is linked to urogenital atrophy. Postcoital spotting and stiffness are also present.

3.3.1.3 Menopause Transition and Mood Changes [13]

According to the Penn Ovarian Aging Study, 26% of perimenopausal women fit the criteria for Clinical Depressive Disorder, while 50% of them experience depression. According to the Harvard Study of Moods and Cycles, perimenopausal women experience nearly twice as many depressive episodes as premenopausal women. The Swan Study reported similar results. But in practice, 83% of women experience perimenopausal transition without mood difficulties. The episodes of depression in menopausal transition are linked to poor physical health, smoking, anxiety disorders, stressful life events, and history of premenstrual syndrome and hot flush.

3.3.1.4 Menopause Transition and Cardiovascular Health

The majority of cardiovascular disease is caused by atherosclerosis in major vessels; risk factors include high blood pressure, smoking, diabetes, obesity, abnormal lipid profiles, and a family history of cardiovascular disease. The beneficial effect of estrogen on capillary endothelial events is the reason for the gender difference in CVA (greater in males than in women) prior to age 40. Endothelial synthesis of prostacyclin and nitric oxide, which is positively impacted by estrogen, is responsible for the vasodilatory and antithrombotic effects. Even in the context of hypercholesterolemia, estrogen shields the vital endothelium process from the negative effects of hypercholesterolemia. In addition to preventing LDL from oxidizing, estrogen shields the endothelium from the harmful effects of oxidized LDL. During menopause transition, all these favorable effects are reduced due to hypoestrogenemia and there is progression of atherosclerosis and similar risk of CVA in women as compared to men.

3.3.1.5 Menopause Transition and Obesity [14]

A rise in total cholesterol, triglycerides, LDL cholesterol, and a fall in HDL cholesterol are all positively connected with central fat distribution and apple-shaped obesity during the menopause transition. Estrogen decrease and insulin resistance are the mediators of this atherogenic lipid profile. Obesity, smoking, and inactivity can all raise triglyceride levels.

3.3.1.6 Menopause Transition and Cognitive & Cerebral Function

The menopause transition is characterized by a decrease in brain white matter volume, myelin degradation, mitochondrial respiration, and glucose metabolism. These alterations are also linked to alterations in neurological function and beta amyloid accumulation in the brain [15]. These alterations result in memory loss and brain fog. The activation of mitochondrial ER-β protects the brain from ischemia by acting on neurons. A systemic inflammatory state marked by systemic proinflammatory cytokines, a change in the cellular immune profile, an increase in the availability of inflammasome protein in the central nervous system, and a proinflammatory microenvironment that makes the brain more vulnerable to ischemia and other stressors is caused by the decline in estrogen during the menopause transition. These proinflammatory mechanisms seem to undermine ER-β's ability to shield the brain from ischemia injury. This stage prepares for neurovascular and neurodegenerative diseases with cognitive dysfunction or decline.

3.3.1.7 Menopause Transition and Skin Changes

Wrinkles are caused by a decrease in skin thickness, suppleness, and collagen content brought on by an estrogen deficit. One of the main risk factors for wrinkles on the face is smoking.

3.4 Effects on Musculoskeletal System

In premenopausal women, estrogen protects bone through its beneficial effect. In menopause transition, with lower estrogen profile, there is considerable decrease in bone density correlated with increasing FSH level and low estrogen level. There is metacarpal and lumbar bone loss. Also, a genetic susceptibility for bone loss is important. There is increased incidence and susceptibility to vertebral compression fracture, colles' fracture head of femur and tooth loss (due to oral alveolar bone loss). Additionally, there is a consistent decline in muscular strength, which is influenced by physical activity level, height, and weight.

3.5 Screening of Healthy Women at Menopause Transition

1. A complete medical history with details of variable cycle length, urinary, vaginal, and sexual problems. Also enquire about food habit, exercise, addiction (alcohol, tobacco, betelnut).
2. Questionnaire through Menopause Rating Scale (MRS)—which is a measure for health-related Quality of life (HRQOL).

Menopause Rating Scale (MRS)

Which of the following symptoms apply to you at this time? Please, mark the appropriate box for each symptom. For symptoms that do not apply, please mark 'none'.

Symptoms:	none	mild	moderate	severe	very severe
Score	= 0	1	2	3	4
1. Hot flushes, sweating (episodes of sweating)	☐	☐	☐	☐	☐
2. Heart discomfort (unusual awareness of heart beat, heart skipping, heart racing, tightness)	☐	☐	☐	☐	☐
3. Sleep problems (difficulty in falling asleep, difficulty in sleeping through, waking up early)	☐	☐	☐	☐	☐
4. Depressive mood (feeling down, sad, on the verge of tears, lack of drive, mood swings)	☐	☐	☐	☐	☐
5. Irritability (feeling nervous, inner tension, feeling aggressive)	☐	☐	☐	☐	☐
6. Anxiety (inner restlessness, feeling panicky)	☐	☐	☐	☐	☐
7. Physical and mental exhaustion (general decrease in performance, impaired memory, decrease in concentration, forgetfulness)	☐	☐	☐	☐	☐
8. Sexual problems (change in sexual desire, in sexual activity and satisfaction)	☐	☐	☐	☐	☐
9. Bladder problems (difficulty in urinating, increased need to urinate, bladder incontinence)	☐	☐	☐	☐	☐
10. Dryness of vagina (sensation of dryness or burning in the vagina, difficulty with sexual intercourse)	☐	☐	☐	☐	☐
11. Joint and muscular discomfort (pain in the joints, rheumatoid complaints)	☐	☐	☐	☐	☐

3. Recording height (to apprehend early osteoporosis), body weight, waist circumference, BMI.
4. Breast examination.
5. Pelvic examination and detection of vaginal pH (pH >4.5 indicates estrogen deficiency), vaginal elasticity, rugae, and vaginal lubrication.
6. Routine laboratory investigation with special stress on blood sugar, lipid profile, thyroid profile.

3.6 Management

A. *Lifestyle Change*:
   1. Avoid caffeine, smoking, other tobacco consumption.
   2. Regular Exercise (Walking, Strength training, Yoga) [16] Exercise has a favorable impact on central thermoregulation unless it is linked to significant vasomotor symptoms, obesity, or perspiration.
   3. Balanced diet rich in fiber, protein, calcium, unsaturated fat, and fresh fruits and vegetables.
   4. Stress management (Meditation, Yoga, Deep Breathing). The typical breathing technique, postures, and relaxation poses of Yoga have been hypothesized to decrease sympathetic arousal. Yoga also reduces perceived stress and neuroticism at menopause transition [17].
   5. Good sleep hygiene.
   6. Positive attitude and resilience.

B. *Medical Options—Hormonal*:

   Hormone therapy has positive effect on hot flush, urogenital symptoms, skin, bone, and muscle texture, mood disorder. Estrogen is the most effective treatment available for hot flash. All preparations starting from oral conjugated equine estrogen / estradiol valerate / estradiol hemihydrate, and transdermal estradiol or estradiol spray are 70–95% effective at reducing hot flush. To avoid endometrial hyperplasia or carcinoma in women with intact uterus, progestogens are added in continuous or cycled manner. Another option to women with uterus is Conjugated Equine Estrogen + Bazedoxifene (Tissue Selective Estrogen Complex). Oral Tibolone may improve libido in case of hypoactive sexual disorder (HSDD). Hormone Therapy improves glucose metabolism, insulin resistance, and lipid profile.

3.6.1 Timing Hypothesis to Initiate Hormone Therapy

Early menopausal women have better blood vessels with intact endothelium; in reaction to estrogen, these blood vessels vasodilate and have general anti-inflammatory effects. Age-related plaque buildup causes the vasculature to become increasingly stenotic, and the injured endothelium exhibits poor vasodilatation.

Hence early initiation of MHT (before 60 years of age or within 6 years of menopause) is advocated.

Once plaques are formed, estrogen can destabilize plaque and lead to adverse events. Oral and transdermal hormone therapy have shown to decrease visceral fat and increase lean body mass, improve abdominal obesity, but no effect on body weight.

3.6.2 Estrogen Preparations for Hormone Therapy

Name	Route	Dose range	Frequency	Equivalent dose
17β Estradiol	Oral	0.5–2 mg	Daily	1 mg
	Patch	0.014–0.1 mg	Once or twice daily	0.05 mg
	Gel	0.25–1.25 mg	Daily	1 mg
	Spray	1–3 spray (1.53 mg per spray)	Daily	2–3 spray
Conjugated equine estrogen	Oral	0.3–1.25 mg.	Daily	0.625 mg
Ethinyl Estradiol	Oral	0.01–0.03 mg.	Daily	0.01–0.015 mg
Estradiol acetate	Vaginal ring	0.05–0.1 mg.	90 days	0.05 mg

Transdermal formulation are preferred in women with hyperlipidemia, diabetes, hypertension, and other risk factors for cardiovascular diseases.

3.6.3 Progestogen Preparations for Hormone Therapy [18]

Name	Route	Dose range	Frequency	Side effects
Micronized progesterone	Oral	100–300 mg	Daily cycled	Somnolence, fatigue, bloating, abdominal pain, nausea, dizziness
Levonorgestrel	IUD	52 mg	5 years	Pain with placement, pelvic pain, breast pain, irregular bleeding and spotting, acne, abdominal pain, nausea, dizziness, headache, fatigue
Drosperinone	Oral	4 mg	Daily	Acne, weight gain, nausea, headache, breast tenderness, low libido, hypokalemia
Medroxy progesterone acetate	Oral	2.5–5 mg 5–10 mg	Daily cycled	Bloating, weight gain, abdominal pain, dizziness, fatigue
Norethindrone	Oral	0.35–0.7 mg	Daily cycled	Nausea, headache, breast tenderness

3.6.4 Alternative Hormone Therapy

When women with intact uterus cannot use progesterone for endometrial protection, they may use oral conjugated equine estrogen + Bazedoxifene—a single dose combination of Estrogen—Estrogen receptor against antagonist (ERAA).

But Hormone Therapy is to be restricted to moderate-to-severe symptoms only.

Low dose E + P combined OC pills are helpful in case of heavy anovulatory bleeding. It reduces the risk of endometrial hyperplasia and neoplasia. But combined OC is associated with higher rate of venous thromboembolism.

Topical estrogens are used for local genitourinary symptoms. They have a safer risk profile than systemic hormone therapy.

C. *Other Treatment Options*:
   1. Vaginal lubricants for sexual activity and moisturizers for regular use are the first-time treatment for genitourinary syndrome of menopause.
   2. Oral ospemifene is the only oral treatment option for GSM. Ospemifene has been shown to improve vaginal dryness, dyspareunia, and vaginal pH. It acts as an estrogen agonist on vaginal and bone tissue, but its effect on breast is neutral to antagonistic. Adverse effects include vasomotor symptoms and venous thromboembolism.
   3. Nonhormonal medications—Antidepressants, antihypertensives, antiatherogenic drugs, and bisphosphonates. Several types of antidepressants—serotonin norepinephrine Reuptake inhibitors (SNRI) like venlafaxine desvenlafaxine and selective serotonin Reuptake inhibitors (SSRI) like paroxetine, fluoxetine, sertraline, citalopram, and escitalopram are known to affect mood, may also impact thermoregulation.

      The optimum results have been with venlafaxine 75 mg SR, Des venlafaxine 100 mg, fluoxetine 20 mg daily, or gabapentin 300 mg twice daily.
   4. Supplements of Calcium, Magnesium, and Vitamin D.
   5. Lycopenes, evening primrose oil, Dong quai, Ginseng, and Isoflavone.

Key Points

1. Menopause transition is marked by declining levels of estradiol, testosterone, inhibin, AMH, and DHEA and increasing level of FSH and LH.
2. There is growing evidence that the menopause transition is proinflammatory and interferes with the neurological system that is regulated by estrogen. A network of ERα and ERβ receptors is how estrogen works. ERβ controls the inflammasomes, a crucial part of the innate immune response. Additionally, estrogen controls the mitochondrial activity of neurons. Menopause transition is therefore perceived as an inflammatory process. Consequently, ovarian failure is accelerated by persistent low-grade inflammation.
3. Menopause transition can be well managed by lifestyle changes including well-balanced diet, regular exercise, stress management, and practicing good sleep hygiene.

4. In moderate-to-severe symptoms hormone therapy helps whereas non-hormonal therapy like antihypertensive, anti-depressant, bisphosphonate may be used as per indication.
5. Genitourinary syndrome is well managed by topical estrogen or oral ospemifene.

Long Answer Questions (LAQs)

1. Describe the common symptoms of Menopause Transition.
2. Explain why Menopause Transition is viewed as proinflammatory.
3. Describe the changes in circulating hormone levels at Menopause Transition.
4. Describe the pathophysiology of altered cerebral function in Menopause Transition.

Short Answer Questions (SAQs)

1. Describe the "STRAW" classification of Menopause staging.
2. Describe the vasomotor symptoms of Menopause Transition.
3. State the mechanism that could result in increased estrogen level at Menopause Transition.
4. Describe the genitourinary changes in Menopause Transition.
5. Describe the pathogenesis of obesity in Menopause Transition.

Multiple Choice Questions (MCQs)

1. Number of ovarian follicles at birth–
   A. 30,000–40,000
   B. 3–4 lakhs
   C. 3–4 million
   D. 3000–4000
2. Menopause occurs when number of ovarian Follicles fall below–
   A. 3000
   B. 1000
   C. 300
   D. 50
3. Menopause Transition stage as per STRAW staging is–
   A. −1 & −2
   B. −1, −2 & +1
   C. −1, & +1
   D. −1, 0, +1

4. Healthy menstrual bleeding in Menopause Transition may occur due to–
   A. progesterone deficit
   B. estrogen deficit
   C. progesterone excess
   D. estrogen excess
5. Vaginal dryness appears at–
   A. early menopause transition.
   B. late menopause transition
   C. both
   D. none
6. In Menopause Transition, irregular cycle length occurs due to varying length of–
   A. Luteal phase
   B. Follicular phase
   C. Both
   D. None
7. Which of the following circulating interleukins is NOT increased in Menopause Transition–
   A. IL—2
   B. IL—3
   C. IL—4
   D. IL—6
8. Greater FSH rising rate starts—years prior to menopause–
   A. 2 years
   B. 4 years
   C. 6 years
   D. 8 years
9. Increased endogenous estrogen level at Menopause Transition is NOT due to–
   A. Obesity
   B. Thyroid disorder
   C. Hypertension
   D. Liver disease
10. Tooth loss at Menopause Transition occurs due to loss of–
    A. Oral alveolar bone
    B. Oral trabecular bone
    C. Calcium
    D. All of the above

Answers

1. B
2. B
3. A
4. D
5. B

6. D
7. B
8. A
9. C
10. A

References

1. Alejandra Elizalde Cremonte, Vasomotor symptoms and sleep disturbances in menopause: menopause live update February, 2024.
2. Caldwell CC, Yao J, Brinton RD. Targeting the prodromal stage of Alzheimer's disease: bioenergetic and mitochondrial opportunities. Neurotherapeutics. 2015;12(1):66–80.
3. Meeta GJ. CPG on menopause 2020: 75–76.
4. Modi M, Dhillow S. The neuroendocrinology of the preoptic area in menopause: symptoms and therapeutic strategies. In: Swaab DF, Kreier F, et al., editors. Handbook of clinical neurology. Elsevier; 2021. p. 455–60.
5. McCarthy M, Raval AP. The perimenopause in a woman's life: a systemic inflammatory phase. J Neuroinflamm. 2020;17:317.
6. Ajacayak E, et al. Role of inflammation and oxidative stress in the etiology of primary ovarian insufficiency. Tusk J Obstet Gynaecol. 2016;13(3):109–15.
7. Raval AP, et al. Sexual dimorphism in inflammasome containing extra cellular vesicles and the regulation of innate immunity in the brain of reproductive senescent females. Neurochem Int. 2019;127:29–37.
8. Edwards BJ, Li J. Endrocrinology of menopause. Periodontology. 2013;61(1):177–94.
9. Giannoni E, et al. Estradiol and progesterone strongly inhibit the innate immune response of mononuclear cells in new borns. Infect Immune. 2011;79(7):2690–8.
10. Broz P, Dixit VM. Inflammasomes: mechanism of assembly, regulation and signaling. Nat Rev Immunol. 2016;16(7):407–20.
11. Unger MS, et al. Microglia prevent peripheral immune cell invasion and promote an anti-inflammatory environment in the brain of APP—PS 1 transdermic mice. J Neuro Inflamm. 2018;15(1):274.
12. Doran MF, et al. Trends in incidence and mortality in rheumatoid arthritis in Rochester, Minnesota, over a 40-year period. Arthritis Rheum. 2002;46(3):625–31.
13. Fritz MA, Speroff L. Clin Gynaec Endocrine and Infert, 10th Ed. Dec 2022.
14. Moccia P, Belda Montessinos R, Monllor Tormos A, et al. Body weight and fat mass across the menopausal transition: hormonal modulator. Gynaecol Endocrinol. 2022;38(2):99–104.
15. Mosconi L, et al. Sex differences in Alzheimer risk: brain imaging of endocrine vs. chronologic aging. Neurology. 2017;89(13):1382–90.
16. Amos Pines, The effect of Yoga on menopausal symptoms: results of RCT, Menopause life update July, 2024.
17. "The 2023 Non-Hormone Therapy Position Statement of the NAMS" 2023;30(6):573–590.
18. Sachin GS. Classification of progestins. Pharmacy Freak. 2023 [cited 2025 Dec 9]. Available from: https://pharmacyfreak.com/classification-of-progestins/.

Menopausal Symptoms and Their Assessment

4

Renuka Malik and Vandana Agarwal

Abstract

This chapter addresses the various subjective and objective methods available to assess menopausal symptoms. The Menopausal rating score, Greene menopausal questionnaire, methods to assess hot flushes, genitourinary symptoms, sleep disorder, cognitive decline, and methods to measure bone health and muscle strength are discussed.

Keywords

Menopausal symptoms assessment · Menopausal symptoms score · Hot flashes assessment · Genitourinary syndrome assessment · Sleep disorder assessment at menopause · Cognitive decline assessment at menopause

4.1 Introduction

Menopause is a retrospective clinical diagnosis following 12 months of FMP (final menstrual period) [1]. It is a hypo estrogenic state. Estrogen receptors are found all over the human body in various organs such as the brain, heart, adipose tissue, bones, skin, and urogenital system. There are three major forms of physiological estrogens in women, estrone (E1), 17β-estradiol (E2), and estriol (E3). Estrogen

R. Malik (✉) · V. Agarwal
Department of Obstetrics & Gynaecology, Atal Bihari Vajpayee Institute of Medical Sciences & Dr. Ram Manohar Lohia Hospital, New Delhi, India

R. Malik et al. (eds.), *Menopause Essentials*,
https://doi.org/10.1007/978-981-95-7498-8_4

acts via two receptors found all over the human body—classical nuclear receptors (ERα and ERβ) and novel cell surface membrane receptors (GPR30 and ER-X).

The symptoms attributed to menopause start 2–10 years before the onset of menopause, in the transition phase. Of these, the vasomotor symptoms may last for about 10 years, post menopause. The genitourinary symptoms may be progressive with time. Untreated osteoporosis and sarcopenia are also progressive and cause fracture and disability. Symptoms related to sleep and sexual arousal may also be progressive. Osteoarthritis on the other hand is a degenerative disease attributed to aging and is not directly due to menopause. The symptoms which are attributed to menopause are the ones which appear around menopause and reflect estrogen deficiency. These are as follows:

1. *Vasomotor symptoms* hot flashes and night sweats
2. *Mood changes* irritability, anxiety, depression
3. *Vaginal dryness* and discomfort during intercourse
4. *Sleep disturbances* and fatigue
5. *Weight gain* or changes in body composition with increase in mid-segment obesity
6. *Body aches* and pain
7. *Memory issues* or "brain fog"

4.2 Methods to Assess Menopausal Symptoms

Menopausal symptoms can be assessed from patient's history. There are various questionnaires which can be used in OPD setting or in research. Out of these MRS questionnaire has been used maximum and has been translated into most local languages. The authors have translated it in India in Hindi and is freely available for use, online [2].

1. *Menopause rating score questionnaire (MRS)*

The first widely accepted attempt to measure the severity of menopausal complaints in women was the Kupperman index. The MRS was developed and validated 20 years ago in German language by Heinemann. Globally, this questionnaire has been translated into more than 20 languages to assess menopausal symptoms. The first translation was done into English language (UK and USA) from the German original scale. The English version (Appendix 4.1) was used as the source language for translations into French, Spanish, Swedish, Mexican/Argentine, Brazilian, Turkish, and Indonesian languages. There are 25 translations of the MRS on its official website. In India, Hindi version has been developed by the authors (Appendix 4.2). A globally uniform common document like MRS, helps in judging postmenopausal issues worldwide as well as improvement with treatment.

Postmenopausal symptoms are graded based on their severity. Menopause rating score questionnaire comprises of 11 symptoms which are divided into 3 subscales—Somatic subscale (hot flashes, heart discomfort, joint, sleep disorder, and muscular discomfort) corresponding to questions 1, 2, 3, and 11, respectively, Psychological subscale (depressive mood, irritability, anxiety, and physical and mental exhaustion) corresponding to questions 4, 5, 6 and 7, respectively, and Urogenital subscale (sexual problems, dryness of vagina, and bladder problems) corresponding to questions 8, 9, and 10, respectively. Patients grade their symptoms in a 5-point Likert scale as none (0), mild (1), moderate (2), severe (3), and very severe as (4). Scores are added and individual subscale score is calculated and graded. The total score varies from 0 to 44. Score of 0–4 is graded as none or minimal menopausal symptoms, 5–8 as mild menopausal symptoms, 9–15 as moderate and 16–44 as severe postmenopausal symptoms.

2. *The Greene Climacteric Scale*

It consists of 21 questions covering 5 domains—anxiety, depression, somatic symptoms, vasomotor symptoms, and sexual function (Appendix 4.3, Table 4.1). Each question is answered on a 4-point Likert scale. This rating method was used in the original factor analysis. It gives greater sensitivity to the measures as compared to the binary present/absent rating. Scores are assigned as follows:

Not at all = 0
A little = 1
Quite a bit = 2
Extremely = 3

Answers of all the questions are summed to give a total quality-of-life measure. A higher score indicates worse quality of life. It typically takes 5 min to score the Greene Climacteric Scale.

3. *Menopause-Specific QOL questionnaire (MENQOL)*

It was published in 1996. Two versions of this questionnaire exist: MENQOL and MENQOL-I (Intervention version). MENQOL consists of 29 items divided into four validated domains (vasomotor, sexual, physical, and psychosocial) [3]. It assesses menopause-related quality-of-life over the past 4 weeks. Subscores on each domain range from 1 (none) to 8 (worst) quality of life. Total MENQOL scores are calculated as the average of the 4 domain subscores.

MENQOL-I-Intervention modifications involved the addition of three items to the physical domain. This modified version was developed in order to ensure that

Table 4.1 Green Climactric scale

Scale	Item numbers	Number of items
Psychological—Anxiety	1–6	6
Psychological—depression	7–11	5
Somatic	12–18	7
Vasomotor	19, 20	2
Sexual function	21	1

the side effects of specific therapies which might adversely affect the quality of life were reflected in the outcome measure.

4.3 Vasomotor Symptoms and Methods of Assessment

Hot flashes (HF) is the most common vasomotor symptom which is reported as feelings of intense warmth along with sweating, flushing, and chills. Sweating is mainly reported in the face, neck, and chest area lasting for 1–5 min. It may also last for as long as an hour. The median duration of symptoms is 4 years, with some lasting for 20 years [4]. Racial and ethnic variations in HF have been seen with Caucasian women reporting the highest prevalence and Asian women the lowest prevalence.

Physiological events of the hot flash include peripheral vasodilatation, shown by elevated skin blood flow and temperature in the face, arms, chest, abdomen, back, legs, and digits. Sweating and skin conductance which are an electrical measure of this, also increase during HF. Core body temperature (Tc) also increases before HF along with a small increase in heart rate of about 7–15 beats/min [4].

Since HF occur majorly in women with natural or surgical menopause, estrogens are clearly involved in its etiology. It is consistent with the fact that estrogen treatment virtually eliminates hot flashes. However, estrogen reduction alone does not explain the occurrence of HF because there is no relationship between these symptoms and the plasma, urinary, or vaginal levels of estrogens. Moreover, there is no difference in plasma estrogen levels in women with and without HF. Prepubertal girls have low estrogen levels but they do not have HF.

Hence, estrogen withdrawal is necessary but not sufficient to explain the occurrence of HF. Elevated brain norepinephrine along with estrogen withdrawal are part of the etiology of HF. Hot flashes are triggered by core temperature (Tc) elevation acting within a greatly narrowed thermoneutral zone in postmenopausal women. Hot flashes consisting of sweating and peripheral vasodilation are provoked when Tc reaches the upper threshold. Tc then declines and shivering occurs when the lower threshold is crossed [4].

Vasomotor symptoms can be assessed by MRS and GREENE scale, subjectively as subscale. To assess vasomotor scoring separately, certain questionnaires are available:

1. *Daily Hot Flash Diary*—A measure of self-reported hot flashes, night sweats and/or severity of hot flashes is recorded typically using a dairy on a 4-point scale: mild, moderate, severe, and very severe to provide a hot flash index (sum of the number of hot flashes multiplied by severity) [5].
2. *Hot Flush Rating Scale*—It is used as a measure of behavioral reactions to VMS. It yields a hot flush frequency score (2 items that each have times/day and days/week summed to give number of hot flushes and night sweats that have caused waking in the past week) and a hot flush problem rating (3 items, each scored 1–10) [6].
3. *The Hot Flash Related Daily Interference scale* is a widely used, psychometrically sound, 10-item, self-report questionnaire assessing the impact of hot flashes

on daily activities in nine specific domains within the past week (work, social activities, leisure activities, sleep, mood, concentration, relation with others, sexuality, and enjoyment of life) and overall quality of life, which is the tenth item. The reporting is from 0 to 10 rating scale, 100 being the maximum.
4. *The 3-item HFI* (interference with sleep, mood, and concentration) is another tool which is of benefit in assessing vasomotor symptoms and response to therapy [7].

Objective Assessment of HF diaries kept by patients suffering from HF have errors in compliance and are major sources of bias. HF occurring during sleep are not accurately reported because recall of these events is usually poor and many HF do not produce awakenings, leading in poor recall.

1. *Increased skin conductance* recorded from the sternum is presently the best objective marker of HF. An increase in this measure ≥2 micro Siemens (μS) within 30 s is recorded as a flash. Conductance recording requires the use of electrodes, Freedman hygrometric HF recorder, an innovative tool, requires neither electrodes nor gel and it can be used to measure HF.
2. *Other methods*: Other objective methods used for assessment of HF are increase in heart rate, finger blood flow, respiratory exchange ratio, skin temperature, and core body temperature.

4.4 Genitourinary Syndrome of Menopause and Methods to Assess Them

In 2013, vulvo vaginal atrophy term was replaced by GSM, which included genital, sexual and urinary symptoms at menopause by North American Menopause Society& International Society for study of sexual health.

GSM symptoms are very frequent, affecting about one-quarter to more than three-quarters of postmenopausal women. GSM is diagnosed based on signs and physical findings Unlike vasomotor symptoms, which also intensify over time, GSM symptoms tend to worsen without treatment. It has a major negative impact on a woman's quality of life. Estrogen deficiency causes several hormonal changes in the vaginal tract, including loss of elasticity resulting in shortening, shrinking, and loss of vaginal rugae. There is a thinning of epithelial layer, reduced vaginal secretion, decreased musculature, and reduced vascularity. Estrogen receptors are present in urethra uptil the trigone of bladder, hence urethral discomfort, dysuria, frequency and recurrent UTI are seen in menopause. A dry vagina causes dyspareunia leading to poor sexual health and decreased QoL.

4.5 Symptoms of GSM

- Vulvar itching, burning, or pain
- Vaginal dryness
- Vaginal discharge
- Dyspareunia, sexual discomfort
- Spotting or bleeding after intercourse
- Dysuria, urinary frequency, urgency
- Recurrent urinary tract infections

4.6 Signs of GSM

- External genitalia-decreased labial size, loss of vulvar fat pad, vulvar fissures, receded, or phimotic clitoris
- Prominent urethra with mucosal eversion or prolapse
- Vagina Introital narrowing
- Loss of elasticity with constriction
- Thin vaginal epithelial lining
- Loss of mature squamous epithelium
- Pale or erythematous appearance
- Petechiae, ulcerations, or tears
- Alkaline pH (>5.5)

There is still no agreement on GSM's objective and measurable markers.

Evaluating a vaginal maturation index (VMI) and measuring the vaginal pH are considered simple, useful, and inexpensive tools for diagnosis. The most bothersome symptom (MBS) method is also useful for diagnosing and assessing treatment response. Currently, the most reliable method of diagnosing GSM is to integrate the MBS approach with a physical examination. The most common assessment tools used to quantify the severity and improvement of GSM are the visual analog scale (VAS) of GSM symptoms, vaginal health index (VHI), female sexual function index (FSFI), and patient-reported outcomes measure (PROM) [8].

1. *Vaginal pH measurement*: It is the most frequently used and recommended since 2003 by the FDA for GSM assessment. It is used as a part of the VHI calculation. A piece of litmus paper is placed on the lateral vaginal wall until moistened in order to assess pH. A pH of 4.6 or greater indicates vulvovaginal atrophy (VVA), ruling out vaginal infections and bacterial vaginosis. Premenopausal women without VVA typically have a pH of 4.5 or less.

2. *Vaginal maturation index (VMI)*: In 2003, FDA recommendation to GSM evaluation was the VMI. VMI has not been that successful in the literature as the VHI, since it is not usually found in most studies assessing GSM [8]. The VMI assesses the relative proportion of parabasal (*P*), intermediate (*I*), and superficial vaginal epithelial cell (*S*) types in a vaginal cytology sample.100 cells are taken from lateral vaginal wall and stained and counted. More than 15% superficial cells are considered to be normal in premenopausal women. However, in postmenopausal women with vulvovaginal atrophy, it is typically less than 5%. The VMI is usually calculated as: Maturation value = (0 × % of parabasal cells) × (0.5 × % of intermediate cells) × (1.0 × % of superficial cells) [8].Another formula uses (0.2X% P + 0.6X%I + 1X%S) [9]. The formula can vary. In vulval atrophy, the score is generally less than 50. Vaginal pH and VMI are not used to diagnose GSM which is diagnosed on basis of symptoms, but are useful in research.
3. *Vulva Health Index*: This evaluates labia, urethra, clitoris, introitus as well as elasticity and pain during intercourse; total score ranges from 0 to 24, with higher scores corresponding with greater vulvar atrophy. If the Vulva Health Index is over 8 or there is score of 3 (severe) in any category, vulvar atrophy is suggested [10].
4. *Ultrasound to measure vaginal thickness*: The use of the endovaginal linear crystal which is straight not curved is used perpendicular to vaginal wall to measure its thickness. This is mainly used in research settings [11].
5. *Vaginal biopsy*: Salvatore et al. [12] performed an ex vivo histological study on the effects of micro ablative fractional CO_2 laser on atrophic vaginal samples from five women. They concluded that laser can produce a remodeling of vaginal connective tissue without damaging the surrounding tissue. Owing to potential complications, pain and high cost, biopsy is seldom used outside research.
6. *Diffuse reflectance spectroscopy (DRS)*: Recently DRS, which uses diffused light to measure vulvar and vaginal health has been used. It uses tissue chromophores in the vulva as surrogate markers, to assess GSM. However more studies are needed to elaborate further on this method [13].
7. *Vaginal Health Index (VHI)*: There is a disagreement on considering VHI as a subjective or objective measure for clinical evaluation [14]. Some authors consider Vaginal Health Index as an objective measure. Four out of the five variables (vaginal elasticity, fluid volume, epithelial integrity, and moisture assessment) are subjective, while vaginal pH measurement is objective (Table 4.2). A score less than 15 is suggestive of vaginal atrophy.

Table 4.2 Vaginal health index

Score	Overall elasticity	Type of fluid secretion & consistency	Vaginal pH	Vaginal epithelial mucosa	Moisture
1.	NONE	None	6.1	Petechiae noted before contact	None, inflamed mucosa
2.	POOR (scanty)	Thin yellow	5.6–6.0	Bleeds with light touch	None, mucosa not inflamed
3.	FAIR (superficial)	Thin white	5.1–5.5	Bleeds with scraping	Minimal
4.	GOOD (moderate)	Thin white	4.7–5.0	Not friable, thin mucosa	Moderate
5.	EXCELLENT	Normal white flocculent	<=4.6	Not friable, normal mucosa	Normal

Adapted from Bachmann et al. [15]

4.7 Methods to Assess Bone and Muscle Health

Osteopenia/porosis—BMD assessment by DEXA SCAN is the most widely used test. It is taken to be a gold standard. T score of less or equal to −2.5 is taken as osteoporosis (Table 4.3).

SCREENING TOOLS- FRAX SCORE with or without BMD is the most commonly used method It was first released in 2008.It is available online. Other questionnaires like GARVAN, OST, and SCORE are also used. FRAX Score is a computer-based equation using 7 clinical risk factors (prior fragility fracture, smoking, alcohol use, oral glucocorticoids, rheumatoid arthritis, parenteral fracture), age, sex, and BMI to estimate a patient's 10-year fracture probability of major osteoporotic fracture and hip fracture. Although it has been validated in the general population, it has few limitations which may cause the underestimation of fracture risk in postmenopausal women (Table 4.4). FRAX Score Interpretations [16] are as follows:

Major Osteoporotic Fracture (MOF) Risk:

- <10%: Low risk.
- 10–19%: Moderate risk.
- ≥20%: High risk; treatment is considered.

Hip Fracture Risk:

- <3%: Low risk.
- ≥3%: High risk; treatment is considered.

Sarcopenia Assessment Subjective questionnaires like SARC F which is a self-administered, five item questionnaire on strength, assistance walking, rising from a chair, climbing stairs and falls. SARC-F score is given for each as 0, 1, or 2 with 4 as cut off. AWGS has added measurement of calf circumference to SARC (SARC-CC). If calf circumference is less than 34 cm (33 cm for women in AWGS2), 10 points are added to SARC score. A score of 11 or more is taken as positive screening for sarcopenia.

The Asian Working Group for Sarcopenia (AWGS) 2014 consensus defined sarcopenia as "age-related loss of muscle mass, plus low muscle strength, and/or low

Table 4.3 WHO classification of postmenopausal osteoporosis

Classification	T -score (SD)
Normal	Equal to −1.0 or higher
Osteopenia (low bone mass)	Between −1.0 and 2.5
Osteoporosis	Equal to −2.5 or lower
Severe osteoporosis	Equal to −2.5 or lower with fracture

WHO Technical Report series 843.1994

Table 4.4 Osteoporosis risk assessment calculators

Risk factors	FRAX	GARVAN	OSTA	Score	OPERA	ORAI	ABONE
Age	✓	✓	✓	✓	✓	✓	✓
Gender	✓	✓	✓	✓ (women only)			
Weight	✓		✓	✓	✓	✓	✓
Height	✓						
Age at onset of menopause					✓		
Use of steroid	✓				✓		
Prior fracture	✓	✓		✓	✓		
Secondary osteoporosis	✓						
BMD data	✓ (Femoral bone only)	✓					
Race				✓			
Rheumatoid arthritis	✓			✓			
Prior hormone therapy				✓		✓	✓
Current smoking	✓						
Hip fracture in parent	✓						
Alcohol use	✓						
Falls		✓					

BMD bone mineral density, *FRAX* Fracture risk assessment tool, *HT* hormone therapy, *OSTA* osteoporosis self-assessment tool, *SCORE* simple calculated osteoporosis risk estimation, *OPERA* osteoporosis prescreening risk assessment, *ORAI* Osteoporosis Risk Assessment Instrument, *ABONE* Age, Body size and Estrogen use

physical performance." AWGS 2019 retains the previous definition but revises <18 kg for women; criteria for low physical performance are 6-m walk <1.0 m/s, Short Physical Performance Battery score ≤9, or 5-time chair stand test ≥12 s. AWGS 2019 retains the original cutoffs for height-adjusted muscle mass: dual-energy X-ray absorptiometry <5.4 kg/m^2 in women; and bioimpedance, <5.7 kg/m^2 in women.

The AWGS 2019 update proposes separate algorithms for community versus hospital settings, which both begin by screening either calf circumference, <33 cm in women, SARC-F (≥4), or SARC-CalF (≥11), to facilitate earlier identification of people at risk for sarcopenia. Skeletal muscle strength and mass are both still considered fundamental to a definitive clinical diagnosis. AWGS 2019 also introduces "possible sarcopenia," defined by either low muscle strength or low physical performance only, specifically to be used in primary health care or community-based health promotion in order to enable earlier lifestyle interventions [17].

Muscle Mass The gold standard for measuring muscle mass is DEXA SCAN. MRI, CT scan, and Bio-impedance are other methods with lower sensitivity. Appendicular skeletal muscle index (ASMI), is a measure of muscle mass which is calculated by DEXA scan. Ultrasound also has low sensitivity. Calf muscle circumference can be used in community settings to assess sarcopenia [18]. The cutoff point for low muscle mass of calf circumference for menopausal women was taken as <33 cm, according to the AWGS 2019.
Muscle strength can be measured by hand held dynamometer. AWGS 2019 recommends low muscle strength diagnostic cutoffs of handgrip <18 kg for women.
Muscle performance can be measured by 4 m gait test, timed up and go test (TUGT), chair stand test which are of two types- 5-time chair stand tests are recommended by CDC.

5-Time Chair Stand Test The five-time chair-stand test ≥12 s indicates poor muscle performance and greater than 10 s showed an increased risk of disability onset, and greater than 13.7 s was associated with increased disability and morbidity. It also tests MCI and specific domains of attention, executive function, and processing speed.

Chair Stand Below Average Scores (CDC): count the number of times the patient comes to a full standing position in 30 s. SCORING 60–64 years <12, 65–69 years <11, 70–74 years <10, 75–79 years <10, 80–84 years <9, 85–89 years <8, 90–94 < 4.

Poor performance of chair stand has been associated with associated with mild cognitive impairment [19].

4.8 Methods to Assess Sleep Disorders

Sleep disturbances are more in women than men and increase with age. Sleep disorders are complex. Insomnia, obstructive sleep apnea, snoring, restless leg syn drome alone or in combination, reduce restorative sleep. Objectively, sleep is measured by polysomnography. Notably, polysomnographic studies are not recommended for routine diagnosis of insomnia, as it is a clinical diagnosis.

There are various subjective tools for assessing sleep disorders in climacteric women out of which some are clinically validated—Insomnia Severity Index, Athens Insomnia Scale, Pittsburgh Sleep Quality Index, Epworth Sleepiness Scale, The Jenkins Sleep Scale, and Basic Nordic Sleep Questionnaire [20]. Objective assessments require sleep lab and equipment which can be used only in research settings. There is often less correlative between subjective assessment and lab reports.

Table 4.5 Jenkins Sleep Score

Assessment of Jenkins sleep score	Interpretation
0	No sleep ddisturbance
1–11	Little sleep disturbance
>11	High sleep disturbance

1. *Jenkins Sleep Scale (JSS)* is noted for its brevity and ease of use, consisting of just four items to assess common sleep problems like difficulty falling asleep and waking up exhausted. While the JSS is advantageous for quick assessments, its simplicity may limit its ability to capture the full extent of sleep disturbances, offering only a general overview without in-depth analysis of sleep quality or the impact on daytime functioning (Table 4.5).

   The questions consisted of evaluation of four elements in the last month, which were difficulty in falling asleep, difficulty to stay asleep, waking up at night and waking up exhausted in the morning. A rating of zero indicates that the event or behavior being assessed never occurs. A rating of one corresponds to a possible occurrence of between 1 and 3 days within a given time frame. A rating of two signifies an occurrence of 4–7 days, while a rating of three represents an occurrence of 8–14 days. A rating of four indicates an occurrence of 15–21 days, and finally, a rating of five signifies an occurrence of 22–28 days. The assignment of a numerical value ranging from 1 to less than 11 represents little sleep disturbance, whereas a score beyond 11 indicates high sleep disturbances.
2. *The Pittsburgh Sleep Quality Index (PSQI)* The 19-item PSQI assesses global sleep as well as 7 components of sleep over the past 4 weeks: sleep quality, sleep latency, sleep duration, habitual sleep efficiency, sleep disturbance, use of sleep medications, and daytime dysfunction. Items use varying response categories and scores are calculated using a computational algorithm. Global scores greater than 5.0 are indicative of poor sleep quality and high sleep disturbances, and global scores ≥ 8 have also been linked to fatigue.
3. *Insomnia Severity Index (ISI)* The 7-item ISI assesses insomnia severity over the past 2 weeks. Participants rate each item on a 0–4 point scale (total ranges from 0 to 28). Cut point scores for severity of insomnia are none (0–7), sub threshold (8–14), moderate (15–21), and severe (22–28).

4.9 Methods to Assess Cognitive Decline

Cognitive function comprises of six key domains, complex attention, executive function, learning and memory, language, perceptual—motor control, and social cognition. Assessment questionnaires include the 6-Item Cognitive Impairment Test (6CIT), Montreal Cognitive Assessment, Mini-Mental State Examination, Trail Making Test, Cambridge Neuropsychological Test Automated Battery, Cognitive Failures Questionnaire and Everyday Memory Questionnaire—Revised [20, 21].

Table 4.6 The 6 CIT scoring

Assessment of Cognitive Impairment	Interpretation
0–7	No cognitive impairment
8–9	Mild cognitive impairment
10–28	Significant cognitive impairment

The 6-Item Cognitive Impairment Test (6CIT) [22] is a brief screening tool which is used to assess cognitive function, particularly in elderly populations, including postmenopausal women who may be experiencing cognitive decline. The test is designed to evaluate memory, orientation, and attention. It consists of six questions that cover:

- Temporal Orientation: Asking about the current year, month, and time
- Memory: Recalling a five-item address (short-term memory recall) and
- Mental Calculation: Counting backward from 20 to 1

Each question is scored based on the accuracy of the response, with a higher total score indicating a greater degree of cognitive impairment (Table 4.6). The 6CIT is valued for its simplicity and efficiency, taking only a few minutes to administer, and has been validated in various settings, including in the context of cognitive decline during menopause. This has been validated after translation in Hindi [23].

The 6 CIT score determines the thought process, knowledge, and judgment. It correlated well with decrease in memory, reduction of performance during reaction time that assess attention with magnitude of effects that ranges from small to medium. Subjective cognitive challenges have been found to be correlated with impairment in verbal memory. A score of less than 7 denotes no cognitive impairment, between 8 and 9 denotes mild impairment, and above 10 denotes significant cognitive impairment.

4.10 Serum Estradiol Measurement and Correlation with Menopausal Symptoms

The research in menopause along with the methods to assess the symptoms of menopause is ongoing. In reproductive years, serum E2 value is 30–400 pg/mL, but after menopause, it falls below 30 pg/mol or 141 pmol/L (vitros). The low serum estradiol values correlate with menopausal symptoms but it is only recommended for research settings as the test is expensive and has to be very sensitive to pick up the low values seen in menopause [24]. Traditional immunoassays such as ELISAs (enzyme-linked immunosorbent assay) and commercial E2 assay suffer from cross-reactions and low reproducibility and are not recommended in clinical setting apart from research.

Key Points

- Menopause is a hypoestrogenic state, marked by various symptoms and changes in a woman's life.
- There are mainly subjective, and few objective tests to assess symptoms at menopause including the most bothersome symptoms and relief with treatment. Patient's symptoms are used to assess the severity, need of treatment and symptomatic relief with treatment in clinical practice.
- In choosing methods to assess symptoms, reproducibility, validity, and reliability are to be considered.
- Clinically, more severe, or most bothersome symptom can be used to decide the need for hormone therapy.

Long Answer Questions (LAQs)

1. What are the methods to assess menopausal symptoms. Which of these can be used in clinical settings?
2. Which methods assess osteoporosis at menopause and response to treatment?

Short Answer Questions (SAQs)

1. What are the methods to assess GSM?
2. What are the methods to assess sarcopenia at menopause?
3. What are the methods to assess cognitive decline?
4. What are the methods to assess sleep disorders?

Multiple Choice Questions (MCQs)

1. The cutoff point for low muscle mass of calf circumference for menopausal women was taken as:

   A. Less than 33 cm
   B. less than 18 mm
   C. less than 35 mm
   D. less than 21 mm

2. Menopausal rating score of 16 corresponds to:

   A. Severe symptoms
   B. Mild symptom
   C. Moderate
   D. No symptoms

3. Vaginal pH in GSM is usually:

   A. 2
   B. Less than 2
   C. More than 5.5
   D. Less than 5.5

4. Low hand grip strength in sarcopenia seen by hand held dynameter in menopausal women is:

   A. Less than 15 kg
   B. Less than 18 kg
   C. Less than 22 kg
   D. Less than 55 kg

5. In DEXA scan, T score required to diagnose osteoporosis is:

   A. Equal or less than −2.5
   B. Less than 2
   C. More than 2.5
   D. More than 5

6. Which of the following is an objective test to diagnose GSM?

   A. Vaginal PH estimation
   B. Vaginal elasticity
   C. Presence of itching
   D. Dyspareunia

7. Serum estradiol in menopause is:

   A. Above 200 pg/mol
   B. Above 100 pg/mol
   C. Below 50 pg/mol
   D. Below 30 pg/mol

8. Which method is not used to assess menopausal symptoms in clinical setting?
    A. Serum estradiol estimation
    B. MRS score
    C. Hot flash diary
    D. Greene climacteric scale
9. MHT is useful in all of the following except:
    A. Flushing
    B. Osteoporosis
    C. Vaginal atrophy
    D. Coronary heart disease
10. Estrogen replacement for post-menopausal symptoms cause an increase in?
    A. LDL
    B. Cholesterol
    C. VLDL
    D. Triglycerides

Answers

1. A
2. A
3. C
4. B
5. A
6. A
7. D
8. A
9. D
10. D

Appendixes

Appendix 4.1: English Version of MRS Score

Menopause Rating Scale (MRS)

Which of the following symptoms apply to you at this time?

(X ONE Box For EACH Symptom) For Symptoms That Do Not Apply, Please Mark "None").

Symptoms:	**none**	**mild**	**moderate**	**severe**	**extremely severe**
Score =	**0**	**1**	**2**	**3**	**4**
1. Hot flashes, sweating (episodes of sweating)	☐	☐	☐	☐	☐
2. Heart discomfort (unusual awareness of heart beat, heart skipping, heart racing, tightness)	☐	☐	☐	☐	☐
3. Sleep problems (difficulty in falling asleep, difficulty in sleeping through the night, waking up early)	☐	☐	☐	☐	☐
4. Depressive mood (feeling down, sad, on the verge of tears, lack of drive, mood swings)	☐	☐	☐	☐	☐
5. Irritability (feeling nervous, inner tension, feeling aggressive)	☐	☐	☐	☐	☐
6. Anxiety (inner restlessness, feeling panicky)	☐	☐	☐	☐	☐
7. Physical and mental exhaustion (general decrease in performance, impaired memory, decrease in concentration, forgetfulness)	☐	☐	☐	☐	☐
8. Sexual problems (change in sexual desire, in sexual activity and satisfaction)	☐	☐	☐	☐	☐
9. Bladder problems (difficulty in urinating, increased need to urinate, bladder incontinence)	☐	☐	☐	☐	☐
10. Dryness of vagina (sensation of dryness or burning in the vagina, difficulty with sexual intercourse)	☐	☐	☐	☐	☐
11. Joint and muscular discomfort (pain in the joints, rheumatoid complaints)	☐	☐	☐	☐	☐

Appendix 4.2: Hindi Translated Version of MRS Score

राजोनिवृति आकलन तालिका (एम आर एस) MRS-H

आप पर इस समय कौनसा लक्षण लागू होते है ? प्रत्येक लक्षण केलिए कृपायौचित कॉलम में सही का निशान(✓) लगाएँ / जो लक्षण लागू नहीं उनके लिए ' कोई नही ' कॉलम पर (✓)निशान लगाए

लक्षण :	कोई नही	हल्का	मध्यम	तीव्र	अत्यंत तीव्र
अंक :	0	1	2	3	4
1. तेज़ गर्मी लगना/ पसीना आना (बार बार पसीना आना)……………….	☐	☐	☐	☐	☐
2. दिल की धड़कन संबंधी शिकायतें (असामान्य रूप से दिल धड़कना, रुक रुक कर दिल धड़कना, तेज़ी से दिल धड़कना, दिल में जकड़न सी महसूस होना)………….	☐	☐	☐	☐	☐
3. नींद संबंधी शिकायतें (नींद ना आना, आराम से नींद ना आना, नींद जल्दी खुल जाना)……………………………	☐	☐	☐	☐	☐
4. उदासी (बहुत उदास, दुखी सा महसूस होना कि आँसू ही निकालने वाले हो, कोई काम करने की इच्छा ना होना)…………………	☐	☐	☐	☐	☐
5. चिड़चिड़ापन (घबरा जाना, मानसिक तनाव, गुस्सा आना)……………………………..	☐	☐	☐	☐	☐
6. चिंताग्रस्त (बेचैनी महसूस होना, चिंतित होना)…………………………….	☐	☐	☐	☐	☐
7. शारीरिक एवं मानसिक थकान (रोजमर्रा के काम करने मे परेशानी महसूस होना, संबंधी कम हो जाना , एकाग्रता में कमी , जल्दी भूल जाने की समस्या होना)…………………..	☐	☐	☐	☐	☐
8. सेक्स संबंधी परेशानियाँ (सेक्स के प्रति इच्छा मे बदलाव, सेक्स क्रिया और संतुष्टि में परिवर्तन)…………………………….	☐	☐	☐	☐	☐
9. मूत्राशय संबंधी समस्या (पेशाब करने में दिक्कत होना, बार- बार पेशाब आना, पेशाब निकल जाना)…………………….	☐	☐	☐	☐	☐
10. योनि में शुष्कता (योनि में सूखापन, जलन महसूस होना, सहवास में परेशानी महसूस होना)..	☐	☐	☐	☐	☐
11. जोड़ों एवं मांसपेशियों की परेशानी (जोड़ों में दर्द , गठिया की शिकायत)……………..	☐	☐	☐	☐	☐

Appendix 4.3: The Green Climacteric Scale

NAME: .... DATE: ....

NUMBER: ....

Please indicate the extent to which you are bothered at the moment by any of these symptoms by placing a tick in the appropriate box.

SYMPTOMS	Not at all	A little	Quite a bit	Extremely	Score 0–3
1. Heart beating quickly or strongly					
2. Feeling tense or nervous					
3. Difficulty in sleeping					
4. Excitable					
5. Attacks of panic					
6. Difficulty in concentrating					
7. Feeling tired or lacking in energy					
8. Loss of interest in most things					
9. Feeling unhappy or depressed					
10. Crying spells					
11. Irritability					
12. Feeling dizzy or faint					
13. Pressure or tightness in head or body					
14. Parts of body feel numb or tingling					
15. Headaches					
16. Muscle and joint pains					
17. Loss of feeling in hands or feet					
18. Breathing difficulties					
19. Hot flushes					
20. Sweating at night					
21. Loss of interest in sex					

P (1–11) = ☐	A (1–6) = ☐
S (12–18) = ☐	D (7–11) = ☐
V (19–20) = ☐	S (21) = ☐

References

1. Peacock K, Ketvertis KM. Menopause. National Library of Medicine. StatPearls Publishing; 2023.
2. Malik R, Pokaria C, Singh S, Khera K. Hindi translated version of menopausal rating score questionnaire: a method to evaluate post-menopausal symptoms in India. Int J Reprod Contracept Obstet Gynecol. 2019;8(8):3102–9.
3. Lewis JE, Hilditch JR, Wong CJ. Further psychometric property development of the menopause-specific quality of life questionnaire and development of a modified version, MENQOL-Intervention questionnaire. Maturitas. 2005;50(3):209–21.
4. Freedman RR. Menopausal hot flashes: mechanisms, endocrinology, treatment. J Steroid Biochem Mol Biol. 2014;142:115–20.
5. Sloan JA, Loprinzi CL, Novotny PJ, Barton DL, Lavasseur BI, Windschitl H. Methodologic lessons learned from hot flash studies. J Clin Oncol. 2001;19(23):4280–90.
6. Hunter MS, Ayers B, Smith M. The hot flush behavior scale: a measure of behavioral reactions to menopausal hot flushes and night sweats. Menopause. 2011;18(11):1178–83.
7. Carpenter JS, Bakoyannis G, Otte JL, et al. Validity, cut-points, and minimally important differences for two hot flash-related daily interference scales. Menopause. 2017;24(8):877–85.
8. Meisels A. The maturation value. Acta Cytol. 1967;11:249.
9. Lumbanraja IL, Siregar MFG, Lumbanraja SN, et al. Association of Vaginal Maturation Index and Vaginal pH with the Most bothersome symptoms of genitourinary syndrome of menopause. J South Asian Feder Obstet Gynaecol. 2021;13(5):288–91.
10. Panay N. Genitourinary syndrome of the menopause–dawn of a new era? Climacteric. 2015;18(Suppl. 1):13–7. https://doi.org/10.3109/13697137.2015.1070564.
11. Bosio S, Barba M, Vigna A, Cola A, De Vicari D, Costa C, Volontè S, Frigerio M. A novel method for the measurement of the vaginal wall thickness by transvaginal ultrasound: a study of inter- and intra-observer reliability. Medicina (Kaunas). 2024;60(3):370.
12. Salvatore S, Leone Roberti Maggiore U, Athanasiou S, Origoni M, Candiani M, Calligaro A, Zerbinati N. Histological study on the effects of microablative fractional CO_2 laser on atrophic vaginal tissue: an ex vivo study. Menopause. 2015;22(8):845–9.
13. Dinish US, Logan S, Balasundaram G, Xinhui VT, Vinod Ram K, Ruochong Z, et al. Diffuse reflectance spectroscopy and imaging for non-invasive objective assessment of genitourinary syndrome of menopause: a pilot study. Sci Rep. 2024;14(1).
14. Mension E, Alonso I, Tortajada M, et al. Genitourinary syndrome of menopause assessment tools. J Midlife Health. 2021;12(2):99–102. https://doi.org/10.4103/jmh.jmh_93_21.
15. Bachmann GA, Notelovitz M, Kelly SJ, Owens A, Thompson C. Long-term nonhormonal treatment of vaginal dryness. Clin Pract Sex. 1992;8:3–8.
16. Schini M, Johansson H, Harvey NC, Lorentzon M, Kanis JA, McCloskey EV. An overview of the use of the fracture risk assessment tool (FRAX) in osteoporosis. J Endocrinol Investig. 2024 Mar;47(3):501–11.
17. Chen LK, Woo J, Assantachai P, Auyeung TW, Chou MY, Iijima K, Jang HC, Kang L, Kim M, Kim S, Kojima T, Kuzuya M, Lee JSW, Lee SY, Lee WJ, Lee Y, Liang CK, Lim JY, Lim WS, Peng LN, Sugimoto K, Tanaka T, Won CW, Yamada M, Zhang T, Akishita M, Arai H. Asian Working Group for Sarcopenia: 2019 consensus update on sarcopenia diagnosis and treatment. J Am Med Dir Assoc. 2020;21(3):300–7.
18. Malik R, Goel H. Clinical validation of calf circumference with DEXA scans as a measure of muscle mass to assess sarcopenia in community settings in Indian postmenopausal women. J Midlife Health. 2024;15(2):99–103.
19. Makizako H, Kiyama R, Nakai Y, Kawada M, Tomioka K, Taniguchi Y, et al. Reference values of chair stand test and associations of chair stand performance with cognitive function in older adults. Aging Health Res. 2022;2(3):100090.
20. Monterrosa-Castro Á, Portela-Buelvas K, et al. Instruments to study sleep disorders in climacteric women. Sleep Sci. 2016;9(3):169–78.

21. Conde DM, Verdade RC, Valadares ALR, et al. Menopause and cognitive impairment: a narrative review of current knowledge. World J Psychiatry. 2021;11(8):412–28.
22. Abdel-Aziz K, Larner AJ. Six-item cognitive impairment test (6CIT): pragmatic diagnostic accuracy study for dementia and MCI. Int Psychogeriatr. 2015;27(6):991–7.
23. Agarwal V, Malik R, Jangid A. Assessment of sleep and cognitive decline using Hindi questionnaire. J South Asian Feder Obst Gynae. 2024;16(Suppl 3):S214–9.
24. Malik R, Pokeria C, Singh S. Correlation of menopausal symptoms with serum estradiol: a study in urban Indian postmenopausal women. J Obstet Gynaecol India. 2022;72(4):322–9.

5 Vasomotor Symptoms in Menopause

Kiran Aggarwal

Abstract

Menopause is associated with declining levels of estrogens. Menopause transition, a time four to six years prior to the Final Menstrual period has fluctuating hormonal levels. Vasomotor symptoms (VMSs) occur more so in late transition and early post menopause. Woman has feeling of warmth, hot flushes, may be chills, anxiety, and night sweats. It affects 40–70% women across the globe with Asian women having a lower incidence. Estrogen withdrawal is associated with over stimulation of neurons of hypothalamic thermoregulatory neutral zone and leads to dysregulation of body temperature. VMS are associated with smoking, obesity, hypertension, and higher cardiovascular disease risks. Frequency and severity of the VMS may be graded. A detailed history and examination is needed to rule out other diseases like hypertension, cardiovascular disease, carcinoid syndrome, etc. These may have a similar presentation. Life style management with cooling environment, less spicy food, cotton clothes may be tried. Cognitive behavioral therapy is helpful. For moderate-to-severe VMS Menopausal hormone therapy is indicated if woman is within 10 years postmenopause or less than 60 years of age. Tibolone is also helpful. Nonhormonal therapy with Selective Serotonin Reuptake Inhibitors (SSRIs) and Serotonin-Norepinephrine Reuptake Inhibitors (SNRIs) is also effective. Neurokinin B antagonists Fezolinetant has been found to be effective. Gabapentin a drug used for neuropathic disorders is also useful. Vasomotor symptoms may be used as one of the risk factors predicting CVD in future for the women.

K. Aggarwal (✉)
Department of Obstetrics and Gynaecology, Lady Hardinge Medical College & Smt Sucheta Kriplani Hospital, New Delhi, India

R. Malik et al. (eds.), *Menopause Essentials*,
https://doi.org/10.1007/978-981-95-7498-8_5

Keywords

Vasomotors symptoms · Hot flushes · Menopause hormone therapy · Neurokinin B antagonists Fezolinetant

5.1 Introduction

Menopause a stage of life is a physiological process encountered by all women. It is associated with depleting follicles in the ovaries and declining levels of estrogens in the body. It is associated with changes in woman's metabolism, fat distribution with a higher propensity towards visceral fat. With declining estrogens in the body there is a higher risk of cardiovascular diseases (CVD) and osteoporosis and fractures.

Menopause is defined retrospectively when a woman has an amenorrhea of 12 months with loss of ovarian function for which no other pathology can be assigned. The last period is called as Final Menstrual Period (FMP). Prior to this FMP there is a phase where these changes begin and waxing and waning of the hormones is seen which finally leads to decline in their levels and Menopause. This is called Menopause Transition (MT) and may vary from 4 to 6 years.

Vasomotor symptoms (VMS) affect women in this menopausal transition more so in late transition and early post menopause.

These symptoms comprise of feeling of warmth or heat associated with vasodilatation in the skin which causes hot flushes. At times women gets up in the night and drenched in sweat addressed as night sweats. It is not associated with fever. Vasomotor changes are associated with mood changes, anxiety, depression, and poor quality of life.

Menopausal hormone therapy is indicated for managing these changes along with other lifestyle therapies. In spite of vasomotor symptoms being prevalent in almost 40–70% women across the globe very few women receive treatment for the same.

In this chapter, we plan to address the magnitude of the problem, clinical presentation and assessment, evaluation and management with hormonal and nonhormonal methods.

5.2 Epidemiology

Vasomotor symptoms (VMS) or "hot flashes" occur in about 70–80% of women undergoing menopause transition [1, 2].

The frequency appears to vary by culture and ethnicity [3].

Inspite of mostly describing their symptoms as moderate-to-severe only 0–30% consult for treatment [4].

Forty percent women in early transition present with VMS and this increases to 60–80% in late transition and early postmenopause stage [4].

Duration and severity of symptoms varies across races and ethnicities. In the Study of Women's Health across the Nation (SWAN), African American and Hispanic women had a median VMS duration of 10.1 years and 8.9 years, respectively, compared to non-Hispanic white, Chinese, and Japanese women with a median VMS duration of 6.5 years, 5.4 years, and 4.8 years, respectively. Asian women have the lowest incidence [5, 6].

In India the prevalence of vasomotor symptoms shows a wide range from 16.5-88% [7].

5.3 Pathophysiology

During the perimenopause or the menopausal transition the hormones begin to fluctuate and this period is recognized by altered frequency and duration of the menstrual cycles.

Vasomotor symptoms may be associated with hormonal changes occurring during menopause transition. The pathophysiological process causing VMS is not clear. Falling estradiol levels and non bound sex hormone binding globulins may be causative. Increase in levels of Follicle stimulating hormone (FSH) is also an important factor [8].

The thermoregulatory center is placed in the preoptic area of the hypothalamus. Hypothalamic thermoregulatory neutral zone regulates body temperature. It is comprised of set of neurons which perform this function. During menopausal transition alterations occur in this thermoregulatory neutral zone which are caused by estrogen withdrawal and its fluctuating levels.

These neurons in the neutral zone are together called as KNDy neurons because they coexpress kisspeptin, neurokininB(NKB), and Dynorphin. These are normally suppressed by estrogens. During MT decreasing estrogen levels causes overstimulation of these neurons thus causing dysregulation of body temperature.

Any internal or external stimuli which cause prevention of heat loss from the body precipitate bodily reactions and these fluctuations in hormones increase the frequency of these changes [9].

Cutaneous vasodilation or vasoconstriction occurs for temperature homeostasis and a feeling of flushing, warmth, reddening of skin, and perspiration occurs [9].

These may be followed by chills also [10].

The thermoregulatory neutral zone narrows down in perimenopause and postmenopause and minor triggers which lead to prevention of heat loss cause altered cutaneous response in the form of vasodilation, constriction, feeling of heat, flush, and perspiration. A woman without vasomotor symptoms elevation of core temperature causes initiation of process to dissipate heat by cutaneous flushing and vasodilatation. However in decreasing estrogen scenario this occurs with a minimal increase in the body temperature. That is, there is a narrowing of the thermal regulatory zone.

Pulses of luteinizing hormone (LH) simultaneously are associated with hot flashes but causation is not seen [11]. The medial preoptic area which is the location for major thermoregulatory area in mammals is in close anatomical relation to high density of Gonadotropin releasing hormone (GnRH) containing neurons. This may indicate simultaneous activation of a burst of GnRH release and thermoregulatory changes. KNDy neurons may cause the LH and thermoregulatory changes which is also one of the possibilities [12].

5.4 Risk Factors

Vasomotor symptoms are more common in certain racial and ethnic groups. African American women have a higher incidence than Caucasians and Japanese and Chinese women report less.

Women with sudden menopause like surgical menopause radiation or chemotherapy have a higher incidence of VMS. Lower socioeconomic conditions Higher BMI, Smoking, metabolic syndrome have been associated with VMS. It is associated with hypertension and women with higher cardiovascular disease risks.

Genetic variants—Women with variations in the gene coding for tachykinin receptor 3 (*TACR3)* are more likely to experience hot flashes [13].

5.5 Clinical Presentation and Assessment

Hot flushes present as feeling of heat over chest and face and then spread to other areas of the body. This lasts for 2–4 min and is followed by perspiration. It may last longer also. This may cause loss of heat and fall in core body temperature and then chills may occur to restore the body temperature. These are at times also associated with anxiety, palpitations, feeling of dizziness, and inability to work.

A woman suffering from night sweats has a feeling of heat and has sweating. She has disturbed sleep. This affects her quality of life and lack of focus at work.

Frequency: The incidence of flushes is variable. In severe cases it may happen number of times in a day to less than once in 2–3 days in infrequent presentations.

As per the SWAN study the frequency of vasomotor symptoms has been described as number of days woman has experienced vasomotor symptoms in past two weeks. This is assessed by self reporting questionnaires.

5.5.1 Grading of Vasomotor Symptoms

To document and compare the symptoms intensity of Vasomotor symptoms have been graded [5] as: Table 5.1.

Grading of the symptoms and frequency should be charted. Menopause rating scale (MRS) may be used. Patient may be asked to keep a diary of the symptoms. Night recall may be difficult at times.

Daily hot flash diary is a measure of self reported hot flashes and night sweats and/ or their severity on a four point scale. This is mild, moderate, severe, and very severe. From this Hot flash index is calculated.

Hot flash related daily interference scale (HFRDIS) is used for psychometric assessment. It assesses the impact of hot flashes on daily activities in past week comprising of 10 items [14].

The vasomotor symptoms are seen maximally in late menopause transition and 2 years post final menstrual period. However, they may last for 10 years after FMP. Persistence later in life till the age of 60–70 years has been reported.

Following surgical menopause: After oophorectomy done surgically a woman may present with vasomotor symptoms and complain of hot flushes and palpitations in postoperative period. A differential of vasomotor symptoms should always be kept in mind.

Diagnosis A detailed History should be taken with description of the episode frequency other menopausal symptoms, assessment of co morbidities. A detailed general and systemic examination should be carried out. Blood pressure, local examination, vaginal ph, assessment of vaginal atrophy should be done.

Routine Investigations Complete blood Hemogram, fasting blood sugar, HbA1c, Thyroid function tests, vitamin D levels, lipid profile, serum FSH (>40 IU/L), urine microscopic examination imaging should be done as required.

5.5.1.1 Differential Diagnosis

The other causes of sweating anxiety palpitations should be assessed.

Carcinoid syndrome hyperthyroidism cardiovascular disease, malignancies, brain tumors, migraine, Hyperhidrosis should be evaluated.

Medications; Calcium channel blockers, Raloxefene, and Tamoxifen, gonadotrophin-releasing hormone (GNRH) agonists, calcitonin, metronidazole, ketocanazole, alcohol can cause hot flushes and palpitations.

Some nonhormonal treatments for hot flushes, such as SSRIs or venlafaxine, can also cause sweating at higher doses.

Table 5.1 Frequency and severity of VMS

Frequency (last two weeks)	Severity
None at all 1–5 days 6–8 days 9–13 days All days *Frequent VMS*: 6 or more days *Infrequent* 1–5 days *And no* VMS	Mild: Feeling of heat without sweating and not affecting routine activity Moderate: Feeling of heat with sweating Severe: Feeling of heat and sweating with disruption of normal physical activity

5.5.2 Management

Menopause Hormone therapy (MHT) is the mainstay for the treatment of vasomotor symptoms. The frequency and intensity both are benefitted by the treatment. Response may be seen within 2–3 weeks time of start of the therapy.

5.5.2.1 Hormonal

For women less than 60 years of age or within 10 years of menopause hormone therapy for moderate-to-severe vasomotor symptoms is recommended. (level A) recommendation.

At times women in this age group have associated problems like diabetes, hypertension, dyslipidaemias, etc. Before prescribing MHT individual case should be assessed in details and cardiovascular risk calculated and accordingly the therapy should be tailored to the individual woman's need.

If a woman already has a cardiovascular disease then non hormonal therapies for vasomotor symptoms may be beneficial.

The lowest dose of estrogen alone or estrogen and progesterone combination should be given. In a hysterectomized woman only estrogen is enough however for endometrial protection in those with uterus progesterone should be added. After starting therapy reassessment should be done at 3 months and the dose should be increased if symptoms not controlled.

Progesterons: Progesterone have to be added to the estrogen in MHT for protection of endometrium. It has been seen that Progesterones alone also may relieve vasomotor symptoms.

5.5.2.2 Contraindications to MHT

They are contraindicated in women with Coronary heart disease, thromboembolic disorders, undiagnosed bleeding from genital tract, and impaired liver function. In women with history of breast cancer nonhormonal treatment should be preferred [15].

5.5.3 Medical Conditions

5.5.3.1 Cardiovascular Disease

If MHT is started in younger women less than 60 years of age or within 10 years of menopause and in women with low risk of cardiovascular diseases it may be cardioprotective. In those who have a coronary artery disease MHT should not be given and non hormonal treatment should be considered [16].

CVD outcomes may also be affected by different routes of administering MHT. Transdermal estradiol being associated with lower CAD-related mortality compared to oral estrogens. Currently, HT is not indicated for primary or secondary prevention of CVD, including CAD.

5.5.3.2 Venous Thromboembolism

There is a high risk of venous thromboembolism in women who are obese and/or who have a previous history of venous thromboembolim (VTE). Lower doses of estrogen and non oral route of delivery are seen to have low risk of VTE.

Low dose estrogens are those which have less than 0.625 mg CEE or an oral estradiol preparation less than 1 mg and transdermal preparation which are less than 50 μg.

In both situations where women is obese BMI >25 kg/m^2 or there is high risk of VTE Transdermal route of estrogens is better [17].

Progesterone acetate which is a synthetic progestogen has a higher risk of VTE as compared to micronized progesterone and dydrogesterone which have a lower risk. As the dose of estrogen increases the risk of stroke increases in the women. Transdermal estrogens has a lower risk of VTE. MHT should be preferably avoided in women with history of breast cancer.

MHT has a favorable effect on lipid profile. It decreases low-density lipoprotein cholesterol (LDL-C) and lipoprotein (a). It also causes increase in high-density lipoprotein cholesterol (HDL-C) [18]. In both women with and without Diabetes Mellitus MHT improves glycemic control and insulin resistance. Cardiovascular disease risk factors also improves with MHT.

5.5.3.3 Hormone Therapy and Routes of Administration

Estrogen is available as oral tablet, transdermal patches, topical gels, lotions and vaginal rings. In women with uterus progesterone should be added. Conjugated equine estrogen in combination with selective estrogen receptor antagonist (for example, bazedoxifene) is useful to prevent the risk of endometrial hyperplasia.

Low dose vaginal estrogens used for vaginal atrophy will not help in vasomotor symptoms.

The lowest effective dose should be used and increased if symptoms are not resolved.

Estrogen products are considered low dose if they contain less than 0.625 mg CEE or 1 mg estradiol for oral formulations and less than 50 μg for transdermal formulations (Table 5.2).

5.5.4 Prescription

If continuous combined regime that is a fixed dose of estrogen and progesterone is given throughout 1 mg of estradiol needs 10 mg of Medroxyprogesterone daily or 100 mg of micronized progesterone. This is to be used in menopausal women. If sequential combined regime is followed where everyday estrogen is used with progesterone added in last 10–14 days given in a cyclical fashion, 200 mg of micronized progesterone in the second half of the cycle will be needed for 1 mg of estradiol given daily. This is preferred in perimenopausal women.

The levonorgestrel intrauterine device also may be used in place of oral progesterones. Cyclical therapy decreases exposure to progesterones and side effect of developing breast cancer.

If a woman has obesity, hyperlipidemia, diabetes, hypertension, mild risk of coronary artery disease, and MHT is needed then transdermal route is preferred. It bypasses hepatic metabolism.

5.5.4.1 Follow Up

Follow up of a women on MHT should be at 1–3 months. Relief of symptoms, any adverse effects should be assessed. Annually reassessment for indications, breast evaluation, and medical checkup should be done. After 6 months to 1 year of therapy the dose may be tapered down and MHT may be gradually stopped.

If symptoms recur then the MHT should be restarted and the dose titrated as per the symptoms. At times with severe symptoms therapy may be needed for a longer time.

5.5.4.2 Tibolone

Tibolone:

It is a compound with estrogenic, progestogenic, and androgenic properties. It is a synthetic steroid. Significant relief of VMS occurs and is associated with decreased breast tenderness as compared to MHT. Dose is 1.25 mg–2.5 mg per day.

The million women study which was UK based showed a higher risk of endometrial cancer in potmenopausal women using tibolone. There may be a higher risk of recurrence in women with history of breast cancer and taking Tibolone. The better thing is that it does not increase breast density [19].

5.5.5 Non Hormonal Management

Women may have contraindications to MHT like high risk for cardiovascular diseases, hormone dependent malignancies etc. They may not want to use it as a personal reason. The clinician should be aware of available nonhormonal treatments.

Table 5.2 Doses of estrogens

Estrogen	Ultra low dose mg/day	Low dose mg/day	Standard dose mg/day
Conjugated equine estrogen	0.3	0.45	0.625
Estradiol	0.25	0.5	1
Transdermal	0.014	0.025	0.0375–0.05

5.5.6 Life Style Management

Layered clothing, cotton clothes, improved ventilation and circulation, hand held fans, change of bedding all provide temporary relief and may be improve sleep quality.

Change in diet by including fruits, vegetables, and soy products may help but there is no documented benefit in moderate-to-severe vasomotor symptoms. Larger studies are needed to address these.

5.5.6.1 Exercise

Exercise including yoga may not provide relief and might also trigger vasomotor symptoms.

There are varied interpretations of benefit of exercise on vasomotor symptoms. Though it may not be much beneficial for vasomotor symptoms but improved sleep and quality of life, including depression is seen. Several Cochrane reviews concluded that there was insufficient or poor evidence to consider exercise as a treatment for VMS [20].

Acupuncture It is one of the modalities of treating vasomotor symptoms. Significant clinical effects were seen after 3 treatments, with maximum effects seen after 8 treatments. A systematic review with meta-analysis was done by Befus et al.

They highlighted significant increases in health-related quality of life outcomes for women undergoing acupuncture therapy [21].

Cognitive Behavioral Therapy

Cognitive behavioral therapy (CBT) is a form of psychotherapy. It is used in conditions like depression and anxiety and also helps in chronic pelvic pain. For this the therapist educates the women about VMS, helps in removing negative perceptions about the symptoms, relaxation, and deep breathing techniques.

In an RCT which studied CBT for menopausal symptoms (CBT-Meno), women who had symptoms of VMS who received CBT reported a significant improvement in their VMS symptom interference and bother due to VMS compared to no active intervention [22].

Paced breathing and relaxation techniques do not have enough evidence to support that they help.

5.5.6.2 Pharmacological Therapies

Nonhormonal drugs have been evaluated for treating VMS. These are Selective Serotonin Reuptake Inhibitors (SSRIs) and Serotonin-Norepinephrine Reuptake Inhibitors (SNRIs), Oxybutynin and Gabapentin.

Few of them have been effective in decreasing the frequency and intensity of the symptoms. Two drugs have been approved by FDA for managing VMS. These are Paroxetine mesylate 7.5 mg daily and fezolinetant 45 mg daily. Typically, the onset of action is within 2 weeks.

Selective Serotonin Reuptake Inhibitors (SSRIs) and Serotonin-Norepinephrine Reuptake Inhibitors (SNRIs)
SSRI and SNRI have been found to be useful in treating vasomotor symptoms. Vasomotor symptoms occur due to hypothalamic thermoregulatory disturbance. SSRI and SNRI increase the concentration of norepinephrine and serotonin and help in alleviating the symptoms of VMS.

Common Side Effects Dry mouth, nausea, constipation, decreased libido, and weight gain are seen. These are dose-dependent.

Paroxtiene: It is a SSRI. 7.5 mg a day as a low dose is US FDA approved non-hormonal drug for treatment of vasomotor symptoms. It can be used in moderate to severe VMS. Both frequency and severity of symptoms show improvement. Sleep duration is improved and negative effect on libido is not seen. After a month of use women with VMS showed almost 33% improvement as compared to 23% for a placebo [23].

Paroxetine should be used with caution in women taking tamoxifem.

Escitalopram, another SSRI, was similarly found to reduce hot flash frequency (44%) and severity compared with placebo.

Venlafaxine, an SNRI, Desvenlafaxine, the major active metabolite of venlafaxine, had a 72% decrease in the frequency of moderate-to-severe hot flashes.

All these drugs have shown statistically significant improvement in VMS in multiple meta-analyses and systematic reviews. Gabapentin is a gamma-aminobutyric acid (GABA) analog. It is an anticonvulsant and is also used for neuropathic disorders. It improves vasomotor symptoms also it binds with the calcium channels in hypothalamus and widens the thermoregulatory zone. It causes dizziness, headache, and disorientation so may be used at bed time (Table 5.3) [24].

Oxybutynin Oxybutynin is an antimuscarinic, anticholinergic drug. It is used for the treatment of overactive bladder and urinary urge incontinence. Doses ranging from 2.5 mg or 5 mg twice daily up to 15 mg extended-release daily significantly improved moderate to severe VMS. Dry mouth is a side effect.

5.5.6.3 Neurokinin B Antagonists

Fall in estrogen levels as in menopause transition cause hyperactivity of KNDy neuron activity and increased levels of Neurokinin B. This triggers VMS.

Fezolinetant is a selective neurokinin B receptor-3 antagonist found to be beneficial in VMS for both severity and frequency [26].

- *Side effects* [27]:
  GI upset, fatigue, headaches, and upper respiratory infections.
  Liver function need to be monitored more frequently.
  Use of Fezolinetant for other symptoms of menopause has yet not been defined.
  Use in women with current breast cancer or history of same has not been defined.
  Quality of life improves due to improvement in sleep and VMS related distress.

Table 5.3 Nonhormonal pharmacotherapy [25]

SSRIs
Paroxetine: 7.5 mg per day
Citalopram: 10–20 mg/day, initial dose may be from 10 mg/day
Escitalopram: 10–20 mg/day
SNRIs Desvenlafaxine 100–150 mg/day, initial dose may be from 25 to 50 mg/day
Venlafaxine 37.5 mg/day
Gabapentinoids Gabapentin 900–2400 mg/day to be given at night. Initial dose may be 100–300 mg/day
Neurokinin B antagonists
Fezolinetant 45 mg/day

- *Contraindications*:
  - Severe renal impairment
  - Liver disease

5.5.6.4 Clonidine

Clonidine is a central-acting alpha-2 agonist known for its hypotensive and sedative effects. Mainly used as an antihypertensive it is also effective in VMS. Has been studied in tamoxifem induced hot flashes and found to be effective.

Stellate Ganglion Block

Stellate ganglion block (SGB) has been investigated in several studies as a potential treatment to VMS.

Herbs and Dietary Supplement

Black cohosh was initially inducted to Western medicine by the Native Americans. It was used remedy for treating pregnancy associated pain and promoting normal delivery and puerperium. Its scientific name is Actaea racemosa L. The assays both in vitro and in vivo demonstrate its estrogen like activity.

Black cohosh may decrease hot flashes and night sweats both by numbers and intensity. The results are mixed. It is a safe herbal medicine but the way it acts is not clear. Currently, there is insufficient evidence to support its use for VMS. (Level I; not recommended) [25].

Isoflavones and Soya Products

In certain regions and ethnic groups phytoestrogens are an important component of dietary intake. Isoflavones are a form of phytoestrogens which are derived from the plants. Weak estrogenic activity is shown by them. Genistein and Daidzein are the major isoflavones seen in Soy products [28]. They also have antioxidant and anti-inflammatory properties. This may benefit menopause issues. These bind to estrogen receptors and have a weak estrogen like effect. Studies using them are with few participants. Currently data on their usage is inconsistent in breast cancer patients and their use is not recommended.

5.6 Conclusions

VMS is a bothersome presentation of menopause transition and postmenopause. It affects quality of life and performance. It is associated with hypertension and cardiovascular disease risks. Women and health care workers should be made aware of available treatments.

In women with moderate to severe symptoms window of opportunity should be used if women is less than 60 years or within 10 years of menopause to prescribe MHT. It provides other benefits also like for cardio protection and bone health.

In women with contraindication to MHT awareness about nonhormonal methods is a must. VMS may be in future used as one of the risk factors predicting CVD in future for the women.

Key Points

1. Moderate-to-severe VMS should be treated. MHT is the drug of choice.
2. Before diagnosing VMS other conditions causing sweating and flushing like hypertension, CAD, hyperthyroidism should be ruled out.
3. In women within 10 years of menopause or less than 60 years of age MHT may be given.
4. Lowest dose of drugs should be preferred.
5. Paroxetine and Fluxetine should not be prescribed with Tamoxifen.
6. Venlafaxine is preferred in breast cancer survivors on tamoxifen.
7. NK3 receptor antagonist Fezolinetant is USA FDA approved.
8. Further research is needed for alternative therapies.

Long Answer Questions (LAQs)

1. Describe the pathophysiology of vasomotor symptoms
2. What are the non hormonal drugs used for VMS

Short Answer Questions (SAQs)

1. Write the hormone therapy for VMS
2. Write a short note on Fezolinetant
3. Use of SSRI and SNRI in VMS

Multiple Choice Questions (MCQs)

1. Following nonhormonal drug is US FDA approved for treatment of VMS
   A. Fezolinetant
   B. clonidene
   C. oxybutynin
   D. reserpine
2. Vasomotor symptoms are associated with following area in the brain
   A. frontal
   B. pons
   C. cortex
   D. Thermoregulatory zone of hypothalamus
3. Dose of Paroxitene for VMS is
   A. 15 mg
   B. 30 mg
   C. 7.5 mg
   D. 10 mg
4. MHT used in VMS is contraindicated in:
   A. joint pains
   B. migraine without aura
   C. controlled hypertension
   D. breast cancer
5. VMS are associated with following:
   A. metabolicsyndrome
   B. obesity
   C. cardiovascular disease
   D. all above
6. Paroxitene is a
   A. SSRI
   B. SNRI
   C. Beta blocker
   D. antimuscarinic
7. Elevated levels in brain of following is seen in VMS
   A. Melatonin
   B. serotonin
   C. Oxytocin
   D. Growth hormone

8. Which of the following is useful in VMS:
   A. Exercise
   B. fatty diet
   C. paced respiration
   D. Cognitive behavior therapy
9. Vasomotor symptoms are most common in
   A. premenopaue
   B. early menopause transition
   C. late menopause transition
   D. reproductive age
10. VMS lasts for average for following duration
    A. 10–15 years
    B. 4–6 years
    C. 0–2 years
    D. 20–25 years

Answers

1. A
2. D
3. C
4. D
5. D
6. A
7. B
8. D
9. D
10. B

References

1. National Institutes of Health. National Institutes of Health state-of-the-science conference statement: management of menopause-related symptoms. Ann Intern Med. 2005;142(12 Pt 1):1003–13. Epub 2005 May 27.
2. Woods NF, Mitchell ES. Symptoms during the perimenopause: prevalence, severity, trajectory, and significance in women's lives. Am J Med. 2005;118(Suppl 12B):14–24. https://doi.org/10.1016/j.amjmed.2005.09.031.

3. Sievert LL, Morrison L, Brown DE, Reza AM. Vasomotor symptoms among Japanese-American and European-American women living in Hilo, Hawaii. Menopause. 2007;14(2):261–9. https://doi.org/10.1097/01.gme.0000233496.13088.24. PMID: 17151510.
4. Randolph JF Jr, Sowers M, Bondarenko I, Gold EB, Greendale GA, Bromberger JT, Brockwell SE, Matthews KA. The relationship of longitudinal change in reproductive hormones and vasomotor symptoms during the menopausal transition. J Clin Endocrinol Metab. 2005;90(11):6106–12. https://doi.org/10.1210/jc.2005-1374. Epub 2005 Sep 6.
5. Avis NE, Crawford SL, Greendale G, Study of Women's Health Across the Nation, et al. Duration of menopausal vasomotor symptoms over the menopause transition. JAMA Intern Med. 2015;175(4):531–9. PMID: 25686030; PMCID: PMC4433164. https://doi.org/10.1001/jamainternmed.2014.8063.
6. Khan SJ, Kapoor E, Faubion SS, Kling JM. Vasomotor symptoms during menopause: a practical guide on current treatments and future perspectives. Int J Womens Health. 2023;15:273–87. https://doi.org/10.2147/IJWH.S365808. PMID: 36820056; PMCID: PMC9938702.
7. Meeta M, Anuradha M, Ashraf AB, Aggarwal K et al. Clinical practice guidelines for menopause: an executive summary and recommendations; Indian menopause society. J Midlife Health. 2026;17(s1):s23.
8. Rapkin AJ. Vasomotor symptoms in menopause: physiologic condition and central nervous system approaches to treatment. Am J Obstet Gynecol. 2007;196:97–106.
9. Deecher DC, Dorries K. Understanding the pathophysiology of vasomotor symptoms (hot flushes and night sweats) that occur in perimenopause, menopause, and postmenopause life stages. Arch Womens Ment Health. 2007;10(6):247–57. https://doi.org/10.1007/s00737-007-0209-5. [DOI] [PubMed] [Google Scholar]
10. Kronenberg F. Hot flashes: epidemiology and physiology. Ann N Y Acad Sci 1990;592:52–86. PMID: 2197954. doi:https://doi.org/10.1111/j.1749-6632.1990.tb30316.x.; discussion 123–33. [DOI] [PubMed] [Google Scholar].
11. Casper RF, Yen SS, Wilkes MM. Menopausal flushes: a neuroendocrine link with pulsatile luteninizing hormone secreation. Science. 1979;205(4408):823–5. https://doi.org/10.1126/science.462193. PMID: 462193
12. Rance NE, Dacks PA, Mittelman-Smith MA, Romanovsky AA, Krajewski-Hall SJ. Modulation of body temperature and LH secretion by hypothalamic KNDy (kisspeptin, neurokinin B and dynorphin) neurons: a novel hypothesis on the mechanism of hot flushes. Front Neuroendocrinol. 2013;34(3):211–27. https://doi.org/10.1016/j.yfrne.2013.07.003. Epub 2013 Jul 17. PMID: 23872331; PMCID: PMC3833827.
13. Crandall CJ, Manson JE, Hohensee C, Horvath S, Wactawski-Wende J, LeBlanc ES, Vitolins MZ, Nassir R, Sinsheimer JS. Association of genetic variation in the tachykinin receptor 3 locus with hot flashes and night sweats in the women's health initiative study. Menopause. 2017;24(3):252–61. https://doi.org/10.1097/GME.0000000000000763. PMID: 28231077; PMCID: PMC5327841.
14. Carpenter JS. The hot flash related daily interference scale: a tool for assessing the impact of hot flashes on quality of life following breast cancer. J Pain Symptom Manag. 2001;22:979–89.
15. The NAMS 2022 Hormone Therapy Position Statement Advisory Panel. The 2022 hormone therapy position statement of the North American Menopause Society. Menopause. 2022;29(7):767–94. https://doi.org/10.1097/GME.0000000000002028. [DOI] [PubMed] [Google Scholar].
16. Boardman HM, Hartley L, Eisinga A, et al. Hormone therapy for preventing cardiovascular disease in post-menopausal women. Cochrane Database Syst Rev. 2015;(3):CD002229. https://doi.org/10.1002/14651858.CD002229.pub4. [DOI] [PMC free article] [PubMed] [Google Scholar].
17. Canonico M, Oger E, Conard J, The ESTHER Study, et al. Obesity and risk of venous thromboembolism among postmenopausal women: differential impact of hormone therapy by route of estrogen administration. J Thromb Haemost. 2006;4(6):1259–65. https://doi.org/10.1111/j.1538-7836.2006.01933.x. [DOI] [PubMed] [Google Scholar]

18. Koh KK, Shin MS, Sakuma I, et al. Effects of conventional or lower doses of hormone replacement therapy in postmenopausal women. Arterioscler Thromb Vasc Biol. 2004;24(8):1516–21. [DOI] [PubMed] [Google Scholar].
19. Formoso G, Perrone E, Maltoni S, et al. Short-term and long-term effects of tibolone in postmenopausal women. Cochrane Database Syst Rev. 2016;10(10):CD008536. https://doi.org/10.1002/14651858.CD008536.pub3. [DOI] [PMC free article] [PubMed] [Google Scholar].
20. Daley A, Stokes-Lampard H, Thomas A, MacArthur C. Exercise for vasomotor menopausal symptoms. Cochrane Database Syst Rev. 2014:CD006108. https://doi.org/10.1002/14651858.CD006108.pub4.
21. Befus D, Coeytaux RR, Goldstein KM, et al. Management of menopause symptoms with acupuncture: an umbrella systematic review and meta-analysis. J Altern Complement Med. 2018;24:314–23.
22. Green SM, Donegan E, Frey BN, et al. Cognitive behavior therapy for menopausal symptoms (CBT-Meno): a randomized controlled trial. Menopause. 2019;26(9):972–80. https://doi.org/10.1097/GME.0000000000001363. [DOI] [PubMed] [Google Scholar].
23. Simon JA, Portman DJ, Kaunitz AM, et al. Low-dose paroxetine 7.5 mg for menopausal vasomotor symptoms: two randomized controlled trials. Menopause. 2013;20(10):1027–35. https://doi.org/10.1097/GME.0b013e3182a66aa7. [DOI] [PubMed] [Google Scholar].
24. Yoon SH, Lee JY, Lee C, Lee H, Kim SN. Gabapentin for the treatment of hot flushes in menopause: a meta-analysis. Menopause. 2020;27:485–93. PubMedGoogle Scholar
25. The 2023 nonhormone therapy position statement of the North American Menopause Society. Menopause. 2023;30(6):573–90. https://doi.org/10.1097/GME.0000000000002200. PMID: 37252752.
26. Archer DF. Nonhormonal management of vasomotor symptoms: understanding the options. Climacteric. 2022;25:113–21.
27. Johnson KA, Martin N, Nappi RE, Neal-Perry G, Shapiro M, Stute P, Thurston RC, Wolfman W, English M, Franklin C, Lee M, Santoro N. Efficacy and safety of Fezolinetant in moderate to severe vasomotor symptoms associated with menopause: a phase 3 RCT. J Clin Endocrinol Metab. 2023;108(8):1981–97. https://doi.org/10.1210/clinem/dgad058. PMID: 36734148; PMCID: PMC10348473.
28. Keshavarz Z, Golezar S, Hajifoghaha M, et al. The effect of phytoestrogens on menopause symptoms: a systematic review. J Isfahan Med Sch. 2018;36:446–59.

Genitourinary Syndrome of Menopause

6

Asna Beg Ashraf

Abstract

The Genitourinary syndrome of menopause (GSM) is a progressive urogenital condition caused by declining estrogen and androgen levels during menopause transition and menopause. Changes in the vulvovaginal and lower urinary tract tissues result in a range of genital, sexual, and urinary symptoms. With increasing life expectancy, the impact of GSM on the quality of life, sexual function, and urogenital health is becoming more evident. Healthcare providers should screen women for symptoms, diagnose, counsel, and treat women with GSM to optimize symptom control. First-line therapies for mild symptoms limited to vaginal dryness or dyspareunia include nonhormonal vaginal lubricants and moisturizers. For moderate-to-severe GSM, low-dose vaginal estrogen therapy, vaginal DHEA, and oral SERM ospemifene are safe and effective options. Vulvovaginal energy-based devices offer a choice to women in whom vaginal estrogen is contraindicated, but long-term safety is not known.

Keywords

Genitourinary syndrome of menopause · Lubricants · Moisturizers · Laser · DHEA · Ospemifene · Local estrogen therapy · Vulvovaginal atrophy · Menopause · Dyspareunia

A. B. Ashraf (✉)
Ujala Medical Center, Lucknow, India

Lucknow Menopause Society, Lucknow, India

Stillbirth Society of India, Lucknow, India

R. Malik et al. (eds.), *Menopause Essentials*,
https://doi.org/10.1007/978-981-95-7498-8_6

6.1 Introduction

Advancements in healthcare and rising life expectancy mean that women may now spend nearly 40% of their lives in menopause [1]. Genitourinary Syndrome of Menopause (GSM) is a broad term encompassing genital, sexual, and urinary symptoms and signs caused by anatomical and physiological changes in the vulva, vagina, and lower urinary tract tissues, primarily due to the progressive reduction and loss of ovarian estrogen production [1, 2]. Reduced androgen levels and aging of urogenital tissues also contribute to its manifestations [3]. It is often referred to as a silent epidemic, with a lack of awareness hindering accurate diagnosis and access to treatment [4]. In contrast to vasomotor symptoms, GSM is a chronic progressive condition that does not resolve spontaneously, and tends to worsen without treatment [1, 5, 6]. It can adversely affect the quality of life (QoL) and effective long-term care for symptom control requires a combination of hormonal and nonhormonal options [5].

GSM may also occur in premenopausal women with primary ovarian insufficiency (POI), hypothalamic amenorrhea, following cancer treatments (bilateral oophorectomy, pelvic radiation, or chemotherapy) that impair ovarian function, or the use of antiestrogenic therapy (aromatase inhibitors, tamoxifen, and GnRH agonists) [5, 7, 8]. Temporary GSM-like symptoms may also develop in postpartum breastfeeding women or women on progestin-only contraceptives [7, 8].

6.2 Terminology

GSM was earlier known as vulvovaginal atrophy (VVA). In 2014, at a consensus meeting of the International Society for the Study of Women's Sexual Health and the North American Menopause Society, the new term "genitourinary syndrome of menopause" was introduced to describe the constellation of urogenital and sexual symptoms arising from the deficiency of estrogen [2]. It was coined to replace "VVA", "vaginal atrophy" and "atrophic vaginitis" because they only described the structural changes in the genital tissues, and not the associated symptoms [2]. Urinary tract changes are also not included in VVA. The word "atrophy" has negative connotations for some women, and "vagina" can be a taboo word in conversations [1]. The aim was to describe more accurately and inclusively the symptoms and signs related to estrogen deficiency in the entire female genitourinary tract, including the labia, introitus, vulva, vagina, clitoris, bladder trigone, and urethra [2, 9]. However, changes in terminology have not significantly improved the recognition and treatment of this condition [4]. Diagnosing GSM remains challenging due to the lack of well-defined, standard diagnostic criteria [6].

6.3 Prevalence and Impact

The reported prevalence of GSM-related symptoms varies due to the nonuniformity of assessment tools and diagnostic criteria. GSM is estimated to affect between 27% and 84% of women in menopause, often leading to notable declines in health, sexual and emotional wellbeing, and QoL [1, 5]. An Indian study reported GSM in 48.7% of women attending menopause clinics, with prevalence increasing across menopause stages, from 28.5% in menopause transition to 57.9% in early postmenopause (<8 years since the final menstrual period) and 71.1% in late postmenopausal women (>8 years since the FMP) [10]. In a systematic review of 27 studies, 13–87% of women reported GSM symptoms, 47–81% were not familiar with GSM as a condition, and 52–91% reported that their lives had been negatively impacted by GSM symptoms. Symptomatic women who sought help from healthcare providers (HCP) varied from 25% in Asia to 52–75% in the EU, US, and Canada, to 92% in Latin America [6].

Many women consider the symptoms of GSM to be a natural part of ageing and, may not report them to HCPs. Women may also refrain from seeking treatment due to embarrassment, cultural or religious beliefs, societal stigma, or a lack of awareness about treatment options [5]. HCPs may hesitate to address GSM symptoms, often due to limited awareness, discomfort with the topic, or time constraints during consultations. Consequently, GSM is frequently under-reported, underdiagnosed, and undertreated [1, 6]. Without appropriate intervention, this condition typically progresses in most women, leading to functional and structural changes in urogenital tissues that may be challenging to reverse [1]. GSM can also lead to anxiety and depression, sexual dysfunctions such as desire, arousal, and orgasm disorders. It may also adversely affect daily activities, reduce QoL, negatively impact self-image, and intimate relationships [1, 8, 10].

6.4 Pathophysiology

The genital and lower urinary tracts in women share a common embryological origin and both express alpha and beta estrogen receptors (ERs) during the reproductive years. After menopause beta-ERs expression declines, but this can be restored by estrogen treatment [2]. Hypoestrogenism leads to anatomical changes in urogenital tissues, including reduced collagen content and hyalinization, decreased elastin, epithelial thinning, alterations in the structure and function of smooth muscle cells, increased connective tissue density, and a reduction in blood vessels within the lamina propria. Decreased strength of vaginal tissues, increased fragility and reduced lubrication can lead to epithelial damage during penetrative sex, causing pain, burning, fissuring, irritation, and spotting or bleeding [2, 11]. Estrogen is crucial for urinary continence through its effects on periurethral vessels, striated musculature, smooth muscle, and pelvic connective tissue. Hypoestrogenism can increase the risk of urgency and urge incontinence [7].

During reproductive years the superficial mucosal cells of the vagina shed approximately every 4 h, releasing large amounts of glycogen, which is metabolized by lactobacilli, into lactic acid, lowering the vaginal pH to 3.5–4.5 and protecting from vaginal and lower urinary tract infections [7]. During menopause since fewer squamous cells are released into vaginal secretions due to thinning of the vaginal epithelium, glycogen levels fall, lactobacilli decrease, and as a result, the vaginal pH increases [2, 4]. The duration of estrogen deficiency plays a key role in the development and severity of GSM symptoms [7].

6.5 Clinical Manifestations and Evaluation of GSM

The diagnosis of GSM is clinical and is based entirely on a thorough medical history and detailed physical examination [1, 12]. Women may exhibit some or all symptoms and signs, which should be distressing and not attributable to any other disease [5]. Genital symptoms include vulval or vaginal dryness; irritation; burning or itching of the vulva or vagina and sometimes vaginal discharge [2, 7, 8]. Urinary symptoms include frequency, nocturia, urgency, and dysuria together known as the lower urinary tract symptoms (LUTS), and recurrent urinary tract infections [2, 8]. Sexual symptoms include discomfort and pain with sexual activity, reduced lubrication, postcoital bleeding or spotting, and decreased libido, arousal, and orgasm [2, 8].

6.5.1 Focused History

HCPs should proactively inquire about genitourinary and sexual symptoms in all perimenopausal and postmenopausal women [5]. A thorough assessment should include symptom onset, duration, severity, associated distress, and impact on quality of life. Sexual history, covering partner relationships, current activity, and how symptoms affect sexual well-being should also be discussed [1]. Potential vulvar irritants, such as tight clothing, synthetic underwear, scented products, and hygiene items, must be considered. Reviewing medications, past surgeries, and other medical conditions is equally important [9]. Discussing the effectiveness of past interventions and any adverse effects is key to guiding management strategies [5].

6.5.2 Physical Examination

A thorough pelvic examination is vital for diagnosing GSM and differentiating it from other vulvovaginal disorders with overlapping symptoms [5].

6.5.2.1 Signs of GSM on Inspection of External Genitalia [2, 5]

There is a reduction of the fat content in mons pubis and labia majora. Labia minora undergo resorption and labial fusion may be seen in severe cases. The urethral meatus may appear prominent. Urethral caruncle, a benign outgrowth of inflammatory mucosal tissue arising from the posterior urethral meatus, is common in postmenopausal women and is related to hypoestrogenism. Vestibular tissue may appear pale. The introitus becomes narrow or even stenotic. Vulvar fissures may be seen in untreated severe cases usually in elderly women.

6.5.2.2 Per Speculum Examination

A narrow introitus, and a short, narrow vagina can make the insertion of a speculum difficult and painful. A well-lubricated smaller size or pediatric speculum should be used to minimize patient discomfort and avoid trauma [5]. Vaginal mucosa may appear pale or erythematous. There is reduced vaginal moisture and elasticity. Due to the loss of vaginal rugae, the mucosa appears smooth and shiny. Alterations in the vaginal microbiome can predispose some women to infections, often presenting as increased vaginal discharge. Vaginal petechiae or bleeding may occur due to mucosal thinning and increased friability, often triggered by minimal blunt trauma from speculum insertion. The cervix may be flushed with the vagina with obliteration of the vaginal fornices [5].

Symptoms do not always align with clinical signs. A woman who is not sexually active may show signs of severe atrophy yet report no symptoms [5]. Conversely, a sexually active woman may experience significant dryness and discomfort during intimacy despite showing minimal signs on examination [4, 5]. An accurate diagnosis depends on both history and physical examination [5].

6.5.2.3 Assessment of Vaginal Health

Assessment tools may be used to accurately assess the severity of urogenital and sexual dysfunction and the response to treatment. While commonly used in research settings, these tests are not necessary to diagnose GSM in clinical practice [12]. Subjective tools, influenced by patient perception, include the Visual Analogue Scale (VAS) for GSM symptoms and various Patient Reported Outcome Measures (PROMs) like the Female Sexual Function Index (FSFI) which assesses six domains of sexuality (desire, arousal, lubrication, orgasm, satisfaction, and pain), Vulvovaginal Symptoms Questionnaire (VSQ), and Day-to-Day Impact of Vaginal Aging (DIVA) questionnaire [8, 12].

Complementary tools such as the Vaginal Health Index (VHI), Vaginal Maturation Index (VMI), and vaginal pH can be used for objective assessment of vaginal health [7]. To assess pH, a piece of litmus paper is placed on the lateral vaginal wall until moistened [12]. A vaginal pH of >5 in the absence of infection or semen can be considered an indicator of vaginal atrophy due to hypoestrogenism in association with symptoms and signs [4, 7].

VHI is a clinician-assessed tool comprising five vaginal parameters evaluated on a 5-point Likert scale, with total scores ranging from 5 to 25. (1 = none, 5 = excellent). Four out of five parameters (vaginal elasticity, fluid volume, mucosal integrity, and moisture) are subjective and one is objective (vaginal pH) [12]. A VHI ≤15 is indicative of vaginal atrophy [8]. VMI offers an objective, cytological measure of estrogen effect on vaginal epithelium; the relative proportions of parabasal, intermediate, and superficial vaginal epithelial cells in a smear from the upper two-thirds of the vagina are calculated [7]. VMI = (% parabasal cells × 0) + (% intermediate cells × 0.5) + (% superficial cells × 1.0). A higher VMI indicates a greater proportion of mature, superficial cells, suggesting higher estrogen levels. If superficial cells are <5% or parabasal cells >75% it indicates GSM [3, 9].

6.5.3 Investigation

Though not essential for the diagnosis, laboratory tests or biopsies can be helpful in the differential diagnosis when the appearance is atypical or the lesion does not respond to treatment [9]. LUTS can often be misdiagnosed as urinary tract infection (UTI). However, some women may develop culture-positive UTIs. Therefore, urinalysis is important, and a mid-stream sample should be sent, for microscopy and culture.

Wet-mount microscopy shows more than one white blood cell per epithelial cell, immature vaginal epithelial cells with relatively large nuclei (parabasal cells), and reduced or absent lactobacilli. Recolonization with a variety of bacteria can occur, including gut organisms commonly linked to UTIs [5]. A vulvovaginal biopsy should be considered if symptoms do not resolve after a trial of vaginal estrogens or DHEA or if there are unusual findings [5].

6.6 Differential Diagnosis

Other vulvovaginal conditions that mimic GSM should be ruled out [5, 7, 9]. As these conditions can coexist with GSM, regular re-evaluation is necessary, especially if symptoms persist, or worsen despite adequate GSM management [7].

Lichen simplex chronicus (a hyperkeratotic plaque, or papule produced by repeated scratching), lichen sclerosus (a chronic inflammatory dermatosis with glistening ivory-white plaques or patches in the vulva and anus which may coalesce), lichen planus (inflamed painful red plaques which can affect the skin, nails, and mucous membranes including the genital area) and allergic contact dermatitis can also cause vulvovaginal symptoms [7, 8].

Vaginitis can be due to desquamative inflammatory vaginitis (vaginal rash and purulent discharge), vulvovaginal candidiasis, and other infections [8].

Vulvar intraepithelial neoplasia (red, white, or dark raised or eroded multifocal lesions) and vulvar cancer (solitary ulcer with raised or indurated edge, a rare malignant disease) both can only be confirmed with a biopsy [7].

Vulvodynia (an idiopathic chronic vulvar pain that lasts more than 3 months), vestibulodynia, chronic pelvic pain, provoked pelvic floor hypertonia (vaginismus), presence of foreign bodies, and trauma are some other etiologies [7, 8].

6.7 Management of GSM

The therapeutic management of GSM should be sequential, considering the age, symptoms, overall health, comorbidities, effect on QoL, and personal preferences.

1. Lifestyle modifications
2. Control of underlying medical conditions
3. Non-hormonal vaginal treatments—lubricants and moisturizers
4. Vaginal estrogens
5. Menopause Hormone therapy
6. Vaginal DHEA
7. Ospemifene
8. Energy-based therapies
9. Pelvic floor muscle (PFM) rehabilitation

6.7.1 Lifestyle Modifications

A balanced diet, sufficient vitamin D and calcium, limiting alcohol consumption and regular physical activity are the first steps for managing mild GSM. A sedentary lifestyle is linked to an increase in the prevalence of urogenital atrophy due to reduced blood flow to the pelvis and estrogen deficiency [11].

Smoking increases the metabolism of estrogen, and smoking cessation may decrease the atrophic effects due to increased capillary refilling. A weight loss of 5–10% of total body weight may improve urinary symptoms. Sexual activity, including masturbation, enhances genital blood flow and provides mechanical stimulation, contributing to the maintenance of urogenital tissue elasticity and integrity [1, 5]. This may mitigate the progression of GSM and support the maintenance of normal vaginal pH [4, 11]. Women should avoid scented hygiene products because they can disrupt the normal vaginal flora.

6.7.2 Control of Underlying Medical Conditions

Women with comorbidities (diabetes, obesity, or hypertension) are more likely to develop GSM. Effective management of comorbid conditions may improve genitourinary and sexual function. Both sexual function and QoL may improve if depression is treated [7].

6.7.3 Vaginal Moisturizers and Lubricants

Vaginal moisturizers primarily consist of water combined with either plant-based or synthetic polymers that help them adhere to the mucosal surface. Excipients in moisturizers provide viscosity, pH buffering and preservation, and other ingredients prevent contamination. They rehydrate tissue and mimic vaginal secretions. The effect lasts for 2–3 days by changing the endothelial fluid content and decreasing the vaginal pH, which maintains vaginal moisture and acidity. They are longer lasting than lubricants and are used to alleviate day-to-day discomfort associated with urogenital atrophy [13]. Hyaluronic acid is a naturally occurring polysaccharide and a key component of the extracellular matrix in various body tissues, including the vaginal epithelium. It possesses notable antioxidant properties. Moisturizers containing hyaluronic acid are safe and effective treatment for GSM [13].

Lubricants, which can be water-, silicone-, or oil-based, are used before intercourse to help reduce vaginal dryness [1]. They provide short-term relief but are less long-lasting than moisturizers. Some lubricants do not list their ingredients, making it difficult to identify the cause of irritation or inadequate effectiveness [13].

The moisturizers and lubricants should be physiologically similar to vaginal secretions in terms of pH (i.e. around 3.5, with a range of 3–5) and osmolality (around 380 mOsmol/kg, with a range of 200–600 mOsmol/kg) [13]. They should be free from parabens, chlorhexidine, and Polyquaternium-15 due to their potential for adverse effects. Commercial moisturizers can vary significantly in composition, and some may cause epithelial irritation due to abnormal pH, osmolality, or additives.

While some women will benefit from non-hormonal treatments, they should be informed about the chronic and progressive nature of GSM and its underlying endocrinological cause [1].

6.7.4 Vaginal Estrogen Therapy

When nonhormonal treatments fail to relieve symptoms, and no other menopausal issues are present, low-dose local estrogen therapy (LET) is considered the gold standard for managing vulvovaginal dryness, irritation, and dyspareunia [5, 8]. It is also recommended in patients with overactive bladder and recurrent UTI [5, 8]. LET increases local blood flow with positive effects on both subjective and objective measures of urogenital atrophy and improves some domains of sexual function. Estrogen is absorbed vaginally in a dose-dependent manner, but low-dose LET maintains serum levels within the postmenopausal range (from undetectable to 10.7 pg/ml) [3]. Since systemic absorption is minimal, there is no need for additional progestogen therapy.

Low-dose LET includes a range of products (vaginal tablets, rings, capsules, pessaries, creams, gels, and ovules) for treating symptomatic GSM, though availability may differ globally [8]. The different molecules are estradiol, estriol, promestriene, conjugated equine estrogens, and estrone. Estradiol (E2) is the primary ovarian estrogen during the reproductive years, and ultra-low dose E2 formulations (4–10 μg), are now most commonly used. Compared to low-dose 25 μg E2, these ultra-low doses significantly improve vaginal cell maturation and pH, and reduce GSM symptoms, while causing less increase in circulating E2 levels [3]. Estriol (E3), a short-acting estrogen of placental origin and the final metabolite of estrogen synthesis, is highly effective when administered intravaginally. It has a preferential affinity for ER-β over ER-α with the advantage of reduced extra-vaginal effects. Estriol vaginal formulations are not available in the US due to lack of FDA approval, insufficient large-scale clinical trial data, and regulatory restrictions. Only estradiol and conjugated estrogens are approved for vaginal use. Low-dose conjugated equine estrogen cream (0.625 mg active ingredient/g) and estriol (0.01% w/w) cream are the available formulations in India.

Promestriene is a synthetic estrogen used as a 10 mg cream or insert, has minimal absorption and acts superficially on the vaginal mucosa. It is safer for women with severe atrophy and estrogen-sensitive cancers while effectively improving urogenital symptoms [3].

Estrone is a weak estrogen formed in visceral fat in postmenopausal women. It is available as a 1 mg/g vaginal cream for short-term use. Due to variable increases in circulating E2, estrone is considered less safe than other low- and ultra-low-dose LET [3].

LET is used daily for 2 weeks, followed by twice-per-week administration. If the vaginal ring is being used, it should be changed every 90 days [3].

Adverse Events vaginal discharge, vulvovaginal candidiasis, vaginal bleeding, and breast pain [5].

6.7.5 Menopause Hormone Therapy

Systemic menopause hormone therapy (MHT) is effective in relieving GSM symptoms in most postmenopausal women. Its main indications are the treatment of vasomotor symptoms and the prevention of postmenopausal osteoporosis [3]. In some patients, systemic MHT alone may not provide sufficient relief from GSM symptoms and a combination of MHT and low-dose vaginal ET may be required, especially in those with severe symptoms [5].

6.7.6 Dehydroepiandrosterone

Dehydroepiandrosterone (DHEA), also known as Prasterone, is a neurosteroid and key precursor to sex hormones, with about 80% being produced by the adrenal glands and 20% by the ovaries [9]. After menopause, it becomes the exclusive source of estrogens and androgens [4]. A low-dose DHEA vaginal insert used daily with an applicator is recommended for the treatment of moderate-to-severe dyspareunia in menopausal women [8]. DHEA significantly improves vaginal maturation index (VMI), normalizes vaginal pH, and alleviates symptoms of dyspareunia and vaginal dryness in menopausal women with GSM [5, 9].

Mechanism of Action DHEA undergoes intracrine conversion within vaginal epithelial cells, where local enzymatic activity transforms it into active estrogens and androgens. This leads to the maturation of parabasal cells into superficial cells, resulting in increased mucosal thickness and secretions. Additionally, androgens derived from DHEA enhance collagen density in the lamina propria and stimulate the underlying muscle by acting on fibroblasts. Active hormones (~95%) are inactivated locally, preventing systemic absorption and endometrial stimulation [4].

Dose 6.5 mg vaginal pessary daily.

Adverse Effects Vaginal discharge is the most common adverse effect [9].

6.7.7 Ospemifene

Ospemifene is an oral selective estrogen receptor modulator (SERM). It is an appropriate choice for women who are not eligible for vaginal ET, or who prefer oral route to any form of vaginal therapy [4]. It has an antagonist effect on the endometrium and breast and can be used in women with a history of breast and endometrial cancer who have completed treatment. However, there is no clinical trial data for use in patients with current breast cancer [4]. Ospemifene has been associated with decreased risk for breast cancer and breast cancer recurrence in preliminary studies [5].

Mechanism of Action It has agonist activity in the vaginal mucosa, decreasing vaginal pH, and improving the VMI, thus reducing symptoms of vaginal dryness and dyspareunia [4, 5].

Dose 60 mg oral tablet daily.

Adverse Effects Vasomotor symptoms are the most common adverse effects.

6.7.8 Energy-Based Therapies

Vulvovaginal energy-based devices including lasers (light amplification by stimulated emission of radiation) and radio-frequency devices, are under investigation as treatments for GSM, but none have FDA approval for this indication [5].

There are two types of laser therapy [4]:

1. CO_2 microablative laser
2. Erbium Yag nonablative photothermal laser therapy

Both laser types are administered every 4–6 weeks for three initial sessions, followed by an annual session.

Mechanism of Action The laser targets the residual water in connective tissue, producing a thermal effect that causes edema, and stimulates collagen-producing fibroblasts. This leads to collagen formation, neovascularization, urogenital tissue restructuring, and an increase in vaginal lubrication, and acidity. The stratified squamous epithelium thickens, with an increase in glycogen and lactobacilli [4]. Using a probe adapted to the vagina, fractional CO_2 vaginal laser therapy induces morphologic changes in the vagina, and data from small studies support improvement in GSM symptoms of vaginal dryness and dyspareunia [5].

Radiofrequency devices are nonablative and emit focused electromagnetic waves that heat the superficial layers of the tissue.

6.7.8.1 Advantages and Disadvantages of Energy-Based Therapies

Laser therapy is an option for women who cannot use hormone therapy or who avoid using existing treatment regimens due to safety concerns, inconvenience, or suboptimal response to treatment [4]. Therapy is delivered less frequently than other options and is independent of sexual intercourse. The primary disadvantage is that vaginal laser treatment is expensive and less cost-effective.

Adverse Events include discomfort during treatments, vaginal scarring, vaginal lacerations on resumption of intecourse and persistent and/or worsening dyspareunia [5].

In 2018, the FDA cautioned that the safety and effectiveness of these devices have not yet been established. Although laser therapy shows promise as a nonhormonal treatment for GSM, more robust evidence from well-designed trials is needed before routine recommendations can be made [4, 5]. A meta-analysis of 7 RCTs demonstrated no statistically significant difference in FSFI, VHI scores, and VAS for dyspareunia, burning, itching, and dysuria between groups, suggesting that CO2 laser may not offer any benefit for GSM [14]. HCPs should counsel patients that current evidence does not support the use of CO_2, ER:YAG laser, or radiofrequency for treating GSM and their use can only be on an experimental basis, based on shared-decision making [8].

6.8 Duration of Therapy and Follow Up

An improvement in GSM symptoms is seen within a few weeks of starting therapy; but treatment for 12 weeks is usually needed for maximum benefit. Low dose vaginal ET may be continued as long as needed to relieve symptoms, if there are no contraindications. Upon discontinuation, objective signs of GSM return to pretreatment levels in about 1 month, while subjective symptoms return in approximately

3–6 months [3]. Clinical trial safety data are limited to1 year, but observational studies have shown safety with long-term use [5].

Patients should be reassessed at regular intervals, for monitoring the response to therapy and any adverse effects [8]. If low or ultra-low doses are insufficient, HCPs may consider increasing the dose or switching to alternative hormonal or nonhormonal therapies [3]. HCPs should also inform the patient that long-term treatment and follow-up may be necessary [8]. After discontinuing vaginal estrogen, Endometrial surveillance is not required with vaginal estrogen, vaginal DHEA or ospemifene [8].

6.9 Pelvic Floor Muscle (PFM) Rehabilitation

It is a safe, non-invasive, low-cost, conservative treatment that can be used alone or in combination with other treatment modalities for women with GSM. PFM rehabilitation includes education, lifestyle modifications, pelvic floor muscle training (PFMT), manual techniques, electrostimulation, and biofeedback under a specialist pelvic floor physiotherapist [15]. PFMT consists of targeted exercises designed to improve pelvic floor strength, endurance, power, and relaxation. These exercises help alleviate vaginismus and muscle hypertonicity often associated with penetration-related pain [4]. PFMT also promotes blood circulation, improves pelvic floor muscle function, and boosts tissue elasticity. PFM rehabilitation can begin at any stage of menopause to alleviate GSM symptoms. Additional randomized controlled trials are necessary to verify its effectiveness [4, 15].

6.10 GSM in Cancer Survivors

In cancer survivors, GSM is one of the main causes of distress and reduced QoL. It is more severe and more prevalent in cancer survivors than in the general population [11]. It is usually undertreated due to the fear of cancer recurrence. Systemic estrogen therapy is contraindicated in breast cancer survivors. Mild-to-moderate symptoms can be treated with lifestyle modifications and nonhormonal options. If nonhormonal treatments have failed to provide relief, after a discussion of risks and benefits, low-dose LET may be used, in breast cancer survivors, including those on Tamoxifen [11]. For patients on Aromatase inhibitors, low-dose LET may be used after shared decision-making between the patient, gynecologist, and oncologist [11]. Larger, high-quality clinical trials with longer follow-ups are needed, for emerging treatment options such as vaginal lasers.

6.11 Genitourinary Syndrome of Lactation

Postpartum breastfeeding women may experience urogenital symptoms similar to menopause due to high prolactin levels inhibiting estrogen and androgen secretion. It can lead to vaginal dryness, dyspareunia, and urinary symptoms. Despite the high prevalence, there are no screening or treatment guidelines. The new term "genitourinary syndrome of lactation" (GSL), has been proposed to raise awareness and guide management [16].

Key Points

- Genitourinary Syndrome of Menopause (GSM) can have a profound and lasting impact on both quality of life (QoL) and urogenital health, and it is essential that women are informed about the progressive effects of estrogen deficiency, as well as the full range of available treatment options.
- First-line therapies for mild symptoms limited to vaginal dryness or dyspareunia include nonhormonal vaginal lubricants used with sexual activity and regular use of vaginal moisturizers along with life-style modifications.
- For women with moderate-to-severe GSM and those who do not respond to lubricants and moisturizers, a safe and effective option is low-dose vaginal estrogen therapy administered daily for 2 weeks followed by twice weekly. Other second-line pharmacotherapies include vaginal DHEA and oral SERM ospemifene.
- Vulvovaginal energy-based devices improve vaginal health and offer a choice to women in whom vaginal estrogen is contraindicated, but long-term safety and efficacy data are lacking.

Long Answer Questions (LAQs)

1. How does GSM affect the quality of life and sexual health of women? Discuss the pathophysiology, clinical manifestations, and evaluation of genitourinary syndrome of menopause (GSM).
2. How does estrogen deficiency affect the vaginal pH and vaginal microbiome? Describe the efficacy and safety profile of low-dose vaginal estrogen therapy in the management of GSM.
3. Give a brief overview of the various treatment options available to treat genitourinary syndrome of menopause. What factors should healthcare providers consider when tailoring a treatment plan for individual patients?
4. What are the benefits and limitations of vulvovaginal energy-based devices in the treatment of GSM, and what is the current understanding of their long-term safety and efficacy?

Short Answer Questions (SAQs)

1. Write a short note on the symptoms and signs of GSM.
2. What are the current tools and methods used to assess GSM severity and treatment outcomes?
3. What is the preferred first line therapy for mild to moderate GSM?
4. What is the role of pelvic floor muscle rehabilitation in managing GSM?
5. What are the special considerations in the treatment of GSM in breast cancer survivors?

Multiple Choice Questions (MCQs)

1. What is the most appropriate management for moderate-to-severe vaginal atrophy in postmenopausal women?
   A. Systemic estrogen therapy
   B. Low-dose vaginal estrogen therapy
   C. Hysterectomy
   D. Oral contraceptive pills
2. A 52-year-old woman with a history of breast cancer treated with aromatase inhibitors complains of severe vaginal dryness and painful intercourse. What is the most appropriate initial management?
   A. Systemic hormone therapy
   B. Low dose vaginal estrogen therapy
   C. Vaginal moisturizers and lubricants
   D. Oral contraceptive pills
3. A 55-year-old woman with an intact uterus is prescribed low-dose vaginal estrogen for GSM. Which of the following statements is most accurate?
   A. Progestogen cotherapy is always required, and long-term use of vaginal estrogen is associated with a high risk of cardiovascular events.
   B. Progestogen cotherapy is not required for low-dose vaginal estrogen, and long-term use is generally considered safe, but data beyond one year are limited.
   C. Progestogen cotherapy is required only in women with a history of endometrial hyperplasia.
   D. Progestogen cotherapy is required if used for more than 6 months, and it is only safe for women under 60.
4. What is the recommended dose and administration frequency for low-dose vaginal estrogen therapy (LET) in treating GSM?

A. Daily for 2 weeks, then twice per week
B. Daily for 1 week, then once per week
C. Twice per week for 2 weeks, then daily
D. Once per week for 1 month, then twice per month

5. Which of the following is a potential adverse effect of vaginal DHEA therapy?

A. Vaginal dryness
B. Vaginal discharge
C. Vaginal itching
D. Vaginal bleeding

6. A 59-year-old woman has been using vaginal estrogen for GSM for 2 years. What is the recommendation regarding endometrial surveillance?

A. Annual endometrial biopsy
B. Pelvic ultrasound every 6 months
C. Routine surveillance is not recommended unless symptomatic
D. Hysteroscopy every year

7. Which of the following is true regarding the mechanism of action of ospemifene in treating GSM?

A. Agonist activity in the vaginal mucosa
B. Antagonist activity in the vaginal mucosa
C. Increases estrogen production
D. Decreases androgen production

8. What is the role of pelvic floor muscle rehabilitation in managing GSM?

A. Reduces estrogen deficiency
B. Improves pelvic floor strength and blood circulation
C. Increases vaginal pH
D. Enhances collagen and elastin production

9. A researcher is planning a clinical trial to test a new intravaginal treatment for GSM. The primary outcome must measure physiological changes in the vaginal environment, while secondary outcomes assess symptom relief and sexual function. Which assessment tools will provide the most robust methodology?

A. Vaginal Health Index (VHI) + Female Sexual Function Index (FSFI)
B. Vaginal Maturation Index (VMI) + Visual Analog Scale (VAS) for dryness
C. Vaginal pH measurement + Visual Analog Scale (VAS) for dryness
D. Vaginal Health Index (VHI) + Vaginal Maturation Index (VMI) + Female Sexual Function Index (FSFI)

10. A 63-year-old postmenopausal woman is embarrassed to discuss vaginal symptoms. What should be the approach of healthcare providers?

A. wait for the patient to bring up symptoms
B. proactively ask about GSM symptoms during consultations

C. only discuss if the patient has urinary symptoms
D. dismiss sexual symptoms as they are not important at this age

Answers

1. B
2. C
3. B
4. A
5. B
6. C
7. A
8. B
9. D
10. B

References

1. Da Silva AS, Baines G, Araklitis G, Robinson D, Cardozo L. Modern management of genitourinary syndrome of menopause. Fac Rev [Internet]. 2021 Mar 3;10. Available from: https://facultyopinions.com/prime/reports/b/10/25/.
2. Portman DJ, Gass MLS. Genitourinary syndrome of menopause: new terminology for vulvovaginal atrophy from the International Society for the Study of women's sexual health and the North American Menopause Society. Climacteric. 2014;17(5):557–63.
3. Nappi RE, Tiranini L, Martini E, Bosoni D, Cassani C, Cucinella L. Different local estrogen therapies for a tailored approach to GSM. Climacteric. Taylor and Francis Ltd. 2023;26:361–6.
4. Briggs P. Urogenital atrophy_ the 'unknown factors' challenging current practice. Post Reprod Health. 2021.
5. Faubion SS, Kingsberg SA, Clark AL, Kaunitz AM, Spadt SK, Larkin LC, et al. The 2020 genitourinary syndrome of menopause position statement of the North American Menopause Society. Menopause. 2020;27(9):976–92.
6. Mili N, Paschou SA, Armeni A, Georgopoulos N, Goulis DG, Lambrinoudaki I. Genitourinary syndrome of menopause: a systematic review on prevalence and treatment. Menopause. 2021;28(6):706–16.
7. Pérez-López FR, Vieira-Baptista P, Phillips N, Cohen-Sacher B, Fialho SCAV, Stockdale CK. Clinical manifestations and evaluation of postmenopausal vulvovaginal atrophy. Gynecol Endocrinol. Taylor and Francis Ltd. 2021;37:740–5.
8. Kaufman MR, Lenore Ackerman A, Amin KA, Coffey M, Faubion SS, Hardart A, et al. Guideline panel staff and consultants systematic review prepared by the Minnesota Evidence-based Practice Center Minneapolis, MN. Investigators. 2025.
9. Cipriani S, Maseroli E, Ravelli SA, Vignozzi L. The vagina as source and target of androgens: implications for treatment of GSM/VVA, including DHEA. Climacteric. Taylor and Francis Ltd. 2023;26:309–15.

10. Ashraf AB, Meeta M, Chitra AB, Pahwa S, Shah J, Mohi M, et al. Genitourinary syndrome of menopause: a multicenter study from the Indian Midlife Registry. Climacteric [Internet]. 2025 May 21;1–8. Available from: https://www.tandfonline.com/doi/full/10.1080/13697137.2025.2496681.
11. López DML. Management of genitourinary syndrome of menopause in breast cancer survivors: an update. World J Clin Oncol. 2022;13(2):71–100.
12. Mension E, Alonso I, Tortajada M, Matas I, Gómez S, Ribera L, et al. Genitourinary syndrome of menopause assessment tools. J Midlife Health. 2021;12(2):99–102.
13. Cox P, Panay N. Non-hormonal treatments for managing vulvovaginal atrophy/genitourinary syndrome of menopause. Climacteric. Taylor and Francis Ltd. 2023;26:367–72.
14. Ni Y, Lian J. Carbon dioxide laser therapy for the management of genitourinary syndrome of menopause: a meta-analysis of randomized controlled trials. Exp Ther Med. 2023;27(1)
15. Mercier J, Dumoulin C, Carrier-Noreau G. Pelvic floor muscle rehabilitation for genitourinary syndrome of menopause: why, how and when? Climacteric. Taylor and Francis Ltd. 2023;26:302–8.
16. Perelmuter S, Burns R, Shearer K, Grant R, Soogoor A, Jun S, et al. Genitourinary syndrome of lactation: a new perspective on postpartum and lactation-related genitourinary symptoms. Sex Med Rev. Oxford University Press. 2024;12:279–87.

7 Osteopenia and Osteoporosis at Menopause

Geeta Mediratta and Sharmistha Garg

Abstract

Postmenopausal osteoporosis is a significant public health concern in India, contributing to fragility fractures, disability, and mortality among women. Estrogen deficiency after menopause disrupts bone homeostasis by enhancing osteoclast activity, resulting in accelerated bone loss and microarchitectural deterioration. Key risk factors include age, low body mass index, nutritional deficiencies, smoking, alcohol, comorbidities, and certain medications. Diagnosis is established through history, clinical examination, laboratory tests, and dual-energy X-ray absorptiometry (DEXA), with the FRAX tool aiding fracture risk prediction. Management strategies emphasize lifestyle modification, adequate calcium and vitamin D intake, fall prevention, and pharmacological therapy such as bisphosphonates, denosumab, selective estrogen receptor modulators, hormone therapy, and anabolic agents in high-risk cases. Regular monitoring of bone mineral density and treatment adherence is essential. Early screening and timely intervention are crucial to reduce the burden of osteoporotic fractures and improving quality of life in postmenopausal women.

Keywords

Postmenopausal osteoporosis · Osteopenia · Fragility fractures · Bone mineral density (BMD) · Dual-energy X-ray absorptiometry (DEXA) · Selective estrogen receptor modulators (SERMs) · Hormone replacement therapy (HRT)

G. Mediratta (✉) · S. Garg
Department of Obstetrics and Gynaecology, Sir Ganga Ram Hospital, New Delhi, India

R. Malik et al. (eds.), *Menopause Essentials*,
https://doi.org/10.1007/978-981-95-7498-8_7

7.1 Introduction

Menopause marks a significant period in a woman's life when ovarian function decreases and estrogen levels decline. This hormonal transition has major implications for bone health. Osteoporosis is a skeletal condition characterized by low bone mass and reduced bone strength leading to increased fracture risk. Low bone mass may be related to inadequate peak bone mass acquisition or ongoing bone loss. Bone loss or fractures can be because of secondary causes such as estrogen deficiency, glucocorticoid exposure or inflammatory or malabsorption condition [1]. During the menopausal transition and early postmenopause, bone mineral density (BMD) declines at an accelerated rate, increasing the risk of developing low bone mass (osteopenia) and eventually osteoporosis. Apart from fractures this condition is also responsible in causing vertebral deformities and poor quality of life so in country like India where life span has increased over the years awareness of this problem, change in lifestyle, and timely intervention is important [2].

7.2 Definition

The World Health Organization (WHO) defined osteoporosis as a "progressive systemic skeletal disease characterized by low bone mass and microarchitectural deterioration of bone tissue, with a consequent increase in bone fragility and susceptibility to fracture" in 1994. The operational description was predicated on a bone mineral density (BMD) T-Score of ≤−2.5.3 because microarchitectural degradation could not be clinically evaluated [3].

Osteopenia Osteopenia is defined as low bone mass which is based on bone mineral density criteria (BMD)as a T score between −1 and −2.5.

Osteoporosis Osteoporosis is defined as low bone mass which is based on bone mineral density criteria (BMD) as a T score ≤2.5, history of fragility fracture or calculated 10-year fracture risk.

Fragility Fracture Fragility fractures are those occurring from a fall from a standing height or less, particularly at the spine, hip, wrist, humerus, and pelvis [4].

The Osteoporosis is a skeletal disorder characterized by compromised bone strength predisposing to an increased risk of fractures. Throughout life, older bone is periodically resorbed by osteoclasts at discrete sites and replaced with new bone made by osteoblasts. This process is known as remodeling. Remodeling is orchestrated and targeted to a particular site that is in need for repair by osteocytes. An oversupply of osteoclasts relative to the need for remodeling or an undersupply of osteoblasts relative to the need for cavity repair are the seminal pathophysiological changes in osteoporosis.

The amount of bone mass acquired by an individual reaches a peak by the third decade of life [5]. Low peak bone mass probably contributes to the development of osteoporosis later in life. However, old age, sex steroid deficiency, lipid oxidation, decreased physical activity, use of glucocorticoids, and a propensity to fall are the most critical determinants of increased fracture risk.

In the menopausal context, osteopenia may be considered a precursor state: bone mass is falling; skeletal microarchitecture is deteriorating, but fracture risk remains lower than the osteoporosis threshold. Progression from osteopenia to osteoporosis depends on the magnitude and rate of bone loss, additional risk factors, and the success of preventive measures [6].

Osteoporosis is characterized by low bone mass, microarchitectural disruption, and skeletal fragility, resulting in decreased bone strength and an increased risk of fracture. Decreased bone strength is related to many factors other than bone mineral density (BMD), including rates of bone formation and resorption (turnover), bone geometry (size and shape of bone), and microarchitecture [6].

The World Health Organization (WHO) has defined diagnostic thresholds for low bone mass and osteoporosis based upon BMD measurements compared with a young adult reference population (T-score) [7].

7.3 Diagnostic Categories for Osteoporosis and Low Bone Mass Based Upon BMD Measurement by DXA [11]

Category	Definition
Normal	BMD within *1.0 SD* of the young adult female reference mean (*T-score* ≥ -1.0)
Osteopenia (low bone mass)	BMD *between 1.0 and 2.5 SD below* the young adult female reference mean (*T-score* < -1.0 *and* > -2.5)
Osteoporosis	BMD *2.5 SD or more below* the young adult female reference mean (*T-score* ≤ -2.5)
Severe (established) osteoporosis	BMD *more than 2.5 SD below* the reference mean *plus one or more fragility fractures*

7.4 Epidemiology and the Menopausal Transition

The highest bone mass attained in a lifetime is known as peak bone mass. Although the exact moment of peak bone mass is unknown, most people experience it around their third decade of life. Variations in timing can be attributed to skeletal location (the type of bone) and the technique used to evaluate bone mineral density (BMD), as well as genetic, hormonal, and environmental factors.

Genetics A portion of the variation in BMD among humans has a genetic basis. Genome-wide association studies have so far identified approximately 518 genetic loci that influence BMD [8]. A remarkable number of these loci are involved in some aspect of Wnt/beta-catenin signaling, the receptor activator of nuclear factor kappa-B (RANK)/RANK ligand (RANKL)/osteoprotegerin (OPG) axis, or in mesenchymal cell differentiation.

Ethnic Variation African Americans have reduced fracture rates at several skeletal locations, such as the hip, clinical vertebrae, upper and lower appendages, and Asian Americans have lower BMD than White Americans. Asian Americans and Hispanic Americans also had lower rates of hip fractures than White Americans, albeit the differential may vary depending on the skeletal site. Crucially, when body size disparities are taken into account, BMD differences typically diminish or disappear [9].

Environmental Factors Acquisition of optimal bone mass is largely a reflection of increases in body size and skeletal loads mainly arising from muscle forces actuating bony levers such that limb muscle mass should be a reasonable measure of skeletal load. As children grow, they gain both body weight and muscle mass, with increasing muscle strength [9].

Osteoporosis-Related Bone Loss The two main causes of osteoporosis are aging and estrogen insufficiency. As a woman's ovarian function abruptly declines at menopause, bone loss occurs quickly. Age-related bone loss starts as soon as bone mass reaches its peak in males and women, however, the majority of bone loss happens beyond the age of 65. Men do not experience an abrupt reduction of estrogens like women do, so they first grow more bone throughout adolescence and then lose less bone as they age [10].

Thus, the menopausal transition is a "window of vulnerability" for skeletal health. Bone is lost at an accelerated rate, many women accumulate risk factors, and yet many are unaware of their skeletal risk until a fracture occurs.

7.5 Pathophysiology of Bone Loss at Menopause

7.5.1 Bone Remodeling Basics

Bone is a dynamic tissue undergoing continuous remodeling: old bone is removed (resorption) by osteoclasts, and new bone is formed by osteoblasts. A balance between these processes maintains skeletal mass and microarchitecture. With aging and hormonal changes, this balance shifts unfavorably.

7.5.2 Effect of Estrogen Deficiency

Estrogen plays a major role in maintaining skeleton integrity:

- It suppresses osteoclastogenesis (via down-regulating RANKL, up-regulating osteoprotegerin).
- It promotes osteoblast survival and function, and reduces apoptosis of bone-forming cells.
- It modulates cytokine production (IL-1, IL-6, TNF-α) by osteoblast/stromal and immune cells, thereby restraining bone resorption [12].
- The decline of ovarian estrogen production in menopause removes this protective effect; the result is increased bone turnover (resorption > formation), net bone loss, thinning of trabeculae, cortical porosity, microarchitectural deterioration, and skeletal fragility [13].

7.5.3 The Menopausal Transition and Rate of Loss

During the late perimenopause and early postmenopause, bone loss is most rapid. The SWAN study and other cohort data show this accelerated phase: for example, annual lumbar spine bone loss of ~2% in the late perimenopause [13]. After this phase, bone loss slows but continues. A lower body weight is associated with higher bone-loss rates [11].

7.5.4 Progression from Osteopenia to Osteoporosis

The trajectory from lower-than-normal bone mass to osteoporosis depends on: the starting peak bone mass, the rate of loss around menopause, additional bone-loss accelerants (secondary causes), and how soon and effectively preventive or therapeutic measures are instituted.

Microarchitectural loss may precede or accompany densitometric decline: trabecular thinning, connectivity loss, cortical thinning, and porosity all contribute [12].

Emerging research suggests that beyond hormonal factors, disturbances in gut-microbiota and immune regulation may modulate post-menopausal bone loss: e.g., increased Th17/regulatory T-cell imbalance, microbiota dysbiosis linked to osteoporosis in postmenopausal women [14].

7.6 Risk Factors

7.6.1 Nonmodifiable Risk Factors

- Female sex (women have smaller bones, lower peak bone mass, and undergo menopause) [15].
- Older age—duration of the postmenopausal period increases cumulative bone loss.
- Early menopause (before ~45 years).
- Family history of osteoporosis or fragility fracture.
- Ethnicity: e.g., Asian women tend to have lower BMD and higher risk relative to some other populations.

7.6.2 Modifiable Risk Factors

- Low body mass index (BMI)/low body weight: less mechanical loading, lower estrogen from adipose tissue, higher bone-loss rates.
- Sedentary lifestyle / low weight-bearing exercise [16].
- Smoking, excess alcohol intake—both negatively impact bone turnover and hormonal milieu [17].
- Inadequate dietary calcium, vitamin D deficiency, malnutrition.
- Secondary causes: hyperthyroidism, glucocorticoid use, rheumatoid arthritis, early oophorectomy, chemotherapy, malabsorption, and other endocrine disorders.

7.6.3 Menopause-Specific Factors

- The rapid decline in estrogen around the final menstrual period.
- The length of time since menopause: the earlier and longer the postmenopausal period, the higher the cumulative bone loss.
- The "bone-loss window" concept: the first 5–10 years after menopause often see the greatest bone-density decline.
- In India and other settings where normative BMD is already lower, the risk may accrue sooner [18].

7.7 Clinical Assessment and Diagnosis

7.7.1 Bone Mineral Density (BMD) Measurement

The standard for diagnosing osteopenia/osteoporosis is measurement of BMD via DXA at key skeletal sites (lumbar spine, total hip, femoral neck). T-score compares the subject's BMD to that of a young healthy adult of same sex. WHO classification for diagnosis based on BMD measurement, is given below (for women ≥50 years) [17]:

- Normal: T-score ≥ −1.0.
- Osteopenia: −1.0 > T-score > −2.5.
- Osteoporosis: T-score ≤ −2.5.

7.7.2 Fracture Risk Assessment

Diagnosis of osteoporosis may also be made in the presence of a fragility fracture (e.g., hip, vertebra, wrist) even if T-score is above −2.5. Tools such as FRAX (fracture risk assessment tool) incorporate clinical risk factors plus BMD to estimate 10-year fracture risk and guide treatment decisions [18].

7.7.3 Clinical History and Physical Exam

- Menstrual/gynecologic history: age at menopause (natural vs surgical), hormone therapy history.
- Risk factor review: family history, smoking, alcohol, medications (glucocorticoids, aromatase inhibitors), comorbidities (thyroid disease, rheumatoid arthritis).
- Lifestyle evaluation: diet, calcium/vitamin D intake, physical activity, fall risk assessment (balance, gait, home environment).
- Physical exam: height/weight (height loss may signal vertebral fracture), signs of kyphosis, previous fractures.

7.7.4 Laboratory and Secondary Cause Evaluation

While primary (postmenopausal) bone loss is common, assessment may include: serum calcium, phosphate, 25-hydroxyvitamin D, thyroid-stimulating hormone, alkaline phosphatase, parathyroid hormone, renal function, liver enzymes. If

Table 7.1 Key differentiating features between osteopenia and osteoporosis

Feature	Osteopenia (low bone mass)	Osteoporosis
Definition	T-score between −1.0 and −2.5	T-score ≤ −2.5 *or* presence of fragility fracture
Bone strength and fracture risk	Elevated fracture risk compared to "normal" but lower than osteoporosis	Significantly increased fracture risk; fractures common
Menopausal impact	Early post-menopausal bone loss may lead to osteopenia	If bone loss continues unchecked and risk factors accumulate → osteoporosis
Typical management focus	Lifestyle interventions + monitoring; pharmacotherapy depending on risk profile	Lifestyle + pharmacotherapy considered standard; higher urgency for fracture prevention
Prognosis	Intermediate stage; potential for stabilization or reversal with appropriate measures	Chronic condition; aim is to prevent further bone loss, reduce fractures, maintain independence

indicated: bone marker tests, testosterone/estradiol (in younger women), bone-turnover markers.

7.7.5 When to Screen

Many guidelines recommend BMD screening in women ≥65 years, or younger women (50–64) with risk factors. Given the accelerated bone loss around menopause, screening near menopause may be considered in high-risk individuals (e.g., early menopause, low BMI, previous low-trauma fracture). The Indian evidence suggests earlier normative lower BMD—thus the screening threshold may need adaptation (Table 7.1) [18].

7.8 Prevention and Management Strategies

LOW BONE MASS: In postmenopausal women with low bone mass [T score between −0.1 and −2.5] with no h/o fragility fracture,the risk of fracture is calculated using FRAX fracture risk assessment tool. The FRAX tool has been developed to evaluate fracture risk. It is based on individualized models that integrate the risks associated with clinical risk factors as well as bone mineral density (BMD) at the femoral neck.

For patients with high estimated fracture risk with prior h/o fragility fracture treatment of osteoporosis is advised whereas patients with low to moderate fracture risk management is decided on individual basis based on patient preferences, expected benefits and risk of drug therapy.

7.8.1 Lifestyle Measures

Lifestyle optimization is fundamental for both osteopenia and osteoporosis, particularly in menopausal women transitioning through rapid bone-loss phases.

- *Calcium and Vitamin D*: all postmenopausal women should take adequate calcium and vit D. Women with adequate calcium intake from diet alone [approx 1200 mg/day] do not need additional supplements in the absence of gastrointestinal malabsorption. However, women with inadequate dietary intake should take supplements [500–1000 mg/day] to reach total of 1200 mg/day is recommended [19].
  Postmenopausal women should ingest 800 IU of vitamin D daily but in the case of gastrointestinal malabsorption or intake of antiseizure medication higher doses may be required.
  Diet: Adequate calorie intake is advised to avoid malnutrition with protein intake of 0.8 gm /kg bodyweight [20].
- *Weight-bearing and muscle-strengthening exercise*: postmenopausal women should undergo 30 min on most days of the week and incorporate muscle strengthening and posture exercised 2–3 days a week [21].
- *Avoiding smoking and excess alcohol*: Cigarette smoking accelerates bone loss and reduce BMD [22]. Smoking one pack per day was associated with a 5–10% reduction in bone density. In women on HRT, smoking negates the effect of HRT. Both smoking and alcohol are independent risk factors for accelerated bone loss.
- *Maintaining healthy weight and muscle mass*: Low BMI is associated with higher rates of bone loss (observed in SWAN).
- *Fall prevention strategies*: As fractures in osteopenia/osteoporosis often result from falls rather than pure bone fragility, interventions to improve balance, home safety (lighting, rails, removing loose rugs), vision/hearing checks, and medication review (to avoid sedatives) are vital.

7.8.2 Pharmacologic Therapy

Pharmacologic treatment is often indicated when fracture risk is sufficiently high (e.g., osteoporosis diagnosis, prior fracture, high FRAX score) but may also be considered in some women with osteopenia who have additional risk factors.

Key pharmacologic classes include:

- Bisphosphonates: Weekly oral bisphosphonates like alendronate, risedronate, ibandronate are preferred because of efficacy, favorable cost and availability of long-term safety data but the limitations include complex dosing regimen and poor long-term adherence [23].

- For women unable to take oral bisphosphonates intravenous zoledronic acid is a good alternative. Periodic measurement of BMD and bone turnover is useful to monitor duration of treatment and determine the next dose [24].
- Denosumab (a RANKL inhibitor)—effective antiresorptive in postmenopausal osteoporosis. Denusomab is an alternative to IV zoledronic acid for women at high risk of fractures who have difficulty with dosing requirements of oral bisphosphonates or who prefer to avoid IV bisphosphonates due to side effects[e.g. acute phase reaction] [25].
- Teriparatide and abaloparatide (parathyroid-hormone analogs)—anabolic therapy for women at very high fracture risk [26].
- Selective estrogen receptor modulators (SERMs, e.g., raloxifene, bazedoxifene)—Raloxifene inhibits bone resorption and reduces the risk of vertebral fracture. Raloxifene also increases thromboembolic events and hot flashes and has no apparent effect on heart or the endometrium. Bazedoxifene is available in Europe and Japan for treatment of postmenopausal osteoporosis and in USA it is available in combination with conjugated estrogen [27].
- Hormone therapy (estrogen with or without progestogen)—in appropriate women (especially younger postmenopausal women <60 years without contraindications), MHT may help reduce bone loss, though the decision must include balance of risks/benefits [28].

Management guidelines emphasize the need to: assess fracture risk, incorporate patient preferences, combine pharmacologic and nonpharmacologic strategies, monitor adherence, side-effects and reassess periodically (e.g., every 3–5 years for bisphosphonates).

7.8.3 Timing and the "Window of Opportunity"

The early postmenopausal period is often described as a "window of opportunity" for preserving bone mass: since bone-loss rates are highest then, initiating preventive or therapeutic measures at this time may yield the greatest benefits in prolonging skeletal health. Some data suggest that hormone therapy initiated near menopause rather than years later confers greater bone protection [29].

7.8.4 Monitoring and Follow-Up

Women diagnosed with osteopenia or osteoporosis require periodic monitoring via DXA scans (often 1–2 year intervals initially, then every 2–5 years depending on risk/therapy), evaluation of adherence to therapy, monitoring of laboratory parameters (e.g., vitamin D status, calcium), reassessment of risk factors (new medications, comorbidities, falls, fractures). Some guidelines also advise for "drug holidays" in certain bisphosphonate users at lower risk after 3–5 years.

7.9 Special Considerations in Menopausal Women

7.9.1 Early Menopause/Surgical Menopause

Women with premature ovarian failure or surgical oophorectomy undergo an abrupt decline in estrogen and are at especially high risk for rapid bone loss. They often warrant earlier screening and intervention.

7.9.2 Ethnic and Geographic Variability

As noted above, normative BMD values vary by ethnicity and geography; e.g., Indian women may have lower peak BMD compared to Western women, and fewer epidemiologic studies address this population comprehensively. Thus, screening strategies must adapt to local populations [22].

7.9.3 Comorbidities and Polypharmacy

Menopausal women may have comorbid conditions (e.g., cardiovascular disease, metabolic syndrome) and may be on medications (e.g., glucocorticoids, aromatase inhibitors, antiepileptics) that accelerate bone loss. Clinicians must consider these when assessing skeletal risk.

7.9.4 Pregnancy/Lactation History

While not always emphasized, lifetime bone accrual, and reproductive history (e.g., multiple pregnancies, lactation) may influence peak bone mass and hence later skeletal risk.

7.9.5 Lifestyle, Nutrition, and Cultural Factors

In many regions including India, dietary calcium intake may be suboptimal, vitamin D deficiency may be common (due to less sun exposure or skin-covering cultural practices), and levels of physical activity may decline postmenopause. All these augment skeletal vulnerability.

7.9.6 Emerging Research Areas

Recent studies point to the role of gut microbiota in bone health in post-menopausal women (e.g., dysbiosis linked to osteoporosis). There is also growing interest in epigenetic regulation, inflammatory signaling and bone-microenvironment interactions beyond classical estrogen–osteoclast/osteoblast pathways [30].

Key Points

1. The WHO defines Osteoporosis as a BMD T-score ≤ -2.5 or the presence of fragility fractures, indicating compromised bone strength and increased fracture risk.
2. The bone loss is accelerated in Menopause due to estrogen deficiency, making the early postmenopausal period a critical window for intervention.
3. Osteopenia (T-score between -1.0 and -2.5) is a precursor state to osteoporosis, with lower bone mass but less fracture risk than osteoporosis.
4. Diagnosis involves BMD measurement via DXA, clinical history, fracture risk assessment (e.g., FRAX), and evaluation for secondary causes.
5. Management includes focus on modifiable risk factors, lifestyle optimization (calcium, vitamin D, exercise, fall prevention), and pharmacologic therapy tailored to fracture risk and patient preferences.

Long Answer Questions (LAQs)

1. Discuss the etiopathogenesis of postmenopausal osteoporosis. Explain the role of estrogen deficiency and the RANKL–OPG system in bone loss.
2. Describe the approach to screening, diagnosis, and risk assessment of osteoporosis in postmenopausal women. Include tools like DEXA, FRAX, and clinical examination findings
3. Explain the pharmacological management of postmenopausal osteoporosis. Include indications, mechanisms of action, dosages, adverse effects, and advantages/disadvantages of commonly used drugs.
4. Outline the non-pharmacological strategies for the management and prevention of osteoporosis in menopausal women. Emphasize dietary and lifestyle recommendations, fall prevention, and vitamin D/calcium recommendations.

Short Answer Questions (SAQs)

1. What are the WHO diagnostic criteria for osteoporosis based on T-scores?
2. List five modifiable and five non-modifiable risk factors for osteoporosis.

3. Define fragility fracture and mention common sites.
4. What is the significance of the "Get up and Go" test in osteoporosis assessment?.
5. Mention two advantages and two disadvantages of bisphosphonates.

Multiple Choice Questions (MCQs)

1. Which of the following is NOT a typical site of osteoporotic fracture?
   A. Hip
   B. Spine
   C. Wrist 6
   D. Humerus
2. Estrogen deficiency in menopause leads to osteoporosis primarily by:
   A. Increasing calcium absorption
   B. Enhancing osteoblast activity
   C. Increasing RANKL expression
   D. Stimulating OPG production
3. Which of the following drugs is an anabolic agent used in osteoporosis?
   A. Raloxifene
   B. Alendronate
   C. Teriparatide
   D. Denosumab
4. Which of the following is the most common cause of secondary osteoporosis?
   A. Vitamin D toxicity
   B. Glucocorticoid use
   C. Diabetes mellitus
   D. Hyperthyroidism
5. FRAX tool calculates the 10-year probability of fractures using:
   A. Only DEXA scan values
   B. Only age and sex
   C. Clinical risk factors ± BMD
   D. Serum calcium and PTH levels
6. Which of the following statements about Denosumab is TRUE?
   A. It is administered orally
   B. It increases osteoclast activity
   C. It is safe in chronic kidney disease
   D. It is taken daily

7. Which is a contraindication for menopausal hormone therapy (MHT)?
   A. 500 mg
   B. 800 mg
   C. 1000 mg
   D. 1200 mg
8. MHT has a definite role to play in all except
   A. VMS
   B. POI
   C. Sarcopenia
   D. GSM
9. T-score of –2.7 in a postmenopausal woman indicates:
   A. Normal BMD
   B. Osteopenia
   C. Osteoporosis
   D. Severe osteoporosis
10. Which SERM reduces vertebral fracture risk and also lowers breast cancer risk?
    A. Alendronate
    B. Tibolones
    C. Raloxifene
    D. Calcitonin

Answers

1. D
2. C
3. C
4. B
5. C
6. C
7. C
8. D
9. C
10. C

References

1. Xiong J, Onal M, Jilka RL, Weinstein RS, Manolagas SC, O'Brien CA. Matrix-embedded cells control osteoclast formation. Nat Med. 2011;17(10):1235–41. https://doi.org/10.1038/nm.2448.

2. Lo JC, Burnett-Bowie SA, Finkelstein JS. Bone and the perimenopause. Obstet Gynecol Clin North Am. 2011;38(3):503–17. https://doi.org/10.1016/j.ogc.2011.07.001. PMID: 21961717; PMCID: PMC3920744.
3. World Health Organization. Assessment of fracture risk and its application to screening for postmenopausal osteoporosis. Geneva; 1994. http://whqlibdoc.who.int/trs/WHO_TRS_843.
4. Johnell O, Kanis JA. An estimate of the worldwide prevalence and disability associated with osteoporotic fractures. Osteoporos Int. 2006;17(12):1726–33.
5. Mora S, Gilsanz V. Establishment of peak bone mass. Endocrinol Metab Clin N Am. 2003;32(1):39–63.
6. Seifert-Klauss V, Link T, Heumann C, Luppa P, Haseitl M, Laakmann J, Rattenhuber J, Kiechle M. Influence of pattern of menopausal transition on the amount of trabecular bone loss. Results from a 6-year prospective longitudinal study. Maturitas. 2006;55(4):317–24.
7. Data from: WHO scientific group on the assessment of osteoporosis at the primary health care level: Summary meeting report, 2004. Geneva: World Health Organization; 2007.
8. Morris JA, Kemp JP, Youlten SE, Laurent L, Logan JG, Chai RC, Vulpescu NA, Forgetta V, et al. An atlas of genetic influences on osteoporosis in humans and mice. Nat Genet. 2019;51(2):258–66.
9. Looker AC, Melton LJ 3rd, Borrud LG, Shepherd JA. Lumbar spine bone mineral density in US adults: demographic patterns and relationship with femur neck skeletal status. Osteoporos Int. 2012;23(4):1351–60. https://doi.org/10.1007/s00198-011-1693-z.
10. Liu W, Qi M, Konermann A, Zhang L, Jin F, Jin Y. The p53/miR-17/Smurf1 pathway mediates skeletal deformities in an age-related model via inhibiting the function of mesenchymal stem cells. Aging (Albany NY). 2015;7(3):205–18.
11. Amarnath SS, Kumar V, Das SL. Classification of osteoporosis. Indian J Orthop. 2023;57(Suppl 1):49–54. https://doi.org/10.1007/s43465-023-01058-3. PMID: 38107823; PMCID: PMC10721754.
12. Lo JC, Burnett-Bowie SA, Finkelstein JS. Bone and the perimenopause. Obstet Gynecol Clin N Am. 2011;38(3):503–17.
13. Barnsley J, Buckland G, Chan PE, et al. Pathophysiology and treatment of osteoporosis: challenges for clinical practice in older people. Aging Clin Exp Res. 2021;33:759–73.
14. Ma Z, Liu Y, Shen W, et al. Osteoporosis in postmenopausal women is associated with disturbances in gut microbiota and migration of peripheral immune cells. BMC Musculoskelet Disord. 2024;25:791.
15. Hsu T-L, Tantoh DM, Chou Y-H, Hsu S-Y, Ho C-C, Lung C-C, Jan C-F, Wang L, Liaw Y-P. Association between osteoporosis and menopause in relation to SOX6 rs297325 variant in Taiwanese women. Menopause. 2020;27(8):887–92.
16. Chang CF, Lee JI, Huang SP, Geng JH, Chen SC. Regular exercise decreases the risk of osteoporosis in postmenopausal women. J Public Health. 2022;10:15 June.
17. Bhatnagar A, Kekatpure AL. Postmenopausal osteoporosis: a literature review. Cureus. 2022;14(9):e29367.
18. Thulkar J, Singh S. Overview of research studies on osteoporosis in menopausal women since the last decade. J Mid-life Health. 2015;6(3):104–7.
19. Eastell R. Treatment of postmenopausal osteoporosis. N Engl J Med. 1998;338(11):736–46.
20. Wengreen HJ, Munger RG, West NA, Cutler DR, Corcoran CD, Zhang J, Sassano NE. Dietary protein intake and risk of osteoporotic hip fracture in elderly residents of Utah. J Bone Miner Res. 2004;19(4):537–45.
21. Brooke-Wavell K, Skelton DA, Barker KL, Clark EM, De Biase S, Arnold S, Paskins Z, Robinson KR, Lewis RM, Tobias JH, Ward KA, Whitney J, Leyland S. Strong, steady and straight: UK consensus statement on physical activity and exercise for osteoporosis. Br J Sports Med. 2022;56(15):837–46.
22. Ward KD, Klesges RC. A meta-analysis of the effects of cigarette smoking on bone mineral density. Calcif Tissue Int. 2001;68(5):259–70.
23. McClung M, Clemmesen B, Daifotis A, Gilchrist NL, Eisman J, Weinstein RS, Fuleihan G e-H, Reda C, Yates AJ, Ravn P. Alendronate prevents postmenopausal bone loss in women

without osteoporosis. A double-blind, randomized, controlled trial. Alendronate Osteoporosis Prevention Study Group. Ann Intern Med. 1998;128(4):253–61.
24. Biennial [corrected] IV zoledronic acid (Reclast) for prevention of osteoporosis. Med Lett Drugs Ther 2009;51(1315):49.
25. Bone HG, Wagman RB, Brandi ML, Brown JP, Chapurlat R, Cummings SR, Czerwiński E, et al. 10 years of denosumab treatment in postmenopausal women with osteoporosis: results from the phase 3 randomised FREEDOM trial and open-label extension. Lancet Diabetes Endocrinol. 2017;5(7):513–23. https://doi.org/10.1016/S2213-8587(17)30138-9.
26. Hodsman A, Scientific Advisory Council of Osteoporosis Canada, Papaioannou A, Clinical Guidelines Committee, Ann Cranney, Writing Group on the Systematic Review of Parathyroid Hormone for the Treatment of Osteoporosis. Clinical practice guidelines for the use of parathyroid hormone in the treatment of osteoporosis. CMAJ. 2006;175(1):–48.
27. Delmas PD, Bjarnason NH, Mitlak BH, Ravoux AC, Shah AS, Huster WJ, Draper M, Cristiansen C. Effects of raloxifene on bone mineral density, serum cholesterol concentrations, and uterine endometrium in postmenopausal women. N Engl J Med. 1997;337(23):1641–7.
28. Rossouw JE, Anderson GL, Prentice RL, LaCroix AZ, Kooperberg C, Stefanick ML, Writing Group for the Women's Health Initiative Investigators, et al. Risks and benefits of estrogen plus progestin in healthy postmenopausal women: principal results from the Women's Health Initiative randomized controlled trial. JAMA. 2002;288(3):321–33.
29. Platt O, Beteman J, Bakour S. Impact of menopause hormone therapy, exercise, and their combination on bone mineral density and mental wellbeing in menopausal women: a scoping review. Front Reprod Health. 2025;7:12 May.
30. Yi S, Zhang, Rui Y, Lei J, Wenjia L. Postmenopausal osteoporosis: a mini review. EMJ Rheumatol. 2019;6(1):90.

Sarcopenia and Menopause

8

Jyoti Bhaskar

Abstract

Movement depends on both bone and muscle function, and the relationships between them are becoming more widely acknowledged and researched. Osteopenia, osteoporosis, and sarcopenia are important musculoskeletal conditions associated with menopause that negatively impact health, leading to poor quality of life and increased morbidity. Taken together, they come under "Osteosarcopenia"—a silent disease that slowly and gradually weakens the bone-muscle unit. Menopause is the time when attention is to be paid to detect, screen, prevent, and treat sarcopenia. This chapter deals with the current definition and methods used to diagnose and treat sarcopenia.

Keywords

Menopause · Sarcopenia · Gait Speed · Muscle Mass · Muscle Strength · Muscle Power

8.1 Introduction

Sarcopenia is a progressive and generalized skeletal muscle disorder that can lead to adverse outcomes such as falls, fractures, physical disability, mortality, and contributes to Frailty. Menopause transition due to decrease in estrogen can lead to accelerated and progressive muscle degeneration.

Movement depends on both bone and muscle function, and the relationships between them are becoming more widely acknowledged and researched [1, 2].

J. Bhaskar (✉)
Cloudnine Noida and Delhi, New Delhi, India

Delhi Menopause Society, Delhi, India

R. Malik et al. (eds.), *Menopause Essentials*,
https://doi.org/10.1007/978-981-95-7498-8_8

Osteopenia, osteoporosis, and sarcopenia are important musculoskeletal conditions associated with menopause that negatively impact health, leading to poor quality of life and increased morbidity. Taken together, they come under "Osteosarcopenia" - a silent disease that slowly and gradually weakens the bone-muscle unit [3].

We all are familiar with the term Osteoporosis, but Sarcopenia is a relative new entity. The Greek words "Sarx," which means flesh, and "Penia," which means loss, are the origin of the phrase "sarcopenia," which was first used by Rosenberg et al. in 1989. It took nearly 30 years for Sarcopenia to be given the status of disease in 2016.

Hence, it goes undiagnosed and untreated leading to increased morbidity and mortality in postmenopausal woman.

8.2 Prevalence

It is a global problem. A comprehensive, multicenter study from nine nations on three continents found that the prevalence of sarcopenia was 15.2% overall [4]. The risk of sarcopenia is 2.99 times higher in postmenopausal women. According to global research, 17.5% of elderly Indians have sarcopenia. Patients with comorbidities are more likely to have sarcopenia, hence secondary sarcopenia must be treated as soon as possible.

8.3 Risk Factors

Identifying the risk factors for sarcopenia is crucial, particularly for postmenopausal women. In addition to the patient, family members, caregivers, and other medical professionals should also provide a thorough medical history. The objective is to identify the causes, risk factors, and consequences of sarcopenia (Table 8.1).

Prevalence of sarcopenia with age and Menopause Muscle makes up around 40% of the body weight. From the age of 30 years, body starts to lose 3–8% muscle mass per decade and after 50 years, it increases to 1–2% per year and by 80 years, there is 30–50% loss of muscle mass. Muscle strength declines even faster at menopause and the decline starts at the rate of 1.5–5% per year so that by age of 70 years, 20–40% of muscle strength is lost. In fact, lean body mass (LBM) dropped by 0.5% and fat mass rose by 1.7% annually throughout the menopausal transition.

Declining Estrogen levels at Menopause has a detrimental effect on muscle mass and strength through decreased estrogen receptors, decrease in sensitivity to GH and IGF, through increased inflammatory infiltrates in the muscle and through effect on muscle metabolism [5].

Table 8.1 Risk factors for Sarcopenia

Disease	Causes
Aging	Age related muscle loss—Primary Sarcopenia
Diseases	Endocrine—Type 1 DM, hypogonadism, early menopause, Paget's disease, thyroid disorders, hypercalciuria Malignancies Organ failure: Heart, lung, liver, kidney, or brain Inflammatory disease—Rheumatoid arthritis
Inactivity	Sedentary behavior—Bedrest, limited mobility Physical inactivity, institutionalized patients
Malnutrition	Malabsorption or undernutrition Excessive alcohol use, smoking, and cachexia Obesity and overnutrition Medication-related anorexia

Table 8.2 SARC-F screen for sarcopenia [7]

Component	Question	Scoring
Strength	How much difficulty do you have in lifting and carrying 10 pounds?	None = zero Some = 1 A lot or incapable = 2
Assistance in walking	How much difficulty do you have walking across a room?	None = zero Some = 1 A lot, use of aids, or incapable = 2
Rise from a chair	How much difficulty do you have transferring from a chair or bed?	None = zero Some = 1 A lot or incapable without help = 2
Climb stairs	How much difficulty do you have climbing a flight of 10 stairs?	None = zero Some = 1 A lot or incapable = 2
Falls	How many times have you fallen in the past year?	None = zero 1–3 falls = 1 ≥4 falls = 2

8.4 Screening for Sarcopenia

The European Working Group on Sarcopenia in Older People (EWGSOP 2) [5] was released in 2018, and the South Asian Working Action Group on Sarcopenia (SWAG SARCO) guidelines were released in 2021 specifically for the South Asian community [6].

A FACS algorithm for identifying cases, diagnosing conditions, and measuring severity in routine clinical practice has been provided by EWGSOP2. This algorithm states that the straightforward SARC F questionnaire should be used to screen for sarcopenia in all individuals over 60 and menopausal women who are sitting in the OPD, in the community, or in assisted living facilities (Table 8.2).

SARC F has a very high specificity to predict low muscle strength. It is a low-cost, opportunistic approach to screening for sarcopenia risk. Since SARC-F is filled by the patient, results represent patient's own opinions of their severity of the condition. Poor outcomes and sarcopenia are predicted by a total score of 4 or higher [7] (Table 8.3).

Dual-energy X-ray absorptiometry (DXA); appendicular skeletal muscle mass (ASM); bioelectrical impedance analysis (BIA); computed tomography, or CT; Magnetic resonance imaging, or MRI; TUG (timed up and go); SPPB (short physical performance battery).

In clinical practice, tests to assess muscle strength should be performed if the SARC F score is more than 4. Treatment should be started if this is determined to be low, and more testing should only be done for scientific grounds.

Although the EWGSOP 2 standards are widely accepted, the South Asian guidelines (SWAG SARCO) [4] were necessary since South Asians have lesser muscular mass and strength than Caucasians. Both undernutrition and overnutrition are problems in this rapidly growing area. The "thin-fat obesity" or sarcopenic obesity, commonly referred to as normal weight obesity and having a similar cardio-metabolic risk to obesity, is the distinctive known phenotype of obesity in South Asians. Additionally, the majority of South Asian nations are low-middle-income nations that struggle with costs and resources.

SWAG SARCO 2021 guidelines differ from EWGSOP2 in following aspects:

- Diagnosis: The loss of any two muscle components (strength, function, or mass), without giving importance to any 1 component over the other.
- It emphasizes the significance of sarcopenic obesity and secondary sarcopenia.
- The SARC F incorporates calf circumference. A cutoff is defined as a calf circumference of less than 34 cm for females and less than 33 cm for males. The Sarc F score is increased by 10 points if the CC is below the cutoff. When evaluating sarcopenia, a score of 11 or higher is taken into consideration.
- Male hand grip strength cutoffs are <27.5 kg, while female cutoffs are <18 kg.

Table 8.3 Clinical tools for measurement of muscle strength, mass, and physical performance

Test	Cut off points for women
1. EWGSOP2 cut off points for low muscle strength by grip test and chair stand test	
Grip Strength	< 16 kg
Chair Stand test	> 15 s for 5 rises
2. EWGSOP2 sarcopenia cut off points for low muscle quantity	
ASM(DXA)	< 15 kg
ASM/height [2]	< 5.5 kg/m^2
3. EWGSOP2 sarcopenia cut off points for low physical performance	
GAIT SPEED	≤ 0.8 m/s
SPPB (Short physical performance battery)	≤ 8 points: poor physical performance
TUG (Timed 'up and go' test)	Cut off > 20 s
400 meter walk test	Noncompletion or > 6 minutes for completion

- It suggests that imaging should preferably be utilized in situations where clinical and biochemical measurements are unable to direct judgments about diagnosis or treatment. Skeletal muscle ultrasonography (USGM) is recommended and the choice of imaging is based on accessibility, price, and availability.
- The 5S algorithm (Suspect, Screening, Secondary Sarcopenia, Severity, and Shared Decision Making) is used.

8.5 Management of Sarcopenia

Treatment goals are:

- Prevent decline in muscle function and performance
- Falls and impairment may be prevented/reduced by early intervention.
- To lower death and hospitalization rates among the impacted

8.6 Components of Management

8.6.1 AMEND Muscle Health

*A*ctivity and exercise Optimization
*M*edical and Metabolic care
*E*nvironmental Optimization
*N*utritional Optimization
*D*rug Therapy

8.6.2 Nonpharmacological (Including Nutritional Supplements)

1. *Lifestyle change*: Quitting drinking and smoking should be aggressively encouraged, and assistance should be given. Caffeine, smoke, and salt should be avoided or consumed in moderation [8].
2. *Exercise*: By increasing BMD, resistance training and high-impact sports like jogging have a favorable effect on bone. Similarly, by directly improving muscles, resistance training has a good impact on sarcopenia [9]. Depending on their level of exercise capacity, patients should be encouraged to perform the recommended exercises on a regular basis (*at least three times per week*). It is important to make sure that there is a *sufficient warm-up* before resistance and aerobic activities as well as a sufficient *cool-down* afterward. To avoid falls, cardiovascular exercises should be preceded by strength, flexibility, and balance training. Depending on the patient's tolerability and sufficient protein intake, the intensity of prescribed exercises should be progressively increased. Exercises which are specific in nature for the secondary causes of sarcopenia (cardiac rehabilitation/weight loss) are also important.

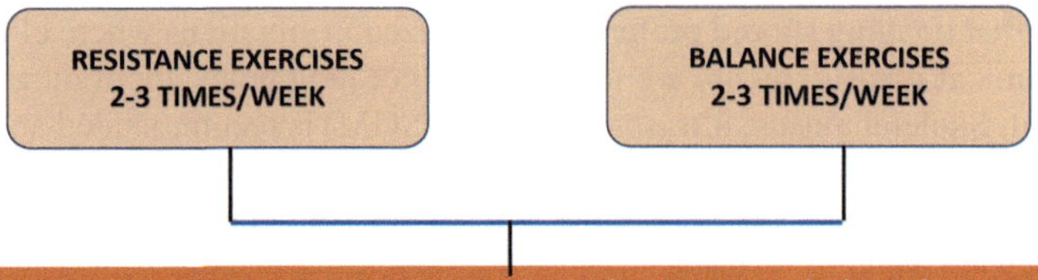

Nutrients that may improve Sarcopenia and recommended intake

Protein	Leucine	HMB	Vit D	Vit E	Vit C	Mg	Se	Ca	Probiotic	Collagen	Polyphenols
1-1.5 gm/kg/day	2.5 gm per meal	3 gm per day	1000-2000 iu per day	400 iu per day	45-90 mg per day	900 mg per day	25-75 Ug per day	1200 mg per day	400 ug per day	50 ml per day	> 500 mg per day

Fig. 8.1 Nonpharmacological and dietary supplements for the Sarcopenia

3. *Medical Optimization of Secondary Causes*: Pharmacological and nonpharmacological treatments (MNT, psychotherapy, exercise, etc.) should be used to address any medical, metabolic, endocrine, and psychological conditions that may be the cause of secondary sarcopenia.
4. *Environmental Optimization*: It consists of three elements: social, psychological, and physical.

   By *installing cameras, wearable and in-home sensors,* and linked gadgets that automatically adapt to the patient's surroundings, the home environment can be made safer. Walking aids (such as walking sticks and frames) *or external orthoses, grab rails, wearable sensors, Western toilets, and toilet chairs can make ADLS simple and safe*. There should be minimal furniture and good lighting in the rooms.
5. *Nutritional Strategies*: All nutritional recommendations should be tailored to the patient's comorbidities, availability, affordability, and food preferences.

   Bone mineral density is slightly increased by dietary calcium and calcium supplements, and it is advised to consume 1000–1300 mg of calcium daily, particularly in the postmenopausal age range [8]. It has also been noted that proteins are crucial for the health of muscles. At least 1.2–1.5 g/kg/day is advised by expert consensus groups, with 2.5–3 g of leucine and 25–30 g of protein every meal. Muscle atrophy was linked to low dietary protein (0.45 g/kg/day) in older adults (65 years of age and older) [10]. By promoting the absorption of calcium and phosphate and supporting calcium-dependent muscular activities, vitamin D plays a critical role in the physiology of bones and muscles. For adults aged 50 years and older, numerous scientific organizations advise consuming at least 1000 IU of vitamin D daily (Fig. 8.1).
6. *Pharmacological*

Menopause Hormonal Therapy

MHT at present is not recommended for the prevention and treatment of Sarcopenia. It is because the results of meta-analysis in 2019 and in 2020 reported only slight

Table 8.4 Pharmacotherapy for the Sarcopenia

Pharmacological Agents	Sarcopenia
Denosumab	No significant effect on muscle function observed [11]. In people with osteoporosis, it improves insulin sensitivity and muscle strength [12].
Testosterone	Testosterone injections can increase muscular mass, strength, and athletic performance in people with lower serum testosterone levels [13].
Growth Hormone	Low growth hormone levels with age contribute to a decrease in lean body mass and an increase in adipose tissue [14].
Antimyostatin Antibodies	(1) A few studies found that Antimyostatin antibodies enhanced muscle hypertrophy and strength [15]. (2) Antimyostatin antibodies may enhance functional measures of muscular power and increase lean mass.

Although there are currently no pharmacologic treatments that explicitly target sarcopenia, denosumab, a RANK ligand inhibitor, has shown positive benefits on bone and muscle

but statistically insignificant effect of MHT on muscle strength and no beneficial effect on muscle mass respectively. The probable reason is that the woman on MHT are less than 60 years of age and have sufficient muscle mass and strength to show any beneficial effect. MHT is not recommended for older woman who have significant sarcopenia (Table 8.4).

8.7 Sarcopenia Prevention

- Sarcopenia prevention should be the aim of every health professional. It can be implemented through the *'Sarcopenia prevention prism'* which starts with *primordial prevention* highlighting the importance of good diet and exercise followed by *primary prevention* which stresses on nutrition and lifestyle, *secondary prevention* on optimal management of secondary causes, *tertiary prevention* in the form of use of assisted devices, physiotherapy, medications, *quaternary prevention* by minimizing over diagnosis and over treatment and lastly, *quinary prevention* by avoiding misinformation and spreading right message for muscle health.

8.8 Conclusion

Sarcopenia is the disease of postmenopausal woman and elderly. It is a progressive debilitating skeletal muscle disorder that increases the morbidity and mortality of the elderly. Every health professional should evaluate their postmenopausal patients for the probable sarcopenia and institute preventive and corrective measures to enhance their quality of life.

Key Points

- Sarcopenia remains underdetected and undertreated. Every postmenopausal woman over the age of 60 years, should be evaluated for Sarcopenia.
- Owing to the high likelihood of co-occurrence of osteoporosis/osteopenia and sarcopenia in older persons, the diagnosis of osteoporosis should initiate an assessment for sarcopenia.
- The use of algorithm of EWGSOP2 should be inculcated in every day practice.
- An effective way to fight sarcopenia is to combine nutritional supplements with resistance and balancing exercises.
- In terms of pharmacotherapies, Denosumab may be beneficial for both bone and muscle health. Further research for new pharmacological modalities is urgently needed.

Long Answer Questions (LAQs)

1. Please elaborate on FACS algorithm in detail.
2. What the tests for physical performance and when should they be done?
3. Write a note on the pharmacological treatment available for Sarcopenia and their benefits.
4. Write in detail about the nutritional supplementation needed for Sarcopenia patients.

Short Answer Questions (SAQs)

1. What are the risk factors for developing Sarcopenia?
2. Elaborate on the importance of exercise and the type and duration of exercise that should be undertaken?
3. What is the role of MHT in management of Sarcopenia?
4. Please elaborate the tests for assessment of the muscle strength.
5. How is the SWAG SARCO guidelines different from the EWGSOP2?

Multiple Choice Questions (MCQs)

1. In SARC F, above which score is Sarcopenia probable

   A. 3
   B. 2
   C. 6
   D. 4

2. Causes of Secondary Sarcopenia are all except

   A. Diabetes
   B. Paget's disease
   C. Malignancies
   D. Hypertension

3. Chair Stand test assesses the

   A. Muscle mass
   B. Muscle strength
   C. Muscle performance
   D. Muscle function

4. The Gold standard for assessment of Muscle Mass is

   A. DEXA scan
   B. BIA
   C. MRI
   D. TUG

5. The treatment for Sarcopenia should be instituted in clinical practisewhen

   A. SARC F score >4
   B. Chair stand test result showing low muscle strength
   C. DEXA scan shows low muscle mass
   D. TUG showing poor performance

6. Full form of FACS is

   A. First Assess Confirm Scan
   B. Find Assess Confirm Severe
   C. Find Accept Confirm Severe
   D. First Accept Concern Scan

7. Protein required per day in elderly

   A. 0.8 gm/day
   B. 1 gm/day
   C. 1. 8 gm/day
   D. 1.2 gm/day

8. MHT has a definite role to play in all except

   A. VMS
   B. POI
   C. Sarcopenia

D. GSM

9. The cut off for Grip strength according to EWGSOP2 for woman is

   A. > 18 kg
   B. > 20 kg
   C. >16 kg
   D. > 14 kg

10. The only drug known to have any benefit in Sarcopenia is

   A. MHT
   B. Denosumab
   C. Testosterone
   D. Raloxifene

Answers

1. D
2. D
3. B
4. C
5. B
6. B
7. D
8. C
9. C
10. B

References

1. Tagliaferri C, Wittrant Y, Davicco MJ, et al. Muscle and bone, two interconnected tissues. Ageing Res Rev. 2015;21:55–70.
2. Kawao N, Kaji H. Interactions between muscle tissues and bone metabolism. J Cell Biochem. 2015;116:687–95.
3. Curtis E, Litwic A, Cooper C, et al. Determinants of muscle and bone aging. J Cell Physiol. 2015;230:2618–25.
4. Dhar M, Kapoor N, Suastika K, Khamseh ME, Selim S, Kumar V, Raza SA, Azmat U, Pathania M, Rai Mahadeb YP, Singhal S, Naseri MW, Aryana IS, Thapa SD, Jacob J, Somasundaram N, Latheef A, Dhakal GP, Kalra S. South Asian Working Action Group on SARCOpenia (SWAG-SARCO) - a consensus document. Osteoporos Sarcopenia. 2022;8(2):35–57. https://doi.org/10.1016/j.afos.2022.04.001. Epub 2022 May 25.
5. Cruz-Jentoft AJ, Bahat G, Bauer J, et al. Sarcopenia: revised European consensus on definition and diagnosis. Age Ageing. 2019;48:16–31.

6. Chen LK, Woo J, Assantachai P, Auyeung TW, Chou MY, Iijima K, et al. Asian Working Group for Sarcopenia: 2019 consensus update on sarcopenia diagnosis and treatment. J Am Med Dir Assoc. 2020;21:300–7.
7. Malmstrom TK, Morley JE. SARC-F: a simple questionnaire to rapidly diagnose sarcopenia. J Am Med Dir Assoc. 2013;14(8):531–2.
8. Meeta M, Harinarayan CV, Marwah R, Sahay R, Kalra S, Babhulkar S. Clinical practice guidelines on postmenopausal osteoporosis: *an executive summary and recommendations—update 2019–2020. J Mid-life Health. 2020;11:96.
9. Liu CJ, Latham NK. Progressive resistance strength training for improving physical function in older adults. Cochrane Database Syst Rev. 2009;2009:CD002759.
10. Castaneda C, Gordon PL, Fielding RA, et al. Marginal protein intake results in reduced plasma IGF-I levels and skeletal muscle fiber atrophy in elderly women. J Nutr Health Aging. 2000;4:85–90.
11. Cummings SR, Martin JS, McClung MR, et al. Denosumab for prevention of fractures in postmenopausal women with osteoporosis. N Engl J Med. 2009;361:756–65.
12. Bonnet N, Bourgoin L, Biver E, et al. RANKL inhibition improves muscle strength and insulin sensitivity and restores bone mass. J Clin Invest. 2019;130:1.
13. De Spiegeleer A, Beckwee D, Bautmans I, et al. Pharmacological interventions to improve muscle mass, muscle strength and physical performance in older people: an umbrella review of systematic reviews and meta-analyses. Drugs Aging. 2018;35:719–34.
14. Rudman D, Feller AG, Nagraj HS, et al. Effects of human growth hormone in men over 60 years old. N Engl J Med. 1990;323:1–6.
15. Camporez JPG, Petersen MC, Abudukadier A, et al. Anti-myostatin antibody increases muscle mass and strength and improves insulin sensitivity in old mice. Proc Natl Acad Sci U S A. 2016;113(8):2212–7.

Sleep and Cognitive Disorders at Menopause

9

Tejas Menon Suri, Jyotsna Suri, and Renuka Malik

Abstract

Sleep disturbances affect nearly half of women undergoing menopause. Hormonal changes, vasomotor symptoms, medical and psychiatric comorbidities, and the aging process all contribute to the development of sleep disorders, including insomnia, obstructive sleep apnea, and restless legs syndrome. Additionally, the menopausal transition is also associated with cognitive decline. Clinicians must assess perimenopausal women for symptoms such as difficulty in initiating or maintaining sleep, snoring, daytime sleepiness, and cognitive challenges. Effective diagnosis and management of sleep disorders during menopause requires close collaboration between the gynecologist and the sleep physician. Diagnostic tools include sleep diaries, actigraphy, and polysomnography. Many nonpharmacological and pharmacological therapies are available for insomnia, OSA, and RLS, and many other therapies are in development. Lifestyle measures, including adequate diet, exercise, sleep hygiene, and stress reduction, remain the cornerstone for preventing cognitive decline during the menopausal period.

Keywords

Menopause · Sleep · Insomnia · Obstructive sleep apnea · Cognitive decline

T. M. Suri (✉)
Department of Pulmonary, Critical Care & Sleep Medicine, All India Institute of Medical Sciences, New Delhi, India

J. Suri
Department of Obstetrics & Gynaecology, Vardhman Mahavir Medical College & Safdarjung Hospital, New Delhi, India

R. Malik
Department of Obstetrics & Gynaecology, Atal Bihari Vajpayee Institute of Medical Sciences & Dr. Ram Manohar Lohia Hospital, New Delhi, India

R. Malik et al. (eds.), *Menopause Essentials*,
https://doi.org/10.1007/978-981-95-7498-8_9

9.1 Introduction

Menopause is a transition period in life characterized by hormonal and other physiological changes that make women vulnerable to various health problems. Sleep health is an essential concern among perimenopausal and postmenopausal women. Sleep encompasses one-third of human life and is vital to physical and mental wellbeing. Approximately half of all peri- and postmenopausal women have sleep disturbances or sleep disorders. In this chapter, we discuss the spectrum of sleep disturbances associated with menopause, their pathophysiological basis, clinical evaluation, and management aspects.

9.2 Spectrum and Epidemiology of Sleep Disturbances and Disorders Associated with Menopause

Among women undergoing menopause, the commonest sleep disturbances include difficulties in initiating and maintaining sleep. Hence, perimenopausal women experience prolonged sleep latency (i.e., time taken to fall asleep), frequent night time awakenings, and increased time spent in wake after sleep onset (WASO) compared to premenopausal women. Salari et al. conducted a systematic review and meta-analysis of the global prevalence of sleep disturbances associated with menopause [1]. They found the overall pooled prevalence of sleep disturbances to be 51.6%. Furthermore, there was an increasing trend in the prevalence of sleep disturbances from premenopausal (46.5%) to perimenopausal (50.3%) to postmenopausal (54.7%) women. The recently published Longitudinal Aging Study in India examined over 28,000 community-dwelling postmenopausal women aged 50 years and above from all over the country and found that the prevalence of sleep problems was 22.3% [2].

Variations in prevalence across different studies may be related to the use of differing tools and questionnaires to determine sleep disturbances; nonetheless, sleep disturbances are widely reported in middle-aged women. In a meta-analysis of 12 studies, the risk factors for sleep problems among postmenopausal women included mood disorders, vasomotor symptoms, comorbid medical disorders, and psychotropic drug use [3].

In contrast, chronic insomnia disorder is defined more narrowly as difficulty initiating sleep, maintaining sleep, or experiencing early morning awakening on at least three occasions per week for more than 3 months, with associated daytime impairments resulting from the sleep disturbances. In the meta-analysis conducted by Salari et al. the global prevalence of chronic insomnia disorder among perimenopausal and postmenopausal women is around 37% [1].

Besides chronic insomnia disorder, other common sleep disorders encountered in the general population include obstructive sleep apnea (OSA) and restless legs syndrome (RLS). OSA is a disorder of repeated collapse of the upper airway during sleep, characterized by loud snoring, cyclical oxygen desaturation, and nonrestorative sleep. OSA is generally more common in males compared to females. However, there is a sharp rise in the occurrence of OSA following menopause. In the Wisconsin Sleep Cohort Study, the odds ratio for OSA in perimenopausal and postmenopausal women was 2.6 and 3.5, respectively, after adjusting for age, body habitus, smoking, and other relevant confounders [4]. In a global meta-analysis, the pooled prevalence of OSA in menopausal women was 30.6% across 13 studies [1].

RLS is characterized by an urge to move the legs during periods of inactivity that is relieved by movement, particularly during the evening hours and just before sleep onset. Patients with RLS often experience abnormal leg movements during sleep, known as periodic limb movements of sleep (PLMS), which can impair sleep quality. There is relatively less data regarding the prevalence of RLS among menopausal women, with the pooled prevalence being 63.8% across 3 studies [1].

9.2.1 Pathophysiology and Consequences of Sleep Disturbances Associated with Menopause

The interplay between two processes regulates sleep in humans: the homeostatic sleep drive and the circadian system. The homeostatic sleep drive is the propensity to feel sleepy after a prolonged period of wakefulness. The supra-chiasmatic nucleus in the hypothalamus orchestrates the circadian system, governing the body's cyclical rhythms that are synced to the environmental day–night cycle. Accordingly, melatonin levels increase with the onset of night and promote sleep.

Sleep disturbances experienced by women during the menopausal transition are multifactorial. The contributing factors include hormonal changes related to menopause itself, vasomotor symptoms, mood changes, medical co morbidities, and the aging process [5].

A decline in estrogen and progesterone levels characterizes menopause. The mechanism by which estrogen deficiency causes sleep disturbance is not fully understood. Estrogen modulates the levels of various neurotransmitters involved in sleep–wake and mood regulation, including norepinephrine, dopamine, and serotonin. Depressive symptoms during menopause may contribute to impaired sleep duration and early morning awakening. Furthermore, estrogen downregulates the hypothalamic kisspeptin/neurokinin B/dynorphin (KNDy) neurons. Estrogen deficit during menopause causes abnormal activation of KNDy neurons involved in thermoregulation, leading to vasomotor symptoms such as hot flashes and night sweats. These symptoms may disturb sleep with frequent nocturnal awakenings. Progesterone is known to have stimulatory activity via the sleep-promoting gamma-aminobutyric acid (GABA) neurotransmitter system.

While menopausal symptoms and hormonal changes precipitate sleep difficulties in predisposed women, these sleep disturbances can perpetuate due to maladaptive behaviors and thoughts, leading to chronic insomnia disorder among perimenopausal and postmenopausal women. Common maladaptations include spending excessive time in bed (which blunts the homeostatic sleep drive), developing conditioned arousal (subconsciously linking bed with wakefulness), and negative thoughts and beliefs about sleep.

Sleep disturbances negatively affect physical and mental health, work productivity, social relationships, and quality of life. The Study of Women's Health across the Nation conducted in the United States, enrolled women between the ages of 42 and 52 and followed them up over 22 years. They found that women with persistent insomnia symptoms and persistently short sleep duration (i.e., around 5 hours per night) had a significantly elevated risk of developing cardiovascular disease [6].

The elevated risk of OSA in postmenopausal women is also likely multifactorial, related to changes in body composition, hormonal status, and upper airway anatomy. Postmenopausal women are known to have increased body mass index, increased visceral fat deposition around the neck, and narrowed upper airway caliber; these features are associated with developing upper airway collapse and OSA [7, 8]. Furthermore, progesterone stimulates breathing and may increase upper airway muscle tone. Consequently, declining progesterone levels in postmenopausal women may exacerbate upper airway collapse during sleep. Notably, OSA may contribute to the increased risk of hypertension, cardiovascular disease, and stroke among postmenopausal women.

9.3 Clinical Evaluation

All women experiencing menopausal symptoms should be asked about sleep difficulties. Some of the common symptoms that need to be elicited include:

- Difficulty in initiating sleep, frequent nocturnal awakening, and early morning awakening, along with their frequency
- Loud snoring, witnessed choking or gasping during sleep (these questions are directed to the patient's bed partner)
- Tiredness, fatigue, difficulty concentrating, or excessive daytime sleepiness
- Unpleasant sensation in legs or urge to move while lying still at night

Physical examination should assess upper airway dimensions, including neck circumference, tongue size, and Mallampati score. The body mass index should be calculated.

Women with features suggestive of chronic insomnia disorder, suspected OSA, or RLS may benefit from a referral to a sleep medicine specialist. Further diagnostic testing may include:

- Sleep diaries or actigraphy: for evaluation of insomnia symptoms
- Polysomnography: a sleep study that monitors multiple physiological variables to diagnose various sleep disorders, including OSA. While polysomnography is typically performed in a sleep lab, a portable sleep study can be conducted at home in select cases.
- Serum iron studies: among women in whom RLS is suspected

9.4 Management of Sleep Disorders at Menopause

In this section, we will discuss the management of menopause-related sleep disturbances, chronic insomnia disorder, Obstructive sleep apnea, and Restless Leg Syndrome.

9.4.1 Menopause-Related Sleep Disturbances and Chronic Insomnia Disorder

Various pharmacological and nonpharmacological strategies have been employed to address difficulties initiating and maintaining sleep among middle-aged women.

Cognitive behavioral therapy for insomnia (CBT-I) is the first-line therapy for chronic insomnia disorder and is preferred over pharmacotherapy for chronic symptoms. CBT-I aims to correct maladaptive behaviors and beliefs that perpetuate insomnia symptoms. The various components of CBT-I include sleep restriction therapy (limiting the time spent in bed to harness the sleep homeostatic drive), stimulus control (getting out of bed when unable to sleep to break the cycle of conditioned arousal in bed), relaxation techniques, and cognitive restructuring. CBT-I is safe and effective among perimenopausal and postmenopausal women. In a randomized controlled trial (RCT) comparing telephone-based CBT-I with routine menopausal education, there were greater improvements in insomnia severity, sleep latency, nocturnal awakenings, sleep efficiency, and sleep quality in the CBT-I arm [9]. Another RCT compared CBT-I, single-component sleep restriction therapy, and sleep hygiene education. At 6-month follow-up, insomnia severity improved with both CBT-I and sleep restriction therapy. CBT-I outperformed sleep restriction therapy in improving sleep maintenance [10]. Other nonpharmacological therapies for which there is limited evidence for an adjunctive role in improving sleep quality among perimenopausal women include yoga and exercise [11, 12].

Menopause hormone therapy (MHT), also referred to as hormone replacement therapy, is indicated for the treatment of moderate-to-severe vasomotor symptoms among otherwise healthy women who are within 10 years of the onset of menopause (or below 60 years of age). Among menopausal women with a uterus, MHT comprises transdermal or oral estradiol therapy combined with intermittent micronized progesterone. Interestingly, MHT has been found to improve sleep disturbances, including "minutes to fall asleep" and "number of awakenings", even after controlling for improvements in vasomotor and depressive symptoms [13]. However, MHT is contraindicated among women with a history of breast cancer, cardiovascular disease, stroke, venous thromboembolism, and liver disease.

Nonhormonal pharmacotherapies that may improve menopausal symptoms, including sleep disturbances, include gabapentin and selective serotonin reuptake inhibitors (SSRIs) such as fluoxetine [14]. However, in some cases, SSRIs can worsen insomnia, and sedating antidepressants (e.g., mirtazapine, doxepin) may be preferred. Hypnotics such as nonbenzodiazepine Z-drugs (zolpidem, eszopiclone) and orexin antagonists (suvorexant, Lemborexant) may be used for short-term treatment (up to a few weeks) of acute insomnia but are associated with significant side effects (e.g., falls, osteoporosis) and potential for dependence over longer-term use [14]. Melatonin supplements have also been used as over-the-counter preparations for insomnia. However, their efficacy in treating insomnia is doubtful.

An emerging pharmacological approach for managing vasomotor symptoms among perimenopausal women is the use of neurokinin-1 (NK-1) and neurokinin-3 (NK-3) receptor antagonists. These antagonists prevent the abnormal upregulation of the thermoregulatory KNDy neurons following perimenopausal decline in estrogenic feedback. Recently published RCTs of fezolinetant (NK-3 receptor antagonist) and elinzanetant (dual NK-1, 3 receptor antagonist) have reported improvements in sleep disturbance as critical secondary outcomes [15, 16]. Further research is needed to delineate the roles of these agents for managing sleep disturbances during menopause.

9.5 Obstructive Sleep Apnea

Perimenopausal women with symptoms of OSA (i.e., snoring, witnessed apneas, or excessive daytime sleepiness) and associated comorbidities (i.e., obesity and systemic hypertension) should be evaluated and managed under the supervision of a sleep physician. Continuous positive airway pressure (CPAP) therapy is the most efficacious and first-line treatment option. In selected cases, alternative treatment options include oral appliance therapy and upper airway surgery. Weight loss interventions, including the newer glucagon-like peptide-1 (GLP-1) agonists, may be beneficial among patients with obesity.

9.6 Restless Legs Syndrome

Women with the diagnosis of RLS may be treated through non-pharmacological and pharmacological approaches. Iron supplementation (oral or parenteral) is indicated among patients with a serum ferritin level below 75 ng/mL. Symptomatic patients may benefit from alpha-2-delta ligand drugs, including pregabalin and gabapentin.

9.6.1 Cognitive Decline During Perimenopause and Menopause

It has been seen that there is a cognitive decline in women which may commence during the late perimenopause, increase at menopause, and further increase in severity in the late post menopause. The important clinical features of this include a decline in memory, brain fogging, inability to communicate effectively, difficulty in focusing on a task, and lack of concentration. Dementia is a severe form of cognitive impairment that is diagnosed when there is a loss of core mental activities, namely,

Table 9.1 Neurocognitive domains [17, 18]

Neurocognitive Domains
1. Complex attention
Sustained attention
Divided attention
Processing speed
Selective attention
2. Executive function
Planning
Decision making
Responding to feedback
Working memory
Inhibition
Flexibility
3. Learning and memory
Free recall
Cued recall
Recognition memory
Semantic & autobiographical long-term memory
Implicit learning
4. Language
Object naming
Word finding
Fluency
Syntax & grammar
Receptive language
5. Perceptual-Motor
Visual perception
Visuoconstructional reasoning
Perceptual motor coordination
6. Social cognition
Recognition of emotions
Theory of mind
Insight

memory, judgment, logic, the ability to perform daily tasks, perception of visual signals, and the ability to focus on a given task. Cognitive function comprises of six key domains (Table 9.1)—complex attention, executive function, learning and memory, language, perceptual-motor control, and social cognition. Cognitive decline may manifest as slowing and difficulty in recalling details and learning new information. It significantly impacts the quality of life.

It is estimated that about 2.1 million women suffer from dementia in India [19]. This huge number translates into a significant social and economic burden. The leading cause of cognitive disorders during menopause is the decline in the estrogen hormone.

9.7 Assessment of Cognitive Decline

Identifying cognitive decline during menopause involves using various tools designed to assess different aspects of cognitive function, including memory, executive function, attention, and overall mental sharpness. Some of the widely used tools are Montreal Cognitive Assessment (MoCA), Mini-Mental State Examination (MMSE), Trail Making Test (TMT), Quick Mild Cognitive Impairment (Q*mci*) screen, CANTAB (Cambridge Neuropsychological Test Automated Battery), and Cognitive Failures Questionnaire (CFQ).

A study by Zhu et al. [20] evaluated the Everyday Memory Questionnaire-Revised (EMQ-R) in menopausal women to gain insights into the phenomenon of "brain fog." The researchers focused on assessing the reliability and validity of the EMQ-R in capturing everyday memory lapses reported by menopausal women. They concluded that the EMQ-R can effectively measure subjective memory complaints and provide valuable insights into cognitive challenges during menopause, thereby guiding potential interventions. The Six Item Cognitive Impairment Test (6CIT) [21] is a widely used test which comprises of seven questions covering three domains (orientation, episodic memory, and attention). It has a total score of 28. A score of more than or equal to 8 is suggestive of cognitive impairment.

9.8 Management of Cognitive Decline at Menopause

The Canadian guidelines strongly recommend, with a high level of evidence, that the first-line treatment for postmenopausal women with complaints of cognitive decline includes lifestyle modifications [18]. These include exercise, especially of aerobic variety, inclusion of fresh vegetables in the diet, and a focus on control of chronic medical conditions such as hypertension, diabetes mellitus, and atherosclerotic disorders. Furthermore, another strong recommendation, albeit with moderate evidence, suggests that MHT is not effective in significantly improving cognitive functions when used over several years [22].

Hormone therapy Estrogen therapy especially when started early in the menopause transition phase may preserve cognitive function and decrease the risk of developing Alzheimer's disease later on. However, if started late it can increase the risk of Alzheimer and dementia. In cases of premature ovarian failure, it is seen as per as research that the cause of cognitive decline is genetic rather than estrogen deficiency. More research is required to see the benefit of menopausal hormonal therapy. The findings of MHT Studies on Neurocognitive functions are shown in Table 9.2.

Menopause generally has been associated mild cognitive impairment. Severe cognitive impairment and Alzheimer's need different management.

Hormone therapy-At present there is no current guideline promoting MHT for prevention or treatment of neurocognitive decline at menopause.

Table 9.2 Randomized clinical trials on hormone therapy and cognition in women [17]

Serial No.	Name of Study	Country	*N* (%)	Age (years)	Hormone treatment	Findings
1.	Women's Health Initiative Memory Study-WHIMS	USA	HT users: 2229. Placebo: 2303	≥ 65	CEE + MPA	HT increased dementia risk
2.	Women's Health Initiative Memory Study-WHIMS	USA	HT users: 1464. Placebo: 1483	65–79	CEE alone	Estrogen alone did not decrease incidence of mild cognitive impairment/dementia
3.	Randomized, double-blind study.	USA	HT users: 187. Placebo: 186	≥ 65	CEE with or without MPA	HT did not affect cognition
4.	Randomized, placebo-controlled, double-blind trial	USA	HT users: 208. Placebo: 209	60–80	Ultra–low dose unopposed transdermal estradiol	Transdermal estradiol did not affect cognition
5.	Women's Health Initiative Study of Cognitive Aging-WHISCA	USA	HT users: 1125. Placebo: 1179	65–80	CEE with or without MPA	HT was associated with worsening global cognitive decline and few specific cognitive domains which persisted after the interruption of HT
6.	Women's Health Initiative Memory Study of Younger Women-WHIMSY	USA	HT users: 696. Placebo: 630	50–55	CEE with or without MPA	HT did not alter global cognitive function or any specific domain of cognition
7.	Cognitive and Affective Study-KEEPS-Cog	USA	HT users: 431. Placebo: 262	Mean: 52.6	CEE + micronized progesterone OR Transdermal estradiol + micronized progesterone	HT did not affect cognition
8.	Early vs Late Intervention Trial with Estradiol Cognitive endpoints-ELITE-Cog	USA	HT users: 284. Placebo: 283	Early postmenopause: 55.6. Late postmenopause: 64.9	Estradiol with or without micronized progesterone	HT did not affect verbal memory, executive function, and global cognition, regardless of whether it was started <6 year or ≥ 10 year after menopause

(continued)

Table 9.2 (continued)

Serial No.	Name of Study	Country	*N* (%)	Age (years)	Hormone treatment	Findings
9.	WHIMSY extended + Women's Health Initiative Memory Study of the Epidemiology of Cognitive Health Outcomes (WHIMS-ECHO)	USA	WHIMSY-HT users: 701. Placebo: 635. WHIMS-ECHO-HT users: 1402. Placebo: 1478	Two groups: 50–54&65–79	CEE with or without MPA	HT prescribed to younger women had no significant effect on cognition in the long term while in older women produced decreased global cognitive function, executive function, and working memory
10.	Kronos Early Estrogen Prevention Study (KEEPS)-Cog trial	USA	HT users: 292. Placebo: 387	Early postmenopause	Oral CEE, tE2both with micronized progesterone or placebo pills and patch	No long-term cognitive effects of short-term exposure to HT started in early menopause versus placebo.

CEE Conjugated equine estrogen, *MPA* Medroxyprogesterone acetate, *HT* Hormone therapy, *tE2* transdermal 17β-estradiol

LIFESTYLE MODIFICATION: Healthy lifestyle with adequate exercise, avoidance of obesity, mental and physical stimulation, control of stress, treatment of medical illnesses and depression, and control of vascular risk factors such as diabetes, hypertension, and hyperlipidemia is suggested to prevent cognitive decline.

Exercise Regular exercise, especially aerobics improves cognition, brain plasticity, and decreases the risk of dementia. There is a marked potential for physical activity and exercise training to improve cognitive function. Women with higher levels of baseline physical activity were less likely to develop cognitive decline. Keeping the brain active by continuing to learn new skills is helpful to build cognitive reserve.

Diet Mediterranean diet rich in fruits, vegetables, grains, nuts, and unsaturated fats is considered to be healthy for brain function. Free radical damages can accelerate the brain aging, so by consuming antioxidants such as vitamin E will help the body quench free radical associated changes. A healthy diet helps prevent hypertension (via reduced saturated fats and sodium), prediabetes (reduce sweets and caloric intake and consume more fiber), and stroke (dietary change to reduce cholesterol).

There is evidence that individuals whose diets are high in omega-3 fatty acids, especially docosahexaenoic acid (DHA), have a 50% reduction in their risk of developing dementia. DHA180 mg daily intake is suggested. However, the evidence is mixed. Optimal Vitamin D level is essential for brain health and may benefit women with cognitive decline.

Control of hypertension Key end-organ pathological mechanisms, for which hypertension is proposed to be causative, include acute and covert cerebral ischemia and hemorrhage, accelerated brain atrophy, cerebral microvascular rarefaction and endothelial dysfunction, disruption of blood–brain barrier and neuroinflammation that affects amyloid pathologies. In addition to the direct-effect of hypertension on brain structure and microvasculature, hypertension is a risk factor for other diseases associated with an increased risk of dementia, most notably chronic kidney disease and heart failure. Mid-life hypertension increases the relative risk of life-time dementia by 20–54%.

Sleep hygiene Improving the quality of sleep via behavioral modification and or medical therapy may help in cognitive function. A regular sleep schedule, a calming nighttime ritual, and an idealized sleeping environment are all examples of good sleep hygiene techniques. Establishing a sleep schedule, creating a sleep-inducing environment by ensuring the bedroom is dark, quiet, and cool with comfortable bedding and practicing relaxation techniques like reading, meditation, or taking a warm bath can help signal the body to wind down. Limiting exposure to electronics and reducing screen time before bed helps maintain melatonin production and circadian rhythm. Avoiding stimulants and heavy meals with regular physical exercise helps in falling asleep faster and enjoy deeper sleep but vigorous activity should be avoided close to bedtime. Managing stress and anxiety also helps to sleep better.

Cognitive training Staying mentally active via activities like solving puzzles, reading, and learning new skills helps in cognition.

Reduction of stress and improvement of Mental health Mindfulness-based stress reduction (MBSR) and Cognitive behavioral therapy (CBT): improves overall wellbeing and cognitive function.

DRUG THERAPY-Menopausal women suffering with mood-related cognitive symptoms may benefit with taking antidepressants. Several studies have shown that acetyl-L-carnitine and choline alphoscerate are able to increase the synthesis and the release of Ach in patients with MCI, Alzheimer-related dementia, cerebrovascular damage, and aging. Certain drugs especially antihypertensive drugs can cause cognitive decline. The opposite evidence of antihypertensive to delay cognitive decline also exists. A study found antihypertensive medications that stimulate (thiazides, dihydropyridine calcium channel blockers, angiotensin type I receptor blockers) vs. inhibit (angiotensin-converting enzyme inhibitors, beta-blockers, non-dihydropyridinecalcium channel blockers, type 2 and 4angiotensin II receptors) had lower rate of cognitive impairment. However, there are no large randomized controlled trials comparing different antihypertensive agents with clinical syndrome of dementia or cognitive impairment as the primary outcome [23].

9.9 Association Between Sleep Disorders and Cognitive Decline at Menopause

The association between sleep and cognition has been supported by studies that have found that persons using sleep aids and benzodiazepines have cognitive impairments [24, 25]. However, the link between the two in the ageing brain is still not elucidated. Interestingly, some studies have suggested that sleep disorders can be the moderators for cognitive functions in postmenopausal women. The brain has estradiol receptors which release neurotransmitters that control the cognitive functions like memory [26]. Estradiol, therefore, has a neuroprotective function that enhances synaptic activity and protects against brain cell apoptosis. The sharp decline in the estrogens at menopause leads to vasomotor symptoms as discussed earlier, leading to sleep disturbance and insomnia; this insomnia could be a mediator between menopause and cognitive disorders. This hypothesis is supported by an extensive cohort study involving 5880 women aged over 50 years from diverse racial and ethnic backgrounds. It concluded that earlier age at menopause was associated with a lower cognitive performance, which was possibly mediated by insomnia [27].

Hence, to conclude, it can be said that the decline in the estrogen hormone levels during menopause leads to sleep disorders and cognitive decline and this in turn has an adverse impact on the quality of life at menopause. These are both modifiable factors which are to be timely addressed by treating physician. In addition public awareness regarding self-management should be done.

Key Points

- Sleep disturbances affect approximately half of perimenopausal women and include difficulties in falling asleep and frequent nocturnal awakenings
- Sleep disturbances associated with menopause are multifactorial and may be related to hormonal changes, vasomotor and/or mood symptoms, medical comorbidities and associated sleep disorders like obstructive sleep apnea and restless legs syndrome
- Cognitive behavioral therapy is the first-line treatment for chronic insomnia disorder in menopausal women, while menopause hormone therapy may also have a beneficial impact on sleep disturbances
- Cognitive decline at menopause is a multifaceted issue which requires early diagnosis and treatment.
- Neurocognitive decline may be transient or long lasting. Preventive strategies like lifestyle modifications, regular exercise, stress management, and pharmacotherapy may help in improving cognitive decline.

Long Answer Questions (LAQs)

1. Write a short note on the epidemiology of sleep disturbances and sleep disorders in postmenopausal women.
2. Briefly describe the interplay between the hormonal changes at perimenopause and the development of sleep disturbances.
3. A 45-year-old perimenopausal woman complains of disturbed sleep and tiredness throughout the day. Briefly describe the clinical approach to the patient.
4. Write a short note on the management of insomnia among perimenopausal women.

Short Answer Questions (SAQs)

1. Describe common sleep disturbances encountered by women during postmenopausal women.
2. What is the indication for iron therapy among perimenopausal women with restless legs syndrome?
3. How is obstructive sleep apnea managed among postmenopausal women?
4. What is the role of pharmacotherapy in the management of insomnia among postmenopausal women?
5. What are common manifestations of cognitive decline at menopause?

Multiple-Choice Questions (MCQs)

1. Which of the following factors contributes to the development of sleep disturbances in postmenopausal women?
   A. Vasomotor symptoms
   B. Mood disturbances
   C. Comorbid medical disorders
   D. All of the above
2. All of the following are symptoms associated with insomnia disorder, except?
   A. Difficulty in initiating sleep
   B. Difficulty in maintaining sleep
   C. Loud snoring
   D. Early morning awakening
3. Which of the following is not a feature of restless legs syndrome?
   A. Urge to move the legs
   B. More during periods of inactivity
   C. Relieved by movement
   D. More in morning hours after awakening
4. Which of the following statements is true regarding the epidemiology of sleep disorders?
   A. Obstructive sleep apnea is more common in males than females
   B. The prevalence of sleep disturbances is lower among postmenopausal women compared to premenopausal women
   C. Approximately half of the women in perimenopausal and postmenopausal age have sleep disturbances
   D. The most common sleep disturbance among postmenopausal women is sleepwalking
5. Which of the following statements regarding chronic insomnia disorder is FALSE?
   A. Chronic insomnia disorder affects less than 5% of postmenopausal women
   B. Women with persistent insomnia and short sleep duration (<5 hours per night) have elevated risk of cardiovascular disease
   C. Spending excessive time in bed is a maladaptive behavior that perpetuates insomnia disorder
   D. Negative thoughts and beliefs about sleep are commonly observed among patients with chronic insomnia disorder
6. All of the following changes at menopause contribute to the development of obstructive sleep apnea, except?
   A. Declining progesterone levels
   B. Increased visceral fat deposition
   C. Narrowed upper airway caliber
   D. Increased lung volumes

7. Which of the following investigations should be performed in perimenopausal women with suspected restless legs syndrome?
   A. Serum ceruloplasmin
   B. Serum ferritin
   C. Serum lead levels
   D. Serum IgE
8. Which of the following is the first line therapy for chronic insomnia among postmenopausal women?
   A. Cognitive behavioral therapy for insomnia
   B. Zolpidem
   C. Yoga
   D. Clonazepam
9. In a recent randomized controlled trial, a new drug felozinetant was found to improve vasomotor symptoms in perimenopausal women. A key secondary result of the trial was an improvement in sleep disturbances. Which of the following is the mechanism of action of felozinetant?
   A. GABA-A receptor agonist
   B. Neurokinin-3 receptor antagonist
   C. Neurokinin-1 receptor antagonist
   D. Dual neurokinin-1, 3 receptor antagonist
10. All of the following have been found to be beneficial for cognitive decline following menopause, except?
    A. Aerobic exercise
    B. Dietary alterations
    C. Control of chronic medical disorders like hypertension and diabetes
    D. Menstrual hormonal therapy

Answers

1. D
2. C
3. D
4. D
5. A
6. D
7. B
8. A
9. B
10. D

References

1. Salari N, Hasheminezhad R, Hosseinian-Far A, Rasoulpoor S, Assefi M, Nankali S, et al. Global prevalence of sleep disorders during menopause: a meta-analysis. Sleep Breath Schlaf Atm. 2023:1–15.
2. Maheshwari V, Mishra S, Basu S. Sleep problems in community-dwelling postmenopausal and older women in India: a country level cross-sectional analysis. Discov Public Health. 2025;22(1):219.
3. Zeng W, Xu J, Yang Y, Lv M, Chu X. Factors influencing sleep disorders in perimenopausal women: a systematic review and meta-analysis. Front Neurol [Internet]. 2025 Feb 7 [cited 2025 May 20];16. Available from: https://www.frontiersin.org/journals/neurology/articles/10.3389/fneur.2025.1460613/full.
4. Young T, Finn L, Austin D, Peterson A. Menopausal status and sleep-disordered breathing in the Wisconsin Sleep Cohort Study. Am J Respir Crit Care Med. 2003;167(9):1181–5.
5. Maki PM, Panay N, Simon JA. Sleep disturbance associated with the menopause. Menopause. 2024;31(8):724.
6. Thurston RC, Chang Y, Kline CE, Swanson LM, El Khoudary SR, Jackson EA, et al. Trajectories of sleep over midlife and incident cardiovascular disease events in the study of women's health across the nation. Circulation. 2024;149(7):545–55.
7. Wang Y, Liu H, Zhou B, Yue W, Wang M, Hu K. Menopause and obstructive sleep apnea: revealing an independent mediating role of visceral fat beyond body mass index. BMC Endocr Disord. 2025;25(1):21.
8. Zhang W, Gao X. A cone beam CT study of upper airway morphology in perimenopausal and postmenopausal women. Int J Women's Health. 2021;13:1129–37.
9. McCurry SM, Guthrie KA, Morin CM, Woods NF, Landis CA, Ensrud KE, et al. Telephone-based cognitive behavioral therapy for insomnia in perimenopausal and postmenopausal women with vasomotor symptoms: a MsFLASH randomized clinical trial. JAMA Intern Med. 2016;176(7):913–20.
10. Drake CL, Kalmbach DA, Arnedt JT, Cheng P, Tonnu CV, Cuamatzi-Castelan A, et al. Treating chronic insomnia in postmenopausal women: a randomized clinical trial comparing cognitive-behavioral therapy for insomnia, sleep restriction therapy, and sleep hygiene education. Sleep. 2019;42(2):zsy217.
11. Newton KM, Reed SD, Guthrie KA, Sherman KJ, Booth-LaForce C, Caan B, et al. Efficacy of yoga for vasomotor symptoms: a randomized controlled trial. Menopause N Y N. 2014;21(4):339–46.
12. Sternfeld B, Guthrie KA, Ensrud KE, LaCroix AZ, Larson JC, Dunn AL, et al. Efficacy of exercise for menopausal symptoms: a randomized controlled trial. Menopause N Y N. 2014;21(4):330–8.
13. Geiger PJ, Eisenlohr-Moul T, Gordon JL, Rubinow DR, Girdler SS. Effects of perimenopausal transdermal estradiol on self-reported sleep, independent of its effect on vasomotor symptom bother and depressive symptoms. Menopause N Y N. 2019;26(11):1318–23.
14. Cheng YS, Tseng PT, Wu MK, Tu YK, Wu YC, Li DJ, et al. Pharmacologic and hormonal treatments for menopausal sleep disturbances: a network meta-analysis of 43 randomized controlled trials and 32,271 menopausal women. Sleep Med Rev. 2021;57:101469.
15. Shapiro CM, Cano A, Nappi RE, Santoro N, English ML, Mancuso S, et al. Effect of fezolinetant on sleep disturbance and impairment during treatment of vasomotor symptoms due to menopause. Maturitas. 2024;186:107999.
16. Pinkerton JV, Simon JA, Joffe H, Maki PM, Nappi RE, Panay N, et al. Elinzanetant for the treatment of vasomotor symptoms associated with menopause: OASIS 1 and 2 randomized clinical trials. JAMA. 2024;332(16):1343–54.
17. Conde DM, Verdade RC, Valadares ALR, Mella LFB, Pedro AO, Costa-Paiva L. Menopause and cognitive impairment: a narrative review of current knowledge. World J Psychiatr. 2021;11(8):412–28.

18. Gross AL, Nichols E, Angrisani M, Ganguli M, Jin H, Khobragade P, et al. Prevalence of DSM-5 mild and major neurocognitive disorder in India: results from the LASI-DAD. PLoS One. 2024;19(2):e0297220.
19. Meeta M, Digumarti L, Agarwal N, Vaze N, Shah R, Malik S. Clinical practice guidelines on menopause: *an executive summary and recommendations: Indian Menopause Society 2019-2020. J Mid-life Health. 2020;11(2):55–95.
20. Zhu C, Thomas EHX, Li Q, Arunogiri S, Thomas N, Gurvich C. Evaluation of the everyday memory questionnaire-revised in a menopausal population: understanding the brain fog during menopause. Menopause. 2023;30(11):1147–56.
21. O'Caoimh R, Molloy DW. Comparison of the six item cognitive impairment test (6CIT) to commonly-used short cognitive screening instruments in a memory clinic population. J Alzheimers Dis Rep. 2023;7(1):299–306. Published 2023 Apr 20.
22. Shea AK, Wolfman W, Fortier M, Soares CN. Guideline No. 422c: menopause: mood, sleep, and cognition. J Obstet Gynaecol Can. 2021;43(11):1316–1323.e1.
23. Malik R, Agarwal V. Neurocognitive decline at menopause. NARCHI Bulletin, March, 2025, Issue 4.
24. Lee JE, Ju YJ, Chun KH, Lee SY. The frequency of sleep medication use and the risk of Subjective Cognitive Decline (SCD) or SCD with functional difficulties in elderly individuals without dementia. J Gerontol A Biol Sci Med Sci. 2020;75(9):1693–8.
25. Stewart SA. The effects of benzodiazepines on cognition. J Clin Psychiatry. 2005;66(Suppl 2):9–13.
26. Morgan KN, Derby CA, Gleason CE. Cognitive changes with reproductive aging, perimenopause, and menopause. Obstet Gynecol Clin N Am. 2018;45(4):751–63.
27. Shieu MM, Braley TJ, Becker J, Dunietz GL. The interplay among natural menopause, insomnia, and cognitive health: a population-based study. Nat Sci Sleep. 2023;15:39–48.

Metabolic Syndrome at Menopause

10

Shobha N. Gudi and Neha Pruthi Tandon

Abstract

Metabolic syndrome is a lifestyle disorder constellation of interrelated risk factors—including central obesity, insulin resistance, Type 2 DM, dyslipidemia, hypertension, and predilection to cancer especially endometrial cancer. Its prevalence rises during the menopausal transition owing to hormonal changes, altered body fat distribution, and aging. Estrogen deficiency contributes to increased visceral adiposity, adverse lipid profile, and reduced insulin sensitivity, thereby amplifying cardiometabolic risk in postmenopausal women. Early recognition of metabolic syndrome at menopause is crucial, as it offers a window for timely lifestyle modification and pharmacological intervention to reduce long-term morbidity and mortality. This chapter reviews the risk factors, diagnostic criteria, and management strategies of metabolic syndrome in menopausal women, emphasizing the importance of multidisciplinary care and preventive approaches tailored to this vulnerable population.

Keywords

Menopause · Metabolic syndrome · Insulin resistance · Cardiovascular risk · MHT

S. N. Gudi (✉)
St. Philomenas Hospital & Consultant, Manipal Sagar and Excel Care Hospitals, Bengaluru, India

N. P. Tandon
Department of Obstetrics & Gynecology, Atal Bihari Vajpayee Institute of Medical Sciences & Dr. Ram Manohar Lohia Hospital, New Delhi, India

R. Malik et al. (eds.), *Menopause Essentials*,
https://doi.org/10.1007/978-981-95-7498-8_10

The Metabolic syndrome is a lifestyle disorder strongly linked to a sedentary lifestyle. It is associated with an increased risk of hypertension, heart disease, type 2 DM, cerebrovascular accidents, and endometrial cancer.

There have been several organizations like World Health Organization (WHO), the International Diabetes Federation(IDF), the National Cholesterol Education Program Adult Treatment Panel III (ATP III), the European Group for the Study of Insulin Resistance (EGSIR), and the American Association of Clinical Endocrinologist (AACE) that have established the criteria for the diagnosis of metabolic syndrome [1] (Table 10.1). The most commonly used are WHO and ATP III.

10.1 Risk Factors for Metabolic Syndrome at and Beyond Menopause

1. *Age*
   Age itself is an independent risk factor for metabolic syndrome. The risk of metabolic syndrome increases by 60% after menopause.
2. A history of diabetes or cardiovascular disease in the family can increase a woman's risk of metabolic syndrome.
3. *Lifestyle Factors*
   The metabolic syndrome results from factors like high caloric unhealthy diet, lack of physical activity, insomnia, poor quality sleep, and smoking.
4. *Central Obesity*
   Increased abdominal fat, particularly around the waist, is a hallmark of metabolic syndrome and is more common in postmenopausal women.
5. *Certain Medications*
   Second-generation antipsychotics, like clozapine and olanzapine, have been shown to have a higher risk of causing weight gain, increased blood sugar, and altered lipid levels, all of which are contributing factors to metabolic syndrome.
6. *Low Vitamin D Levels*
7. *Women with PCOS*- As PCOS women reach perimenopausal age they present as metabolic disorder. The spectrum of disorder includes insulin resistance, energy expenditure problems, type 2 DM, hypertension, obesity, dyslipidemia cardiovascular disease, and cancer.
8. *Other Factors*- nonalcoholic fatty liver disease, hyperuricemia, and obstructive sleep apnea have significant associations.

Clinicians should recognize that this condition encompasses a range of subtle endocrine and metabolic abnormalities that significantly increase the risk of cardiovascular disease, type 2 diabetes, obesity, and cancer.

Table 10.1 Criteria for diagnosis of Metabolic syndrome

Criteria	WHO (1998)	IDF (2005)	ATP III (2001, revised 2005)	EGIR (1999)	AACE (2003)
Central Obesity	Waist: Women->85 cm or BMI- 30 kg/m^2	Required. Waist: Ethnic-specific (e.g., Europid Women ≥80 cm)	Waist: Women >88 cm (optional, as any 3 of 5 risk factors suffice)	Waist ≥80 cm in women; BMI-30 kg/m^2 or just waist measurement	Not required; presence increases suspicion
Glucose Abnormality	Impaired Glucose Tolerance (FPG ≥110), Diabetes, or Insulin Resistance	Fasting Glucose ≥100 mg/dL 5.6 mmol/L) or diagnosed diabetes	Fasting Glucose ≥100 mg/dL 5.6 mmol/L) or on glucose- lowering meds	Fasting insulin above the 75th percentile for nondiabetic individuals. (FPG ≥110)	Impaired fasting glucose (FPG ≥110), impaired glucose tolerance, or diabetes
Blood Pressure	≥140/90 mmHg or on antihypertensives	≥130/85 mmHg or on antihypertensives	≥130/85 mmHg or on antihypertensives	≥140/90 mmHg or on antihypertensives	≥130/85 mmHg or on antihypertensives
Triglycerides	≥150 mg/dL	≥150 mg/dL	≥150 mg/dL	≥150 mg/dL	≥150 mg/dL
HDL Cholesterol	<39 mg/dL 1.0 mmol/L (women)	<50 mg/dL 1.29 mmol/L (women), or specific treatment	<50 mg/dL 1.29 mmol/L (women), or specific treatment	<39 mg/dL 1.0 mmol/L (men only, women excluded)	50 mg/dL (women), or on treatment
Insulin Resistance	Required	Not required	Not required	Required (estimated via fasting insulin)	Clinical judgment; considered core abnormality
Other Factors	Microalbuminuria Urinary albumin-to-creatinine ratio: 30 mg/g, or albumin excretion rate: 20 µg/min.	None	None	None	Other risk factors: PCOs, Family history, Sedentary lifestyle, age > 40 yrs
Diagnostic Threshold	Glucose abnormality plus 2 of: obesity, dyslipidemia, hypertension, microalbuminuria	Central obesity + any 2 of: raised TG, low HDL, raised BP, raised glucose	Any 3 of: abdominal obesity, raised TG, low HDL, raised BP, raised glucose	IR 2 of: central obesity, hypertension, high TG, low HDL	No minimum number; based on overall risk evaluation by the clinician

10.2 Prevalence and Epidemiology

The prevalence of metabolic syndrome increases with age and shows a higher incidence in peri and postmenopausal women.

An alarming fact that has emerged is that midlife women show a prevalence of metabolic syndrome up to 20–30%. It is commoner in women, with varying prevalence from 7% to 46% from various sources. An increased risk of metabolic syndrome in postmenopausal women is now well recognized, and we can rely on data from cross-sectional studies as a prevalence of 32.6–41.5% [2].

The risk of metabolic syndrome, its consequences, complications, and severity are higher in midlife women than in men. This is because of the menopause transition, the depletion of sex steroid hormones leads to a higher risk of disease in hormone-sensitive tissues like the bones, brain, and cardiovascular system. The onset of menopause occurs due to estrogen deficiency.

The following mechanisms have been considered for a higher risk of metabolic syndrome in midlife:

1. Estrogen plays a crucial but poorly understood role in regulating insulin sensitivity. That is why impaired glucose metabolism, after the decline in estrogen levels, results from increased insulin resistance, which can cause hyperglycemia. Also, estrogen deficiency induces changes in the body which include: abdominal obesity, insulin resistance hypertension, dyslipidemia (increased total cholesterol and triglycerides, decreased HDL, increased low-density lipoprotein, increased lipoprotein), decreased insulin secretion, decreased insulin elimination, impaired vascular function, increased factor VII and fibrinogen, reduced sex-hormone binding globulin and reduction in lean mass [3].
2. During menopause, abdominal fat tends to increase, serving as a key risk factor for metabolic syndrome. This fat acts as a metabolically and endocrinologically active tissue, releasing hormones and inflammatory mediators that promote insulin resistance, hypertension, and other elements of metabolic syndrome [4].
3. A decreased level of the hormone adiponectin, which is involved in regulating glucose and lipid metabolism, may also play a role in the development of metabolic syndrome.

The most important alert in postmenopausal women is the risk of cardiovascular disease which is higher if women have PCOS. There is also a higher incidence, a predisposition for arterial hypertension in women with PCOS even after adjusting for age and BMI, which is perhaps explained by IR and hyperandrogenism The impaired carbohydrate and lipid metabolism, chronic inflammation, (elevated levels of inflammatory markers), obesity, and the hypertensive state adds to the risk of cardiovascular disease.

10.3 PCOS and Menopausal Transition

Women with PCOS undergoing menopausal transition are at a higher risk of metabolic syndrome as compared to women without PCOS. The principal hormonal change at menopause transition is a dramatic fall in estrogen levels but a stable or even mild increase in androgen levels. The source of androgens is from both the ovary and adrenals in premenopausal women, as women approach menopause there is a decline in ovarian secretion of androgens whereas the adrenal source remains normal. In women with PCOS, however, the ovarian androgen secretion remains elevated till the late reproductive years and well into menopause and adds to the adrenal source which also remains pronounced well into menopause. This protracted hyperandrogenic state worsens the features of IR, visceral adiposity, chronic inflammation, and dyslipidemia, thereby increasing their life-long health risks in midlife [5]. The following clinical and biochemical parameters are different in women with PCOS attaining menopause as against menopausal women without PCOS:

1. Persistent hyperandrogenemia: There is a fall in androgen levels normally at menopause, but in women with PCOS the fall is less significant and levels remain above normal for some indefinite period. So, to quote a particular study, postmenopausal women with PCOS showed up with average serum testosterone levels of 47 ng/dL, androstenedione levels of 205 ng/dL, and DHEAS levels of 143 mcg/dL, while postmenopausal women without PCOS had corresponding serum levels of 37 ng/dL, 107 ng/dL, and 60.2 mcg/dL for testosterone, androstenedione, and DHEAS, respectively. The higher levels of androgens are associated with lower SHBG levels in women with PCOS at menopause. One interesting longitudinal cohort study of 30 years duration with 118 age-matched controls and 33 women with PCOS beginning at 50 years of age serum androgens to be higher in PCOS than controls until approximately age 70 years and declined to similar levels by a mean age of 81 years [6].
2. Diagnosis of Metabolic Disorders in Higher degree of IR: Women with PCOS, just before and even after menopause, express higher baseline insulin levels and higher insulin response to oral glucose tolerance test, representing increased Insulin resistance in this cohort. This was again demonstrated in increased Homeostatic Model Assessment for IR (HOMA-IR) in PCOS menopausal women as compared with controls with no PCOS.
3. A variation in age at menopause: On average a delay of 2–4 years has been observed in various studies. The reason is not exactly known but may be due to the originally higher number of follicles in the ovaries at birth or differentials in the rates of apoptosis and atresia in the follicles
4. Higher AMH levels: In contrast to younger women the higher AMH level co-relates well with Antral follicular count
5. Lower FSH levels at menopause: S-FSH levels <50 IU/L are common in women with PCOS.

10.4 Metabolic Syndrome (MS) in Menopausal Women with PCOS

There are some subtle differences in the MS manifestation in menopausal women with PCOS as compared to menopausal women without PCOS.

Dyslipidemia, Obesity, hyperinsulinemia, and an abnormal lipid profile a hallmarks of PCOS as already mentioned above: at menopause, there is further worsening of triglyceride levels (higher) and there is further lowering of HDL levels though LDL cholesterol levels will remain similar in derangement as earlier to menopause. This fact is indeed supported by other longitudinal studies showing worsening lipid profile (e.g., elevated triglycerides and reduced HDL concentrations) and increasing waist circumference, BMI >30, and HOMA, and higher incidence of type 2 DM in postmenopausal women with the syndrome [7].

The other manifestations will persist: as central obesity: Waist-to-hip ratio: >0.85, hypertension, microalbuminuria, higher C-reactive protein concentrations (CRP: reflecting chronic inflammatory status), greater insulin response to an OGTT compared with controls with higher insulin area under the curve

Cardiovascular and other vascular accidents: So far, there is no evidence of increased risk of CVD-related morbidity and mortality in menopausal women with PCOS. Further studies are needed to establish and determine whether the increased cardiovascular risk in reproductive life persists in later life for women with PCOS. However, one notable exception is a subgroup where PCOS women maintain hyperandrogenemia after menopause, i.e., when MS persists it is almost always with a higher incidence of CVD. Therefore, longitudinal cohort study data show more common hypertension and hypertriglyceridemia in the PCOS group, myocardial infarction, stroke, diabetes, cancer, and mortality prevalence was similar in the two cohorts with similar BMI.

Symptoms of menopausal transition: Though the BMI, WHR, and incidence of endocrinopathies like Type 2 Diabetes and hypothyroidism remain similar to controls, the following differences in the symptomatology of menopausal transition have been found in women with PCOS as compared to controls:

1. The episodes of vasovagal symptoms (hot flushes and sweating) are less frequent than in control women due to the persisting hyperandrogenism, and secondary to the related beneficial effects on libido, sense of well-being, and positive mood.
2. A higher reporting of vaginal dryness and related dyspareunia and genitourinary symptoms, again secondary to more frequent sexual experiences (higher libido, FAI).
3. A major concern is the persisting well beyond the FMP, the cosmetic challenge of hirsutism and alopecia, and even baldness due to long-lasting elevated androgen levels, during the transition. This unfortunate situation impacts the woman's body image and self-esteem at a very critical phase of life. It needs dermatological and esthetic interventions and is seen when PCOS is poorly managed during the transition.

10.5 Menopausal Women

History and Physical Examination Women are considered postmenopausal after a 12 consecutive month absence of menses. History of weight gain, particularly redistribution of body fat, accumulation of visceral fat, increase in waist circumference, and changes in body shape in perimenopausal women and menopausal women is important. Abdominal obesity increases IR, and, consequently, the risk of diabetes and MS.

Information that could be found through physical examination includes

- Body Mass Index: Weight (kg)/square of height (m)
- Waist Hip Ratio: WC (cm)/hip (cm)
- Waist Circumference—measurement be made at the approximate midpoint between the lower margin of the last palpable rib and the top of the iliac crest. The woman stands with arms at the sides, feet positioned close together, and weight evenly distributed across the feet.
- Blood pressure -the diagnostic criteria are considered to be met if 130–140 mmHg or more for systolic, 85–90 mmHg or more for diastolic, or if the patients are taking antihypertensive drugs

10.5.1 Investigations

- *Fasting Blood Glucose*: it is a key component of the metabolic syndrome diagnosis.
- *Lipid Profile*: Assessment of Total cholesterol, LDL cholesterol, HDL cholesterol, and triglycerides is done to evaluate dyslipidemia.
- *Hormone Levels*: Estrogen plays a role in lipid metabolism and glucose tolerance. Understanding estrogen levels can help evaluate the impact of menopause on metabolic health. It has no role in the diagnosis.
- *Other Tests*: May include a complete blood count (CBC), thyroid function tests, and serum creatinine, depending on individual needs and risk factors.
- *Markers of metabolic syndrome*: Metabolic syndrome is undoubtedly a pro-inflammatory, prothrombotic state, and elevated levels of inflammatory markers: C-reactive protein (CRP), interleukin (IL)-6, and plasminogen activator inhibitor (PAI)-1 when found may indicate a risk for subsequent CVD and type 2 diabetes, but a causal association is yet to be established and the tests for markers continues to have optional status.
- Imaging

  (a) Transvaginal ultrasound (TVS) in women with metabolic syndrome: especially for women with features of hyperandrogenism,

  Ovaries may show multiple cysts, persist for a few months/years, and avascular inclusion cysts mistaken for follicles with a confusing picture of PCOS.

Ovarian tumors secreting Androgens: Sertoli—Leydig cell tumors and Leydig cell tumors.

(b) Rarely CT or MRI for the Adrenal gland to exclude androgen-secreting adrenal tumors (adenoma or carcinoma) is needed.

Management of Metabolic Syndrome in menopausal women: The focus is mainly on preventive measures, after a thorough risk assessment and evaluation of existing disease burden and planning for the ideal therapeutic approach to these problems.

Aims of management

1. Addressing the underlying drivers of metabolic syndrome such as obesity, physical inactivity, diet, and nutrition through LSM(Lifestyle modification).
2. Optimal therapy for dyslipidemia, hypertension, DM, and cardiovascular problems.
3. Prevention of cancer and osteoporosis and Menopause hormone therapy as dictated by the situation.

Lifestyle modification Intensive lifestyle interventions have been shown to significantly improve key markers of metabolic syndrome, including waist-hip ratio, triglyceride levels, HDL cholesterol, blood glucose control, blood pressure regulation, and insulin sensitivity—ultimately lowering the risk of cardiovascular events. A network meta-analysis of randomized clinical trials found that lifestyle changes were more effective in resolving metabolic syndrome than standard care. Notably, controlling hypertension emerged as the most impactful factor in reducing cardiovascular risk. Additionally, lifestyle modifications have been proven to lower the risk of developing type 2 diabetes in women with metabolic syndrome, with these benefits lasting for up to 15 years.

The following lifestyle modifications LSM should be recommended:

1. *Weight reduction*: Weight reduction, is the mainstay of lifestyle modification as it has a direct impact on insulin sensitivity.

Optimally achieved with a multimodality approach that includes diet, exercise, and, for selected patients, pharmacologic therapy, or surgical intervention.

1. *Increased physical activity*: Regular exercise is highly recommended for MS Exercise along with dietary changes will augment weight loss and help in maintaining the achieved weight, especially by reducing the abdominal fat.
   A. Women should be encouraged to adopt a sustainable exercise routine, including 30 minutes of moderate-intensity brisk walking daily, complemented by aerobic activities, yoga, and resistance training. Evidence supports the inclusion of resistance training for its positive impact on metabolic parameters

such as body weight, waist-hip ratio, glycemic control, triglyceride levels, and the prevention of cardiovascular events.

There are situations of osteoarthritis, chronic knee joint pain, peripheral neuropathies, previous fragility fractures and osteoporosis, cardiac disease with poor effort tolerance, etc. which limit the activity. In such cases encourage any activity level within their physical limitation and effort tolerance.

1. When intensive LSM cannot be sustained and weight loss is not achieved to beget risk reduction for CVD and stroke, then pharmacotherapy for weight loss or bariatric surgery can be considered.
2. *Diet planning* and modification with restricted fats, carbohydrates, and salt. The following diet plans have shown benefits in markers of MS: weight reduction, lipid profile, glycemic control, lowered BP, inflammatory markers, and endothelial dysfunction. The type of diet advised must be matched to the socio-economic constraints and cultural norms of the patient's immediate family.
3. Mediterranean diet (high in fruits, vegetables, nuts, whole grains, and olive oil)
4. Low-fat diet for weight reduction associated with reductions in all-cause mortality
5. The Dietary Approaches to Stop Hypertension (DASH) diet (daily sodium intake limited to 2400 mg and higher dairy intake)
6. Low glycemic index diet: replacing refined grains with whole grains, fruits, and vegetables, may be particularly beneficial for patients with metabolic syndrome.
7. A high-fiber diet (≥30 g/day)—can have equivalent results to the use of more complex diets for e.g. as recommended by AHA with fruits, vegetables, whole grain, high fiber, lean animal and vegetable proteins.
8. Intermittent fasting: An eight-hour time-restricted eating schedule can reduce all components of metabolic syndrome [8].

4. Smoking cessation.
5. Avoid excess alcohol intake.
6. Cultivating a new intellectual engagement as a new hobby or a career change.
7. Managing restful sleep of 8 hours is preferable to a continuous stretch.

Management of independent modifiable cardiovascular risk factors to lower all-cause mortality:

1. Aggressive treatment of hypertension, Patients with metabolic syndrome benefit from a lower blood pressure target than the general population. The choice of the drug must be in collaboration with the physician in charge for all her medical comorbidities and Calcium channel blockers, ACE inhibitors, and ARB agents. Thiazide diuretics are less suitable as they affect glycemic control and lipid profile.

2. Prevention of type 2 diabetes, Patients who have persistent insulin resistance despite attempts at lifestyle changes may benefit from Metformin and other pharmacotherapy.
3. Lowering of serum cholesterol and hypertriglyceridemia: All women with MS must have an assessment for future ASCVD (atherosclerotic cardiovascular disease) and evidence-based doses of moderate-to-high intensity statins must be initiated

MHT: Menopause hormone therapy Current evidence does not support hormone therapy (HT) as a standalone preventive strategy for metabolic syndrome during menopause, as no treatment has proven more effective than lifestyle modification. However, careful individualization may guide the use of menopausal hormone therapy (MHT), particularly transdermal estrogen, to help prevent chronic diseases after menopause. In well-selected patients, MHT has the potential to improve metabolic syndrome parameters and reduce all-cause mortality.

Women with MS with hyperlipidemia Most women with PCOS and MS have dyslipidemia. In general, MHT in women with dyslipidemia will lower total cholesterol and LDL has the desirable effect of increasing HDL but also slightly increasing the triglycerides. This effect favorably compares with statins, as statins do not show any benefit on HDL, with almost equivalent effect on total cholesterol, LDL, and triglycerides. A combination therapy of MHT and statins must be carefully planned for the best outcomes.

Women with MS with coronary heart disease (CHD) Statins should be the first choice for lipid-lowering therapy as MHT has no role in secondary prevention. This is known now as evident from the lack of cardiovascular protection noted in the Women's Health Initiative (WHI) and Heart and Estrogen/Progestin Replacement Study (HERS) trials. In women with intact uterus, it is mandatory to add progesterone, (to diminish the risk of endometrial hyperplasia cancer). Though some of the beneficial lipid effects of estrogen are attenuated by the addition of progesterone, the net effect of oral estrogen plus progesterone on serum HDL cholesterol is still beneficial.

This issue about which progesterone is good for women with MS was best addressed in the Postmenopausal Estrogen/Progestin Interventions (PEPI) trial, an RCT of 875 women allocated to placebo or one of the four treatment arms: conjugated estrogen (0.625 mg/day) alone, CE with MPA continuous, CE with MPA cyclic, and CE with cyclic micronized progesterone (200 mg/day for 12 days per month). The trial revealed micronized progesterone as the lipid-friendly option with the most favorable effect on serum HDL rise and fall of plasma Lipoprotein a. The regime can be continuous or cyclic combined, and the effects were equivalent to the two regimens. Oral estrogen therapy with or without progestin can potentially raise triglyceride concentrations by about 25%, although transdermal estrogen preparations do not raise triglyceride concentrations [9].

Women with MS and hypertension In women with well-controlled hypertension, MHT can still be used as evinced in the PEPI trial which found that estrogen, with or without progestin, did not affect blood pressure. A transdermal route for estrogen is preferred.

Women with MS with high BMI In women with PCOS/MS at menopause who are obese, MHT can be prescribed for standard indications, provided efforts to lose weight with lifestyle modification are continuously in place. In a prospective cohort study of 651 women followed up for 15 years: the Rancho Bernardo cohort: found that estrogen therapy had no effect on absolute body weight, and it also has a neutral or favorable effect on body fat distribution, favoring the pear-shaped rather than the apple-shaped visceral adiposity.

Women with MS and Diabetes Mellitus Both the landmark studies HERS and WHI concluded that combined HT appears to reduce the risk of type 2 diabetes mellitus, possibly mediated by a decrease in insulin resistance. However, the effect is not strong enough to recommend HT as a diabetes prevention strategy in women with CHD. In the group most likely to take HT, 50–59 years, a 5-year study period revealed 11 fewer cases per 1000 women. (for both estrogen–progestin and estrogen alone) [10].

Considering all the evidence together, when women with PCOS and the varying manifestations of MS are nearing or attain menopause, they will benefit from MHT for the standard indications, with the added benefit of primary prevention of cardiovascular disease and an improved lipid profile and also better musculoskeletal health which is so essential for the critical lifestyle interventions and the exercise schedule mandatory for menopausal care. Though transdermal or oral estradiol both are effective equally in women with hypertriglyceridemia, the transdermal route is preferred.

Menopausal women with MS with established cardiovascular disease The menopausal women with MS and established cardiovascular disease will not benefit from MHT, in other words, MHT has no role in the secondary prevention of myocardial infarction, stroke, or heart failure. In this cohort for relief of vasomotor symptoms, nonhormonal therapy is advised. Some of such interventions are:

1. CBT(Cognitive-behavioral therapy),
2. Drugs like SSRI (selective serotonin reuptake inhibitors), SNRI (serotonin-norepinephrine reuptake inhibitors), gabapentin, fezolinetant (Level I); oxybutynin (Levels I-II);
3. Weight loss,
4. Stellate ganglion block (Levels II-III)

10.6 Conclusion

With increasing female longevity, an aging population, and declining lifestyle habits metabolic syndrome will inevitably pose a significant burden on our healthcare system.

Metabolic syndrome is highly prevalent among postmenopausal women due to hormonal changes that influence fat distribution, insulin sensitivity, and lipid metabolism. This condition significantly increases the risk of cardiovascular disease and type 2 diabetes in this population. Metabolic syndrome in menopause is a lifestyle disorder and is a preventable entity. Early identification and lifestyle modifications are crucial for prevention and management. Hormone replacement therapy may offer benefits but must be carefully considered on an individual basis. Overall, a multidisciplinary approach is essential for improving long-term outcomes.

Key Points

- Menopause increases the risk of metabolic syndrome due to hormonal changes, especially estrogen decline.
- Metabolic syndrome includes central obesity, hypertension, insulin resistance, and dyslipidemia.
- Postmenopausal women show a higher prevalence of metabolic syndrome compared to premenopausal women.
- Early screening and diagnosis using waist circumference, lipid profile, glucose, and BP are essential.
- Lifestyle changes and targeted therapy can effectively manage and prevent metabolic syndrome in menopausal women.

Long Answer Questions (LAQs)

1. Define Metabolic Syndrome. What are the risk factors for Metabolic Syndrome at and beyond menopause?
2. Discuss the Management of Metabolic Syndrome in menopausal women
3. Discuss the long-term metabolic and cardiovascular implications of Polycystic Ovary Syndrome (PCOS) in women transitioning to menopause.

Short Answer Questions (SAQs)

1. List diagnostic criteria for metabolic syndrome in women according to WHO.
2. Mention two benefits and two risks of using hormone replacement therapy (HRT) in postmenopausal women with metabolic syndrome.

Mutiple Choice Questions (MCQs)

1. Which of the following is NOT a component of metabolic syndrome as per ATP III criteria?
   - A. Elevated waist circumference
   - B. Elevated triglycerides
   - C. Low HDL cholesterol
   - D. Elevated TSH
2. At menopause, which of the following factors increases the risk of metabolic syndrome?
   - A. Estrogen deficiency
   - B. Increased progesterone levels
   - C. Decreased insulin levels
   - D. Decreased LDL cholesterol
3. The most common change in lipid profile in postmenopausal women is:
   - A. Increased HDL
   - B. Decreased triglycerides
   - C. Increased LDL
   - D. Decreased total cholesterol
4. Which of the following Waist-to-hip ratio is used in Indian women for diagnosing central obesity (a component of metabolic syndrome)?
   - A. >0.88
   - B. >0.80
   - C. >0.90
   - D. >0.85
5. Metabolic syndrome increases the risk of which major health condition in postmenopausal women?
   - A. Osteoporosis
   - B. Dementia
   - C. Cardiovascular disease
   - D. Endometriosis
6. Which hormone's decline at menopause plays a central role in the development of insulin resistance and abdominal obesity?
   - A. Progesterone
   - B. Estrogen
   - C. FSH
   - D. Cortisol

7. The diagnostic criteria for metabolic syndrome include all EXCEPT:
   A. Fasting glucose ≥100 mg/dL
   B. Triglycerides ≥150 mg/dL
   C. HDL ≥60 mg/dL
   D. Blood pressure ≥130/85 mmHg

   (Note: Low HDL < 50 mg/dL in women is a risk factor, so ≥ 60 is not a diagnostic criterion.)
8. What is the preferred initial management of metabolic syndrome in postmenopausal women?
   A. Hormone replacement therapy (HRT)
   B. Bariatric surgery
   C. Lifestyle modification
   D. Statin therapy
9. Hormone Replacement Therapy (HRT) in metabolic syndrome:
   A. Is universally recommended
   B. Has no effect on metabolic parameters
   C. May improve insulin sensitivity in some women
   D. Worsens lipid profile
10. Which of the following is NOT a modifiable risk factor for metabolic syndrome in menopausal women?
   A. Smoking
   B. Physical inactivity
   C. Age
   D. Diet

Answers

1. D
2. A
3. C
4. D
5. C
6. B
7. C
8. C
9. C
10. C

References

1. Tsai SS, Chu YY, Chen ST, et al. A comparison of different definations of metabolic syndrome for risk of atherosclerosis nd diabetes. Diabetol Metab Syndr. 2018;10:56.
2. Chedraui P, Hidalgo L, Chavez D, Morocho N, Alvarado M, Huc A, et al. Quality of life among postmenopausal ecuadorian women participating in a metabolic syndrome screening program. Maturitas. 2007;56:45–53.
3. Lobo RA. Metabolic syndrome after menopause and the role of hormones. Maturitas. 2008;60:10–8.
4. Bermingham KM, Linenberg I, Hall WL, Kadé K, Franks PW, Davies R, Wolf J, Hadjigeorgiou G, Asnicar F, Segata N, et al. Menopause is associated with postprandial metabolism, metabolic health and lifestyle: the ZOE PREDICT study. EBioMedicine. 2022;85:104303.
5. Millán-de-Meer M, Luque-Ramírez M, Nattero-Chávez L, Escobar-Morreale HF. PCOS during the menopausal transition and after menopause: a systematic review and meta-analysis. Hum Reprod Update. 2023;29(6):741–72.
6. Markopoulos MC, Rizos D, Valsamakis G, Deligeoroglou E, Grigoriou O, Chrousos GP, Creatsas G, Mastorakos G. Hyperandrogenism in women with polycystic ovary syndrome persists after menopause. J Clin Endocrinol Metab. 2011;96(3):623–31.
7. Sánchez-Ferrer ML, Arense-Gonzalo JJ, Prieto-Sánchez MT, Gómez-Carrascosa I, Hernández-Peñalver AI, Mendiola J, Torres-Cantero AM. Anthropometric characteristics of polycystic ovary syndrome and their associations with insulin resistance and lipid profile. Appl Sci. 2021;11(12):5395.
8. He M, Wang J, Liang Q, et al. Time-restricted eating with or without low-carbohydrate diet reduces visceral fat and improves metabolic syndrome: a randomized trial. Cell Rep Med. 2022;3:100777.
9. Bontempo S, Yeganeh L, Giri R, Vincent AJ. Use of MHT in women with cardiovascular disease: a systematic review and meta-analysis. Climacteric. 2023;27(1):93–103. https://doi.org/10.1080/13697137.2023.2273524.
10. Santen RJ, Allred DC, Ardoin SP, et al. Postmenopausal hormone therapy: an Endocrine Society scientific statement. J Clin Endocrinol Metab. 2010;95:s1.

Cardiovascular Risks and Events at Menopause

11

Rajat Mohan

Abstract

Cardiovascular diseases (CVD) is an important cause of mortality in women. The cardiovascular events occur approximately 10 years earlier than men. Premenopausal women have a lower incidence of coronary artery disease (CAD) then men due to protection given by estrogens. Changes in body fat distribution, lipid profile, impaired glucose tolerance, hypertension, and increased inflammatory markers start from menopause transition (MT) are linked with estrogen deficiency. These cause endothelial dysfunction causing higher CVD risks. This causes nonobstructive coronary artery disease in women. There is increase in Total cholesterol (TC) levels, Low density lipoproteins (LDL-C), and decreased High density lipoproteins (HDL) during menopause transition. Hypertension, Impaired glucose tolerance, increases over menopause stages and are risk factors for CVD. Oral or Transdermal MHT does not increase the risk of heart disease if given within 10 years of menopause or before the age of 60 years in low risk women for CVD. MHT can alleviate the majority of CVD risk factors to varying degrees, including visceral obesity, dyslipidemia, and glucose homeostasis. MHT is not recommended for the primary prevention of cardiac diseases. WHO ISH risk prediction charts, Framingham's risk score calculator, PREVENT: Predicting Risk of Cardiovascular Disease events's are various scores to assess cardiovascular risks. Lifestyle management, exercise, adequate sleep, healthy diet, and managing stress are important. Visceral adiposity, Diabetes, Hypertension Dyslipidemias should be addressed early and prevention should be the aim.

R. Mohan (✉)
Department of Cardiology, Sir Ganga Ram Hospital, New Delhi, Delhi, India

R. Malik et al. (eds.), *Menopause Essentials*,
https://doi.org/10.1007/978-981-95-7498-8_11

Keywords

Cardiovascular disease risk · Dyslipidemias in menopause · CVD risk scores · Framingham · PREVENT

11.1 Introduction

Cardiovascular diseases (CVD) are one of the most common Noncommunicable diseases (NCD) in India. They are the leading cause of death worldwide and in India. As per WHO NCD were the cause of 63% of all fatalities in 2016 and 27% of these were due to CVD in India [1–3].

With rising global aging population, it is important to address cardiovascular diseases and their risks in women as they are leading cause of mortality in women. The cardiovascular events occur approximately a decade later than the age at which highest incidence is seen in men.

Estrogens protective effect in premenopausal women cause a lower incidence of CVD than men.

Menopause is defined retrospectively when women has cessation of menstrual cycles for a duration of 1 year with loss of ovarian function and follicles with no other pathology associated with it. In the western countries average age is 52 years whereas as per Indian Menopause Society data it is 46–47 years for Indian women.

There are changes in body fat distribution, lipid profile, impaired glucose tolerance, hypertension and increased inflammatory markers which start occurring from menopause transition (MT) and are linked with estrogen deficiency also. Estrogen deficiency evoked endothelial dysfunction in postmenopausal women causes higher cardiovascular morbidity and mortality.

The SWAN study showed that when observed longitudinally Low density lipoproteins which are not good fats increased in women over MT and menopause as compared to premenopause [4]. These changes in metabolic profile are the cause of rise in CAD postmenopause as compared to younger women.

11.2 Epidemiology

Cardiovascular diseases comprises of various types of heart diseases like coronary heart disease, vascular diseases, arterial and deep venous thrombosis etc. These are leading cause of mortality and morbidity in men and women in developed countries. Increased prevalence of coronary artery disease in men have a correlation with low estrogen levels. Atherosclerotic heart disease are most common cause of myocardial ischemia.

CVD contributed to 25% of total deaths in India. In Asians, the incidence of CVD is average 10 years earlier as to other countries.

In this chapter, we address these changes which occur at menopause transition and menopause. Routine screening for women is important and counseling should be done so that those at high risk for CVD may take preventive measures and appropriate treatment in time.

Modifiable risk factors Half the cardiovascular deaths in India occur young in less than 70 years of age.

The modifiable risk factors for CVD like overweight, visceral fat, hypertension, diabetes mellitus and deranged lipid profile, high Homocysteine levels, low HDL (High Density Lipoprotein) cholesterol, lower apolipoprotein level, and low physical activities are on the rise. They are seen more in urban areas as compared to rural areas.

Low socioeconomic and poor nutrition are also factors contributing to higher CVD risks

11.3 Pathophysiology

11.3.1 Changes at Menopause Transition and Menopause

11.3.1.1 Blood Vessels and Endothelial Function

Estrogen has anti-inflammatory and antioxidant action. It releases Nitrous oxide at the endothelium of the blood vessels. This causes vasodilatation. Fall in levels of estrogens as in MT cause oxidative stress. Increase in levels of Endothelin 1which is a vasoconstrictor and inflammatory marker is also seen with decreasing estrogens levels [5]. Nitric oxide causes inhibition of smooth muscle propagation. This provides cardioprotection. Oxidative stress enhances vasomotor symptoms like hot flashes and night sweats at menopause [6].

Aging in both men and women causes increasing stiffness of arterial walls. There is a decreased dilatation of the vessels. This increases systolic blood pressure. Though these changes occur with age they happen rapidly at MT and postmenopause in women and increase the cardiovascular disease risks.

By decreasing oxidative stress and enhancing vasodilatation estrogens are neuroprotective also.

In women endothelial dysfunction may cause nonobstructive coronary artery disease as compared to obstructive disease.

Coronary endothelial dysfunction may be measured by cardiac magnetic resonance imaging. In this cross-sectional area of coronary arteries and blood flow through them is measured in response to exercise like hand grip [7].

11.3.1.2 Changes in Lipid Profile

Adverse changes in lipids occur around final menstrual period and in menopausal transition. Endothelial dysfunction is reflected by deranged lipid profile and increases risk of atherosclerotic heart disease. There is increase in (HDL). Serum

Cholesterol and Low density lipoproteins values increase and High density lipoproteins levels decrease.

Lipoprotein (a) (Lp (a)) levels also increase around menopause. Its particles penetrate the endothelium and cause increased chances of atherosclerotic changes in the vessels increasing the cardiovascular risks [8]. These changes in lipid profiles are different from the changes seen prospectively with aging. Increased levels of Serum FSH are seen with elevated levels of cholesterol and LDL-C levels. When menopausal hormone therapy (MHT) is given levels of FSH decrease. With this decrease improvement in lipid levels is seen [9].

Other markers

Homocysteine: It is an essential amino acid. Increased levels are independent risk factor for CVD and its levels increase with age, menopause, smoking, folic acid, and Vit B12 deficiency. Raised inflammatory markers like C Reactive proteins are associated with increased risk of Cardiovascular diseases.

11.3.1.3 Diabetes

Diabetes is a strong risk factor for CVD, doubling the risk. It also increases the risk of stroke.

With menopause, impaired glucose tolerance is seen. Increased incidence of type II Diabetes mellitus is also seen. Hyperglycemia is a risk factor for cardiovascular disease. It is generally associated with altered lipid profiles and obesity. Menopausal hormonal therapy improves sugar levels and lipid profiles. Hormone therapy improves glucose levels due to increased lipid oxidation. Central obesity also shows improvement [10].

11.3.1.4 Metabolic Syndrome

Increase in BMI, Central adiposity, deranged lipid profile is seen at menopause. Metabolic syndrome is a group of conditions associated with increased waist circumference (>80 cms), indicating visceral adiposity, high blood pressure (higher or equal to 130/85), increased fasting blood glucose levels, low levels of HDL Cholesterol, and increased Triglycerides. It signifies changes in metabolism which is unhealthy and its presence is an increased risk for cardiovascular disease.

Metabolic syndrome is seen almost 2–3 times in postmenopausal women as compared to premenopausal women. HDL decreases and Triglycerides increase by about 10–15%. Knowledge of this guides to incorporate healthy life style and take preventive measures [11, 12].

11.3.1.5 Age at Menopause

Women who have a early menopause have a higher risk of suffering a cardiovascular event as compared to those who attain menopause at 50–51 years of age because of early decline in estrogen levels. They usually suffer a nonfatal cardiac event before 60 years of age. Age at menopause may be an important marker to predict cardiovascular disease. A study with 301,438 women demonstrated that premature menopause was associated with a significantly higher risk of CVD compared to those women with normal age of menopause. It showed that CVD events were related to the age of onset of menopause [13].

11.3.1.6 Hypertension

Hypertension is seen less in younger women. As compared to premenopause hypertension is twice more prevalent in postmenopause. Endothelial dysfunction is seen with borderline hypertension and moderate hypertension aslo. This dysfunction is seen more in women as compared to men with similar hypertensive range [14].

Asystemic analysis and metanalysis revealed that higher risk of arterial hypertension is seen in women with early menopause (<45 years) as compared to those with menopause after 45 years [15]. This happens probably due to declining estrogen levels which increase production of endothelin and angiotensinogen which are vasoconstrictors. The androgen levels also increase [16].

Persistent hypertension leads to enhanced cardiovascular risks. The ideal targeted blood pressure should be below 120/80 mm of Hg. Therapeautic life style management should be counseled. Healthy weight as per population specific guidelines should be aimed. Excerise, meditation, high fiber diet with less fat and salt should be emphasized. Drugs should be prescribed if Blood pressure is higher or equal to 140/90 and if target organ damage is there then at 130/80 mmHg.

11.4 Hormone Therapy and Cardiovascular Risks

Menopausal Hormone therapy (MHT) is indicated for moderate-to-severe vasomotor flushes and night sweats. The other indications are prevention of osteoporosis, genitourinary syndrome of menopause, and premature ovarian insufficiency.

MHT is not indicated for primary prevention of cardiovascular disease and prevention of memory loss.

During the reproductive years, estrogen has a protective effect on lipid metabolism and vascular endothelium. The protective effect on the cardiovascular system is due to the promotion of angiogenesis and vasodilatation. Oxidative stress is decreased, and mitochondrial function is enhanced. Vasomotor symptoms are associated with symptoms like anxiety, palpitations, sleep disturbances, and poor quality of life. These symptoms have an overlap with presentation of a cardiovascular disease. Therefore it is important that patient should be fully evaluated to rule out cardiovascular disease [17].

MHT comprises of only estrogen (Estrogen Therapy ET) in women who do not have uterus. In women with uterus both estrogens and progesterone (EPT) should be given. Progesterone is to be given for endometrial protection to prevent endometrial hyperplasia and neoplasia. Progesterones should be in adequate dose and duration when supplemented along with estrogens for endometrial protection. 52 mg Levonorgestrel intrauterine system, dydrogesterone may be used for this.

Menopause hormone therapy should be individualized. Lowest dose of hormones for relief of symptoms should be used for least period of time needed. MHT should be prescribed after evaluating the comorbidities which will help in deciding the need, route and dose. The therapy should be individualised.

Vasomotor symptoms call for hormone therapy. Careful assessment of individual risk and benefits should be done the risk of venous thromboembolism is related to the dose therefore. Lowest doses shoudl be used as they decrease the risk of venous thromboembolism (VTE) [18].

For relief of vasomotor symptoms with hormone therapy it may take a time of 6-8 weeks. various available estrogens for use are oral conjugate equine estrogen (CEE) 0.3 mg, 17 beta estradiol 0.5mg and estradiol gel.

MHT whether oral or transdermal is safe if given to women with low risk for CVD within 10 years of menopause or before 60 years of age. Lower doses of hormones when used early that is less than 60 years of age have been shown to be cardioprotective. However they cannot be used only for this use. Progression of the thickness of the carotid media intima layer of carotid artery may be delayed by use of MHT. This increase in thickness causes atherosclerosis and coronary calcification [19].

The risk of thromboembolism and stroke is increased by a dose-dependent increase and not by the type of formulation of the hormone therapy. This applies to both Oral and Transdermal MHT [20].

MHT can improve many cardiovascular disease risk factors. Improvement in metabolic changes like visceral fat, lipid changes and impaired glucose tolerance is seen. Fall in levels of Total cholesterol, low density lipoproteins is seen along with increase in levels of beneficial high density lipoprotein cholesterol [21].

There are two types of receptors where Estrogens act. The classical receptors are nuclear (ERα and ERβ). The other is novel cell surface membrane receptors (GPR30 and ER-X) [22].

The action of estrogens is through different receptors at various tissues. These various actions bring out different effects at different organs. Estrogens in brain act through the membrane receptors both on cell surface and nuclear receptors and are neuroprotective. However, the action of estrogens on reproductive system such as in puberty, fertility, estrous cycle are mainly through nuclear receptors [22].

11.5 Anti-Müllerian Hormone (AMH)

AMH levels are recently been used as biomarkers for reproductive aging. Ultrasensitive AMH levels along with age may help in predicting the onset of menopause. They can help to assess when a woman is going to undergo final menstrual period that is menopause. It may be better than FSH levels as a predictor of Final Menstrual period [23].

Cardiovascular Changes and Risks at Menopause		
Cardiovascular Parameter	At MT and later	outcome
LDL cholesterol	Increases	increases atherosclerotic cardiovascular disease risk
HDL cholesterol	Decreases	↑ CVD risk
Triglycerides	Increases	↑ Cardiometabolic risk
Blood pressure	Increases	↑ Hypertension, and stroke risk with other end organ damages
Insulin resistance	Increases	impaired glucose tolerance, metabolic syndrome, and increased CVD risk
Weight/Fat distribution	Central (abdominal) obesity females WC greater than or equal to 80cm	↑ Metabolicrisk, impaired glucose tolerance and increased inflammatory markers, causing increased CVD risk
Endothelial function	Impaired	↑ Vascular aging, atherosclerosis
Plaque progression	Accelerated	increased ischaemic heart disease and stroke

11.6 Assessment by Clinician/Gynecologist/ Menopause Specialist

1. Detailed socio demographic history including age, education, socioeconomic strata. Residence urban/rural should be documented.
2. Gynecological details, age at menarche, menopause,
3. History of Gestational diabetes mellitus, Gestational hypertension, preeclampsia, PCOS, smoking, exercise, dietary history should be taken.
4. Personal and family history of NCD, malignancies should be elicited.
5. Detailed physical, systemic, and gynecological examination should be done.

11.7 Assessment of Cardiovascular Risks

1. *WHO/ISH cardiovascular risk prediction charts.*

   WHO updated the CVD risk charts in 2019. Risk-prediction charts have been provided for different ethnic-geographic regions. Two variants are available. One which uses total cholesterol (TC) and blood sugar values and the other without the laboratory investigations. It is externally validated in numerous studies Risk distribution assessed in datasets representing 79 countries.

2019 WHO CVD risk charts

- Age range which is studied in WHO risk prediction charts: 40–80 yrs
- If total cholestrol values and blood sugar values are there, then use charts catering to: Age, sex, smoking, Systolic blood pressure (SBP), TC, DM
- If investigations are not there then use charts with Age, sex, SBP, smoking, BMI

- These charts give us a 10-yr risk of fatal and nonfatal CVD (CHD or stroke)

Management of Total CVD risk: WHO Package of essential noncommunicable (PEN) disease interventions for primary health care (WHO PEN protocol)

This protocol guides to various management options as per the risk calculated.
Risk (<10%)
Nutritional and diet counseling
Encourage physical activity
Counsel to stop smoking
Stop excessive use of alcohol
Risk 10% to <20%
Counsel as above
If hypertension is there with persistent Blood Pressure (BP ≥140/90 mmHg) consider antihypertensive drugs.
3–6 monthly follow up should be done.
Risk >20%
Life style management as above.
However, antihypertensives to be given at levels of Persistent BP ≥130/80
Statins should be given for lipid lowering
Follow up should be earlier at 3 months

If the patient does not improve or cardiovascular disease risks persists then referral should be done to the next level.

Practical Tips
Patient with known cardiovascular disease, renal disease, and Diabetes mellitus the risk is >20% if:

If there is left ventricular hypertrophy, retinopathy, or albuminuria signifying end organ involvement
If BP is raised persistently ≥160/100 mmHg
If cholesterol levels are equal to or more than 320 mg/Dl these women should be referred to a specialist for further assessment and management.

Follow up
Enquire about any complaints or new problems.
Ask for lifestyle management adherence.
Whether drugs have been taken regularly.
Do a detailed physical examination
Assess CVD risks
Refer if needed.

2. Framingham risk score: This has been one of the most widely used risk assessment score following the Framingham study.

   It can also be used for the 10 year risk assessment for CVD in asymptomatic women without CVD or Diabetes. It is widely used. Major risk factors for CVD are cigarette smoking, hypertension (Blood pressure 140/90 mm Hg or on anti-hypertensive medication), high LDL > 100 mg/dl, low HDL cholesterol < 50 mg/dl, family history of premature CHD. Followed by this 10 year risk is calculated. According the scores further preventive management should be started.

ASCVD (Atherosclerotic cardiovascular disease) risk calculator: (American college of cardiology)
It calculates 10 year risk for atherosclerotic disease and helps to decide for statin therapy.

The ASCVD risk calcualtor is used for women without any history of atherosclerotic heart disease in the past.

Risk is divided as follows:

Low risk <5%
Border line risk (5–7.4%)
Intermediate risk(7.5–19.9%)
High risk (>20%)

Ten year risk is calculated for patients between age 40 and 79 years and lifetime risk is for age 20–59 years.

Additional questions for 40–79 years takes to advice tabs.

3. SCORE 2

   This predicts 10 year CVD risk in patients without prior CVD or Diabetes.
4. PREVENT: Predicting Risk of Cardiovascular Disease EVENTs

   Predicts 10- and 30-year risk of CVD and CVD subtypes in patients aged 30–79 without known CVD.

11.8 Management and Treatment

11.8.1 Lifestyle Management

Woman should be asked to stop Smoking.

Exercise: 30 min/day five times a week moderated intensity exercise. This should include strength and resistance training

Diet and nutrition: High fiber, fresh fruits, nuts, and seeds with high protein diet should be consumed with recommended calorie intake. Locally available food items should be counselled

Targeted ideal weight for the age should be counseled.
Management of stress and depression.

Targets
Adequate sleep. 7–8 h of sleep per day.
Optimal lipid targets
Total cholesterol <160 mg/dl
LDL <100
HDL > 50 mg/dl
Triglycerides <150 mg/dl
Wasit circumference: < 80 cm/31 inches for women
BMI: < 23 kg/m^2
BLOOD PRESSURE <130/85
<120/80 with end organ or diabetes or heart failure.
HBA1c < 7.0

11.9 Conclusion

Menopause is an important pivotal point in women's health. Changes occur in fat distribution with increasing central obesity, dyslipidemias, increased chances for Diabetes and Hypertension. The risk of coronary heart disease and CVD increases which become an important cause of morbidity and mortality.

Addressing these changes and adapting preventing measures is important. Women who have preeclampsia, gestational diabetes mellitus, PCOS, and family history of these diseases need to exercise more caution.

Appropriate preventive care and regular checkup will go a long way for healthy aging.

Key Points

1. Menopause is associated with changes in body composition, weight, glucose tolerance, and altered lipid profile.
2. Woman develops higher chances of coronary heart disease.
3. Vasomotor symptoms are associated with cardiovascular risks
4. MHT can be given in well selected cases after cardiovascular risk estimation
5. Lowest dose for least time of MHT should be given
6. Preventive measures should be adapted in time and lifestyle management is a must for healthy cardiovascular health

Long Answer Questions (LAQs)

1. What are the key physiological changes in the cardiovascular system during menopause
2. How does menopause impact endothelial function and arterial stiffness
3. what are the effects of Menopause hormone therapy on cardiovascular status.

Short Answer Questions (SAQs)

1. Why does cardiovascular risk increase more rapidly after menopause
2. What therapies are available to mitigate menopause-related cardiovascular changes

Multiple Choice Questions (MCQs)

1. Average of menopause in Indians is
   - A. 55 years
   - B. 40 years
   - C. 46 years
   - D. 35 years
2. Vasomotor flushes are associated with
   - A. Rheumatoid arthritis
   - B. Low bodyweight
   - C. Higher education
   - D. Hypertension
3. Ideal value for Low density lipoproteins is:
   - A. <180
   - B. <60
   - C. <100
   - D. <200
4. True for Transdermal estrogens
   - A. First pass hepatic metabolism is bypassed
   - B. Can be used in women with breast cancer
   - C. Does not need progesterone in women with uterus
5. Ideal waist circumference for women in India is:
   - A. <88 cm
   - B. <80 cm
   - C. <89 cm
   - D. <95 cm
6. Estrogens increase the risk of following in dose-dependent way:
   - A. Diabetes
   - B. Psoriasis
   - C. Hypertension
   - D. Stroke
7. Framingham risk score is for
   - A. Women with diabetes
   - B. Women with hypertension
   - C. Women with CAD
   - D. Asymptomatic women without diabetes or hypertension
8. MHT is safe in women before
   - A. 80 years
   - B. 60 years

    C. 40 years
    D. 70 years
9. Menopause is associated with
    A. Higher waist circumference
    B. Metabolic syndrome
    C. Higher risk of ischemic heart disease
    D. All of the above
10. Estrogens can be prescribed in all except
    A. Women less than 60 years
    B. Women with past history of breast cancer
    C. Women with vasomotor symptoms
    D. Women with past liver disease

Answers

1. C
2. D
3. C
4. A
5. B
6. D
7. D
8. B
9. D
10. D

References

1. World Health Organization. Cardiovascular diseases (CVDs). Geneva: World Health Organization; 2021. https://www.who.int/news-room/fact-sheets/detail/cardiovascular-diseases-(cvds).
2. World Health Organization. Noncommunicable diseases country profile. Geneva: World Health Organization; 2014. https://www.who.int/. [Google Scholar].
3. World Health Organization Cardiovascular Diseases India. Accessed on 11 Jan 2025. Available online: https://www.who.int/india/health-topics/cardiovascular-diseases.
4. Derby CA, Crawford SL, Pasternak RC, Sowers M, Sternfeld B, Matthews KA. Lipid changes during the menopause transition in relation to age and weight: the study of women's health across the nation. Am J Epidemiol. 2009;169(11):1352–61. https://doi.org/10.1093/aje/kwp043. Epub 2009 Apr 8. PMID: 19357323; PMCID: PMC2727246.
5. Stanhewicz AE, Wenner MM, Stachenfeld NS. Sex differences in endothelial function important to vascular health and overall cardiovascular disease risk across the lifespan. Am J Physiol Heart Circ Physiol. 2018;315(6):H1569–88. https://doi.org/10.1152/ajpheart.00396.2018. [PMC free article] [PubMed] [Google Scholar].
6. Kronenberg F. Hot flashes: epidemiology and physiology. Ann N Y Acad Sci. 1990;592:52–86. https://doi.org/10.1111/j.1749-6632.1990.tb30316.x. [PubMed] [Google Scholar].

7. Mathews L, Iantorno M, Schär M, Bonanno G, Gerstenblith G, Weiss RG, Hays AG. Coronary endothelial function is better in healthy premenopausal women than in healthy older postmenopausal women and men. PLoS One. 2017;12(10):e0186448. https://doi.org/10.1371/journal.pone.0186448. [PMC free article] [PubMed] [Google Scholar].
8. Yan XN, Jin JL, Hong LF, et al. Lipoprotein(a) is associated with the presence and severity of new-onset coronary artery disease in postmenopausal women. J Women's Health. 2020;4:503–10. [DOI] [PubMed] [Google Scholar].
9. Serviente C, Tuomainen TP, Virtanen J, Witkowski S, Niskanen L, Bertone-Johnson E. Follicle-stimulating hormone is associated with lipids in postmenopausal women. Menopause. 2019;26:540–5. [DOI] [PMC free article] [PubMed] [Google Scholar].
10. Paschou SA, Marina LV, Spartalis E, et al. Therapeutic strategies for type 2 diabetes mellitus in women after menopause. Maturitas. 2019;126:69–72. [DOI] [PubMed] [Google Scholar].
11. Hallajzadeh J, Khoramdad M, Izadi N, et al. Metabolic syndrome and its components in premenopausal and postmenopausal women: a comprehensive systematic review and meta-analysis on observational studies. Menopause. 2018;25:1155–64. [DOI] [PubMed] [Google Scholar].
12. Choi Y, Chang Y, Kim BK, et al. Menopausal stages and serum lipid and lipoprotein abnormalities in middle-aged women. Maturitas. 2015;80:399–405. [DOI] [PubMed] [Google Scholar].
13. Zhu D, Chung HF, Dobson AJ, et al. Age at natural menopause and risk of incident cardiovascular disease: a pooled analysis of individual patient data. Lancet Public Heal. 2019;4:553–64. [DOI] [PMC free article] [PubMed] [Google Scholar].
14. Newson L. Menopause and cardiovascular disease. Post Reprod Heal. 2018;24:44–9. [DOI] [PubMed] [Google Scholar].
15. Anagnostis P, Theocharis P, Lallas K, et al. Early menopause is associated with increased risk of arterial hypertension: a systematic review and meta-analysis. Maturitas. 2020;135:74–9. [DOI] [PubMed] [Google Scholar].
16. Salpeter SR, Walsh JM, Ormiston TM, Greyber E, Buckley NS, Salpeter EE. Meta-analysis: effect of hormone-replacement therapy on components of the metabolic syndrome in postmenopausal women. Diab Obes Metabol. 2006;8:538–54. [DOI] [PubMed] [Google Scholar].
17. Thurston RC, Sutton-Tyrrell K, Everson-Rose SA, Hess R, Matthews KA. Hot flashes and subclinical cardiovascular disease: findings from the study of women's health across the nation heart study. Circulation. 2008;118(12):1234–40. https://doi.org/10.1161/CIRCULATIONAHA.108.776823. [PMC free article] [PubMed] [Google Scholar].
18. Canonico M, Plu-Bureau G, Lowe GD, Scarabin PY. Hormone replacement therapy and risk of venous thromboembolism in postmenopausal women: systematic review and meta-analysis. BMJ. 2008;336(7655):1227–31. https://doi.org/10.1136/bmj.39555.441944.BE. [PMC free article] [PubMed] [Google Scholar].
19. Oppermann K, Colpani V, Spritzer PM. Risk factors associated with coronary artery calcification in midlife women: a population-based study. Gynecol Endocrinol. 2019;35:904–8. [DOI] [PubMed] [Google Scholar].
20. Oliver-Williams C, Glisic M, Shahzad S, et al. The route of administration, timing, duration and dose of postmenopausal hormone therapy and cardiovascular outcomes in women: a systematic review. Hum Reprod Update. 2019;25:257–71. [DOI] [PubMed] [Google Scholar].
21. Anagnostis P, Paschou SA, Katsiki N, Krikidis D, Lambrinoudaki I, Goulis DG. Menopausal hormone therapy and cardiovascular risk: where are we now? Curr Vasc Pharmacol. 2019;17:564–72. [DOI] [PubMed] [Google Scholar].
22. Cui J, Shen Y, Li R. Estrogen synthesis and signaling pathways during aging: from periphery to brain. Trends Mol Med. 2013;19:197–209. [DOI] [PMC free article] [PubMed] [Google Scholar].
23. Finkelstei JS, Lee H, Karlamangla A, et al. Antimullerian hormone and impending menopause in late reproductive age: the study of women's health across the nation. J Clin Endocrinol Metab. 2020;105:E1862–71. [DOI] [PMC free article] [PubMed] [Google Scholar].

Skin Changes and Its Care in Menopause 12

Jaismine Kaur Kohli and Ananta Khurana

Abstract

Menopause marks a significant physiological transition in a woman's life, characterized by the cessation of ovarian function and a sharp decline in estrogen levels. This hormonal shift has profound effects on the skin, contributing to visible and functional changes that impact both appearance and quality of life. Estrogen plays a crucial role in maintaining skin integrity by regulating collagen synthesis, elasticity, hydration, pigmentation, and barrier function. Its decline leads to a range of dermatological concerns, including xerosis, thinning, increased wrinkling, impaired wound healing, and heightened sensitivity. Additionally, hormonal imbalance during menopause contributes to conditions such as acne, hirsutism, and female pattern hair loss, and the genitourinary syndrome of menopause (GSM). Understanding these changes is essential for comprehensive care. Management strategies include general lifestyle modifications, targeted dermatological treatments and in some cases, hormone replacement therapy (HRT). This chapter explores the multifaceted impact of menopause on the skin and offers evidence-based guidance for clinicians to address these challenges through individualized and holistic care.

Keywords

Menopause · Estrogen · Female pattern hair loss · Acne · Hirsutism

J. K. Kohli · A. Khurana (✉)
Department of Dermatology, Venereology and Leprosy, Atal Bihari Vajpayee Institute of Medical Sciences and Dr Ram Manohar Lohia Hospital, New Delhi, Delhi, India

R. Malik et al. (eds.), *Menopause Essentials*,
https://doi.org/10.1007/978-981-95-7498-8_12

12.1 Introduction

Menopause is an inevitable part of a woman's life marking the end of her reproductive years. It is defined as the cessation of menstrual periods for 12 months due to permanent loss of ovarian function, which brings about a sharp decline in estrogen levels [1]. Among the many effects of menopause, skin changes are particularly noticeable and impactful; affecting the person both physically and emotionally. This low estrogen state has implications on the structure and function of the skin, with as many as 64% of women attending menopause clinics reporting skin problems [2].

12.2 The Effect of Estrogen on Skin

Estrogen, the primary female sex hormone, plays a critical role in maintaining the overall health and appearance of the skin. It exerts its effect through estrogen receptors (ER)α and β, both having equal affinity to estradiol. However, ER-β is more widely distributed in the skin and hair [3]. The effects of this hormone are far-reaching, influencing skin structure, hydration, elasticity, and pigmentation. To understand the connection between estrogen and skin health, it is essential to understand how estrogen directly impacts various aspects of skin function.

12.2.1 Collagen Production

Collagen is a critical protein in the dermis, responsible for maintaining the skin's structure, strength, and elasticity. Estrogen plays a pivotal role in regulating collagen production, stimulating the synthesis of both collagen and elastin, which are essential for skin firmness. However, as estrogen levels decline during menopause, the production of collagen, particularly types I and III, decreases [4]. This reduction leads to diminished skin elasticity, and overall structural integrity. Research has shown that collagen loss is more strongly associated with postmenopausal age than with chronological age itself [2]. Furthermore, estrogen hormone replacement therapy (HRT) has been shown to restore skin collagen levels to those typically seen in premenopausal women, offering a potential strategy to prevent further collagen degradation [2]. Notably, a significant increase in collagen content and skin thickness has been observed as early as 3 months after initiating HRT, and this effect is consistent across different methods of estrogen administration [2].

Impact of Estrogen Decline The reduction in collagen production results in visible skin changes, including sagging, the formation of fine lines, and more pronounced wrinkles, particularly around the eyes, mouth, and jawline. Following menopause, women may lose up to 30% of their collagen within the first 5 years, with a subsequent annual decline of approximately 2.1% over the next 15 years [4].

12.2.2 Skin Thickness and Elasticity

Estrogen also affects the thickness and elasticity of the skin. Estrogen increases the mitotic activity of the epidermal keratinocytes [5]. When estrogen levels are high, the skin tends to be thicker, more supple, and less prone to wrinkles. However, as estrogen levels drop, skin elasticity is decreased due to elastic degeneration and connective tissue loss. Compared to women who get topical estrogen, which thickens elastic fibers, increases their quantity, and improves their orientation in the papillary dermis, early postmenopausal women may have a 1.5% annual decline in skin elasticity [4].

Effect of Low Estrogen As estrogen levels fall after menopause, skin becomes thinner and less resilient. This thinning can make the skin more prone to bruising, tearing, and irritation, as well as the formation of wrinkles and sagging.

12.2.3 Moisture Retention and Barrier Function

Estrogen has an important role in maintaining skin moisture and the barrier function. It does it by promoting sebum secretion; primarily by regulating the expression of insulin-like growth factor receptors and increasing the production of insulin-like growth factors from fibroblasts which in turn induces lipogenesis in human sebocytes and leads to moisture retention [6]. Estrogen also stimulates the production of hyaluronic acid, a molecule that is known for its water retention properties [7]. Hence, once menopause sets in, dryness of the epidermis is noted due to an increase in trans epidermal water loss & decreased sebum production. This in turn disrupts the barrier function of the skin and makes women more prone to eczemas and pruritus.

Further establishing this, studies have shown estrogen therapy thickens the epidermis, with an increase in keratinocyte volume and more defined rete ridges, elevates the levels of mucopolysaccharides and hyaluronic acids in the dermis to keep the skin hydrated, which improves the barrier function of the stratum corneum and optimizes the surface area of corneocytes [8].

12.2.4 Skin Regeneration and Healing

The estrogen also supports the skin's natural repair mechanisms. It accelerates the regeneration of skin cells, helping to repair damage from environmental stressors like sun exposure or pollution. In wound healing models, estrogen reduces wound size and stimulates matrix deposition in both human and murine skin [9]. Furthermore, numerous studies have demonstrated that estrogens influence the inflammatory response, promote granulation tissue formation, speed up re-epithelialization and control proteolysis, all of which contribute to the various stages of wound healing [10]. With reduced estrogen levels, the skin's ability to regenerate and heal slows down, meaning that cuts, bruises, or acne may take longer to heal.

Slower Skin Recovery The decline in estrogen slows down the process of skin repair and recovery, which can contribute to increased duration of wound closure and potential risks of chronic wounds.

12.2.5 Pigmentation

Estrogen influences melanin production, which is responsible for the skin's pigmentation. During times of hormonal fluctuation, such as pregnancy or menopause, changes in estrogen levels can lead to uneven pigmentation, such as melasma, linea nigra, and pigmentation of areola seen in pregnancy while solar lentigo, melasma, or general skin discoloration can be seen after menopause. Estrogen also has some protective role against UV radiation. This is also a contributing factor in making women more susceptible to pigmentation in postmenopause [11].

Hyperpigmentation Lower estrogen levels can increase the visibility of hyperpigmented areas or melasma, especially when coupled with sun exposure. Estrogen's decline can also make the skin more vulnerable to the effects of UV radiation, leading to solar lentigos and hyperpigmentation.

12.2.6 Skin Sensitivity and Reactivity

Estrogen helps maintain the skin's barrier function, which protects it from environmental pollutants and pathogens. When estrogen levels drop, this barrier can become compromised, leading to increased skin sensitivity, redness and irritation.

Heightened Sensitivity Skin that is less resilient due to low estrogen is more likely to react to certain skincare ingredients, environmental changes, and allergens. This increased sensitivity can cause discomfort, redness, or flare-ups of conditions like eczema or rosacea.

12.2.7 Oil Production and Acne

Estrogen has a balancing effect on oil production in the skin. It helps to regulate sebum (oil) production, keeping the skin moisturized without being overly greasy. However, when estrogen levels decrease, the relative levels of androgens (male hormones) can increase, leading to an overproduction of sebum [12]. This can contribute to acne, especially along the jawline and chin. The patient may present with open and closed comedones, papules, pustules, and even cystic lesions of acne. Delayed healing due to hypoestrogenic state may worsen the condition [10].

Acne and Oil Imbalance The hormonal imbalance that accompanies menopause often leads to an increase in acne, particularly in women who did not experience acne during their younger years. Women with menopausal acne commonly exhibit deep-seated inflammatory papules or nodules, often with a predominant perioral distribution [13]. Furthermore, these individuals tend to have increased skin sensitivity, which results in a higher incidence of postinflammatory erythema, as well as hyperpigmentation, hypopigmentation, and scarring [14].

12.2.8 Hair Growth and Loss

Estrogen promotes healthy hair growth, while a decrease in estrogen can lead to thinning hair and changes in hair texture. Certain studies have shown that estrogen decreases the resting phase of the hair and prolongs the growing phase of the hair [14]. Hence, hair may become finer, drier, and more brittle, leading to hair loss or thinning, particularly around the scalp and temples. A study reported that up to 26% women suffered from diffuse hair loss after menopause [15].

12.3 Female Pattern Hair Loss (FPHL)

Female pattern hair loss (FPHL) is a patterned hair loss characterized by reduced hair density over the crown and frontal scalp with retention of the frontal hairline (Figs. 12.1 and 12.2). Up to 52.2% of females may suffer from FPHL after their menopause [16]. Trichoscopy is an important tool to make clinical diagnosis esp. in mild cases (Fig. 12.3).

An increased prevalence of FPHL postmenopause suggests a possible hormonal influence. The decrease in the level of estrogen after menopause leads to increase in sensitivity to the circulating androgens, which might contribute to hair follicle miniaturization and conversion of terminal hair into vellus hair [17].

12.3.1 Hirsutism

Hirsutism is defined as excessive terminal hair that appears in androgen-dependent areas (ie, in a male pattern) in women, such as on the chin, upper lip, and abdomen [18].

Hirsutism is a common problem seen in postmenopausal women. The entity is mild in the majority of cases and a part of the normal aging process. It occurs due to a fall in estrogen levels along with the relative rise in circulating androgens. Also with age, there is a decline in sex hormone binding globulin (SHBG), which leads to a rise of circulating free androgens, which is responsible for the conversion of vellus hair into terminal hair [19].

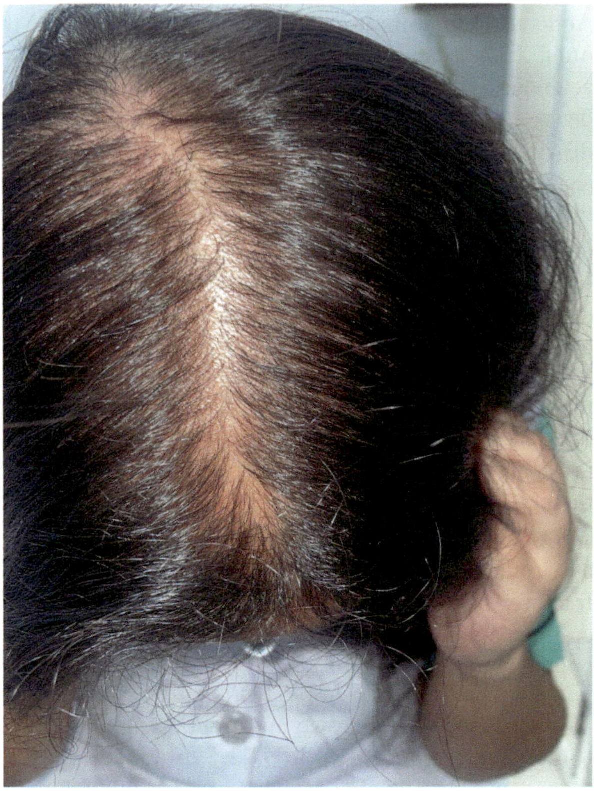

Fig. 12.1 Female pattern Hair Loss Grade 1(Ludwig scale) in a 54 year postmenopausal women before treatment showing reduced hair density in the crown and frontal scalp

12.3.2 The Genitourinary Syndrome of Menopause

It is a collection of symptoms that postmenopausal women suffer mainly vaginal dryness, dyspareunia, and urine characteristics like frequency and urgency. All of these symptoms are linked to a drop in estrogen levels, which causes structural alterations in a woman's genitourinary system [20]. An observational study conducted by Moral et al. identified vaginal dryness as the most common and troubling symptom, impacting up to 93% of women. The study further indicated that this symptom is classified as moderate to severe in intensity in 68% of the instances [21]. The patient presents clinically with findings including loss of labial and vulval thickness, reduced vaginal discharge, diminished pubic hair, and decreased subcutaneous fat in the labia majora. Additionally, there is dry and thin vaginal epithelium, narrowing of the vagina, and a reduction in pelvic floor strength and control [22].

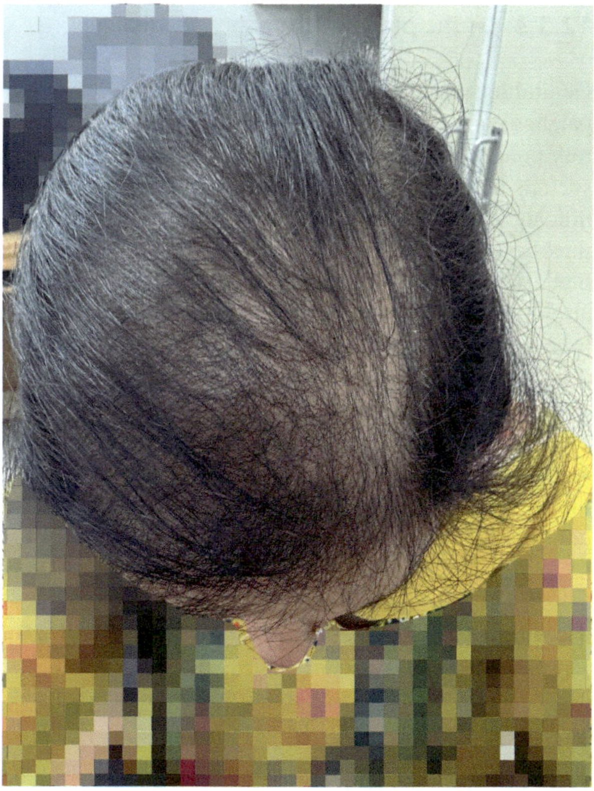

Fig. 12.2 Female pattern Hair Loss Grade 2 (Ludwig scale) showing more severe hairloss

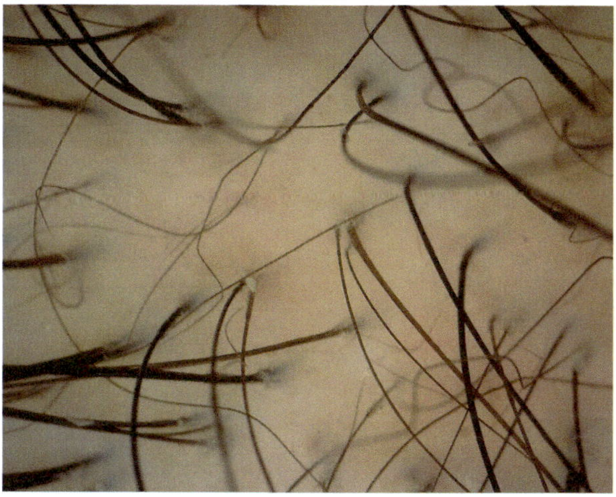

Fig. 12.3 Trichoscopy of FPHL demonstrating high degree of anisotrichosis (hair diameter variability) and single hair follicular units

12.3.3 Leukoplakia Vulva

Genital leukoplakia, a term used for clinical description, refers to white, thickened patches on the genital mucosa, often resulting from chronic irritation or inflammatory conditions. It is a nonhistological term and may be associated with conditions such as lichen sclerosus or squamous cell carcinoma in situ. Estrogen plays a significant role in maintaining the health of genital mucosa by promoting epithelial thickness, elasticity, and vascularization. In conditions like genital leukoplakia, particularly in postmenopausal women, reduced estrogen levels can lead to mucosal atrophy, decreased lubrication and increased susceptibility to irritation and microtrauma. This hormonal deficiency may contribute to the development or exacerbation of chronic inflammatory conditions such as lichen sclerosus, which are associated with leukoplakic changes.

These lesions cause pruritus, burning, and stinging. Diagnosis requires histopathological evaluation to rule out premalignant or malignant changes. Early recognition and appropriate management are essential to prevent progression and complications.

12.4 Skin Problems Seen After Menopause [2]

The following dermatoses are seen in postmenopausal women (Table 12.1).

Table 12.1 Dermatosis in postmenopausal women

General dermatoses
1. Xerosis
2. Pruritus
3. Atrophy
4. Wrinkling
5. Sagging
6. Easy bruising
7. Hyperhydrosis
8. Impaired wound healing
9. Asteatotic eczema
10. Acne
11. Hyperpigmentation
Hair disorders
1. Hirsutism
2. Female pattern hair loss
Genital dermatosis
1. Lichen planus
2. Lichen sclerosis
Oral dermatosis
1. Lichen planus
2. Burning mouth syndrome
3. Xerostomia

12.4.1 Skin Care Practices for Menopausal Women

12.4.1.1 General Measure

Healthy lifestyle choices are essential for general health as well as for preserving good skin after menopause. A nutritious diet that places a focus on getting enough omega-3 fatty acids, vitamin D, and antioxidants (vitamins C and E) are essential.

Regular exercise, drinking enough water, smoking cessation, and getting enough sleep are necessary. Menopausal stress and anxiety might worsen skin aging and aggravate dermatosis. Yoga and meditation are examples of stress-relieving techniques that can aid with distress and help one in staying healthy.

12.4.1.2 Gentle Cleansing

A mild cleanser is crucial during menopause, as harsh soaps can strip the skin of its natural oils, exacerbating dryness and disrupting normal skin barrier. Prescribe a gentle, hydrating cleanser that is sulfate-free and designed for sensitive skin.

12.4.1.3 Hydration and Moisture Retention

- *Use of Emollients and Humectants*: Regularly applying moisturizers that contain humectants (like glycerine and hyaluronic acid) can help attract moisture to the skin and prevent excessive dryness. Emollients containing ceramides can help create a barrier to lock in moisture and prevent transdermal water loss.
- In case of sensitive and eczema prone skin it is advised to apply fragrance free moisturizer without any active ingredients, multiple times during the day, especially soon after the bath to trap in the moisture.

12.4.1.4 Sun Protection

- *Daily Broad-Spectrum Sunscreen*: As the skin becomes thinner and more susceptible to oxidative damage due to hypo estrogenic state, daily sun protection may be advised if there is regular high sun exposure. Using a broad-spectrum sunscreen with SPF 30 or higher can help protect against UVA and UVB rays, which cause skin aging due to collagen loss, hyper pigmentation, and increase the risk of skin cancer (although the risk is low in Indian skin). Women should be advised to reapply sunscreen every 2 hours, when outdoors at times of high UV flux (e.g. high altitude, sea-side, etc). Sunscreen is to be applied not only on face, but also in areas not covered by clothing like neck, chest, arms, and hands.
- *Sun Protective Clothing*: In addition to sunscreen, women are encouraged to wear hats, sunglasses, and protective clothing when in areas with high UV flux.

12.4.1.5 Anti-Aging Skincare

- *Topical Retinoids*: Retinoids, including retinol, are commonly recommended to combat fine lines, wrinkles, and skin texture issues. They help stimulate collagen production and cell turnover. However, these products should be used cautiously, as they can increase skin sensitivity.
- *Antioxidants*: Although there is no significant literature backing, topical antioxidants like Vitamin C, Vitamin E, and niacinamide are claimed to lower free radi-

cals, promote collagen synthesis and protect the skin from environmental damage, thereby improving skin tone and texture.
- *Peptides and Growth Factors*: These ingredients may support collagen production and enhance skin regeneration.

12.4.1.6 Professional Treatments

- *Chemical Peels*: Chemical peel is an office-based procedure performed by dermatologists by applying a chemical of known concentration on the skin. This intentional epidermal damage leads to removal of the superficial layer of the epidermis, promotes collagen production, and improves the appearance of pigmentation and fine lines. A chemical peel can offer potential benefits for various skin conditions in postmenopausal women including acne vulgaris, melasma, wrinkles, actinic keratosis, photodamage, photoaging, and pigmentation disorders. Moreover, they lead to increased neo collagen content in upper dermis after regular sessions.
- *Microneedling*: Microneedling is a technique in which controlled microtrauma is given to the skin which stimulates collagen production and can help improve skin texture, minimize scarring, and reduce the appearance of fine lines.
- *Laser Treatments*: Laser resurfacing treatments can be beneficial for improving skin elasticity, reducing wrinkles, and treating pigmentation issues. Popular laser treatments include fractional CO2 lasers and intense pulsed light (IPL) therapy.
- A more recent therapeutic technique called high-intensity focused ultrasound (HIFU) employs sound waves to heat and remodel tissues, which is advantageous for antiaging effects.

12.4.1.7 Hormone Replacement Therapy (HRT) and Skin

- Hormone replacement therapy (HRT) can improve skin appearance by replenishing estrogen levels and supporting collagen production. However, it is important to weigh the benefits and risks of HRT, and this treatment should only be considered under the guidance of a healthcare provider.
- Topical estrogens also have a role in increasing epidermal and collagen thickness.

12.5 Management of Specific Concerns

Treatment options for various postmenopausal dermatological manifestations are as follows [2] (Table 12.2)

12.5.1 Hirsutism

Hirsutism is most commonly observed on the chin and neck. While mild hirsutism can be considered normal, it is essential to exclude both tumorous and nontumorous causes when other signs of virilization are present. Virilization refers to the development of male secondary sexual characteristics, such as male-pattern hair loss, severe

Table 12.2 Treatment of dermatosis in postmenopausal women

General dermatoses	Treatment
1. Xerosis, pruritus	1. Reduce bathing time 2. Post bath application of emollients 3. Avoidance of irritants and hard soaps
2. Wrinkling, Sagging	1. Gentle cleansing and application of emollients 2. Application of sunscreen 3. Topical retinoids, peptides and growth factors 4. Chemical peels, microneedling, fractional lasers, HIFU
3. Easy bruising	1. Use of gentle cleansers 2. Oral vitamin-C supplementation
4. Asteatotic eczema	1. Regular application of emollients 2. Use of gentle cleansers 3. Mild to medium potency topical steroids as needed
5. Acne	General measures: Life style modification in form of exercise and diet 1. Local: antibiotics, antibacterial, retinoid, and salicylic acid 2. Systemic: Antibiotics (Doxycycline, erythromycin, Minocycline etc), retinoids (Isotretinoin) 3. Antiandrogen drugs like spironolactone 4. OCP (oral contraceptive pills) with caution.
6. Hyperpigmentation	1. Application of sunscreen 2. Depigmenting agents 3. Chemical peels and Q-switch laser
Hair disorders	
1. Hirsutism	1. Conventional hair removal methods or laser 2. Antiandrogen drugs like spironolactone 100–200 mg once daily Flutamide 250–500 mg/day Cyproterone acetate 100 mg per day 5–15 day of menstrual cycle (premenopausal women) 3. Surgical removal of androgen producing tumor
2. Female pattern hair loss	1. Local: Minoxidil 2% solution twice daily, Minoxidil 5% once daily 2. Systemic: Finasteride 1–5 mg once daily Dutasteride 0.5–2.5 mg daily, A/D Spironolactone 100–200 mg once daily Cyproterone acetate 100 mg per day 5–15 day of menstrual cycle (premenopausal women) 3. Adjuvants: Platelet rich Plasma (PRP) 4. Surgical. Hair transplant
Genital dermatosis	
1. Lichen planus	1. Local: Topical corticosteroid and calcineurin inhibitors 2. Systemic: corticosteroids, retinoids, antimalarials, immunomodulators like ciclosporin and methotrexate for severe erosive disease Adjuvant: lidocaine jelly for pain and vaginal dilators to prevent synechiae formation 3. Surgery for scarring sequelae
2. Lichen sclerosis	1. Local: Potent topical corticosteroid,calcineurin inhibitors 2. Systemic: corticosteroids, methotrexate and retinoids 3. Phototherapy 4. Surgery for scarring sequelae

(continued)

Table 12.2 (continued)

General dermatoses	Treatment
Oral dermatosis	
1. Lichen planus	1. Local: Corticosteroids un gels/paste/drops twice daily: clobetasol propionate 0.05%, triamcinolone acetonide 0.1%; 2. Intralesional corticosteroid injections, 3. Calcineurin inhibitors: tacrolimus 0.1%, pimecrolimus 1% twice daily; 4. Retinoid: Isotretinoin 0.05%, 0.1%, or 0.18% cream gel or ointment once daily 5. Ciclosporin: topical or rinse twice daily 6. Systemic: Methotrexate 2.5–12.5 mg week, oral corticosteroids for short course, Mycophenolate mofetil 0.5–3 g/day, Azathioprine 100–150 mg/day, Dapsone 50–100 mg/day
2. Burning mouth syndrome	1. Topical clonazepam 1 mg for 3 min three times daily 2. Alpha lipoic acid (ALA) 200 mg thrice daily 3. Gabapentin 300 mg/day up to 300 mg three times daily for 2 months
3. Xerostomia	1. No topical therapy 2. Hormone replacement therapy (HRT)

acne, deepening of the voice, and clitoromegaly. In such cases, it is crucial for clinicians to rule out underlying ovarian and adrenal gland tumors, which can lead to an increase in androgen production [19]. Diagnostic evaluation should include measuring serum testosterone, sex hormone-binding globulin (SHBG), dehydroepiandrosterone sulfate (DHEA-S), androstenedione, and inhibin B levels, especially in postmenopausal women who exhibit signs of hyperandrogenism [19]. This is critical for determining the underlying etiology of the condition. Treatment usually depends on the cause and in physiological age-related hirsutism lifestyle changes like exercise and diet modification are generally advised along with conventional hair removal methods or laser. Antiandrogens, such as spironolactone are mostly beneficial although the results take many months to become apparent. In cases of malignancy, surgical removal of the tumor is the only resort.

12.5.2 Acne

Most patients with isolated menopausal acne do not exhibit other signs of clinical hyperandrogenism and are classified as normoandrogenic. However, the presence of virilization may indicate severe insulin resistance, androgen-secreting tumors or the use of androgenic substances. In such cases, a comprehensive laboratory panel, including measurements of free and total testosterone, dehydroepiandrosterone sulfate, androstenedione, luteinizing hormone, and follicle-stimulating hormone, as well as transvaginal and abdominal ultrasounds, should be conducted [12]. Unlike teenage acne, postmenopausal acne requires milder treatment. Topical treatment includes: antibiotics, antibacterial, retinoid, and salicylic acid. In severe cases, oral antibiotics and retinoids may also be prescribed. Additionally, spironolactone can be used as it exerts antiandrogenic effects. OCPs can also be used but they come with safety issues in older women like an increased risk of cardiovascular diseases, hypercoagulability and breast and endometrial cancer.

12.5.3 Female Pattern Hair Loss

After menopause, many women notice thinning of hair. This may first present with a widened central part while some notice a receding hairline (Fig. 12.2). For better management, it is always a good idea to start treatment early. According to Singal et al. [17] management of FPHL typically involves a combination of pharmacologic treatments, cosmetic interventions and in some cases, surgical procedures. The first-line treatment recommended is minoxidil, both 2% and 5% have been shown to be useful. For more severe cases and in hyperandrogenism, antiandrogenic medications such as spironolactone or finasteride may be prescribed. Other adjunctive treatments, such as low-level laser therapy, platelet-rich plasma (PRP) therapy and hair transplant surgery, may be considered alongside. Additionally, proper counselling and support are crucial in helping women manage the emotional and social challenges associated with hair loss.

12.5.4 Genitourinary Syndrome

Management of the genitourinary syndrome of menopause (GSM) encompasses both non-pharmacologic and pharmacologic strategies aimed at alleviating symptoms and enhancing quality of life. First-line nonpharmacologic interventions include lifestyle modifications and the use of vaginal moisturizers, lubricants, and gels. When nonhormonal treatments fail to provide adequate symptom relief, pharmacologic options may be considered. These include vaginal estrogen therapy (VET), ospemifene, local androgens, intravaginal dehydroepiandrosterone (prasterone), and laser therapies such as erbium or CO_2 lasers [22]. It is important to note that while these treatments have demonstrated effectiveness, their safety profiles, especially in specific populations like breast cancer survivors, require careful consideration. Early detection and individualized treatment plans are essential in managing GSM effectively. Addressing both vaginal and urinary symptoms can significantly improve the quality of life for affected women.

Key Points

1. *Estrogen's Role in Skin Health*: Estrogen plays a vital role in maintaining skin structure, hydration, elasticity, and collagen production. As estrogen levels decline during menopause, women experience visible skin changes, such as decreased collagen, thinner skin, and less elasticity.
2. *Skin Changes during Menopause*: Menopause leads to skin changes such as sagging, dryness, wrinkles, and a decrease in skin thickness. Skin becomes more

prone to bruising, irritation, and sensitivity, partly due to reduced moisture retention and barrier function.
3. *Impact on Hair*: Estrogen loss during menopause can cause thinning hair, especially around the scalp and temples. Female Pattern Hair Loss (FPHL) and hirsutism (excessive hair growth) are common concerns during this time due to hormonal changes.
4. *Pigmentation and Sensitivity*: Declining estrogen levels can lead to increased skin sensitivity, redness, irritation, and pigmentation issues like melasma. The skin becomes more vulnerable to UV damage, increasing the risk of hyperpigmentation.
5. *Skin Care Recommendations*: Postmenopausal women should focus on hydration, gentle cleansing, sun protection, and using antiaging products like retinoids and antioxidants. Hormone Replacement Therapy (HRT) and professional treatments like chemical peels, microneedling, and laser therapies may also help manage skin changes.

Conflicts of Interest None

Long Answer Questions (LAQs)

1. Explain in detail the role of estrogen on skin.
2. Enumerate and explain skin problems in postmenopausal women.
3. Write a note on healthy skin care practices in postmenopausal women.
4. Explain in detail the management of the following skin concerns in postmenopausal women
   (a) Hirsutism
   (b) Acne
   (c) Female pattern hair loss
   (d) Genitourinary syndrome

Short Answer Questions (SAQs)

1. What are the two estrogen receptor subtypes found in the skin, and which one is more predominant in distribution?
2. Name two nonpharmacologic treatment options used in the management of Genitourinary Syndrome of Menopause (GSM).
3. What is the most commonly used first-line pharmacologic agent for treating Female Pattern Hair Loss (FPHL) in postmenopausal women?
4. How does estrogen deficiency contribute to increased skin dryness after menopause?
5. List two dermatological procedures that can improve skin texture and collagen production in postmenopausal women.

Multiple Choice Questions (MCQs)

1. What is the primary cause of menopause-related skin changes in women?
   A. Increase in testosterone
   B. Decline in estrogen levels
   C. Decrease in progesterone
   D. Increase in cortisol
2. Which histological changes in skin are most characteristic in postmenopausal women not receiving hormone therapy?
   A. Increased rete ridges and mucopolysaccharide accumulation
   B. Epidermal thinning, reduced keratinocyte volume, and collagen degradation
   C. Hyperplasia of sebaceous glands and increased melanocyte density
   D. Increased subcutaneous fat deposition in the dermis
3. Which estrogen receptor subtype is more widely distributed in the skin and hair and mediates many of the cutaneous effects of estrogen?
   A. ER-α
   B. ER-β
   C. ER-γ
   D. GPER1
4. What percentage of collagen can women lose in the first 5 years after menopause?
   A. 10%
   B. 20%
   C. 30%
   D. 50%
5. Which skin manifestation is commonly observed due to estrogen decline and increased UV sensitivity?
   A. Melasma and solar lentigo
   B. Erythema nodosum
   C. Rosacea
   D. Psoriatic plaques
6. What mechanism best explains the occurrence of hirsutism in postmenopausal women?
   A. Estrogen-induced overproduction of androgen precursors
   B. Loss of SHBG and a rise in free circulating androgens, converting vellus hair to terminal hair
   C. Enhanced activity of ER-β in sebaceous glands
   D. Inhibition of 5α-reductase due to low progesterone levels
7. What clinical finding is most consistent with early-stage Female Pattern Hair Loss (FPHL) postmenopause?
   A. Frontal hairline recession with temple balding
   B. Central part widening with preserved frontal hairline
   C. Circular bald patches across the scalp
   D. Complete hair loss in occipital regions

8. What is the first-line nonhormonal approach to managing genitourinary syndrome of menopause (GSM)?
   A. Oral antibiotics
   B. Hormone replacement therapy
   C. Vaginal lubricants and moisturizers
   D. Laser therapy
9. Why might high-intensity focused ultrasound (HIFU) be particularly beneficial for menopausal skin?
   A. It delivers topical estrogen directly to basal keratinocytes
   B. It promotes epidermal thickening via thermal ablation of the stratum corneum
   C. It remodels deeper tissue layers by stimulating collagen through thermal injury
   D. It reduces melanin concentration, improving pigmentation balance
10. In cases of postmenopausal acne with signs of virilization, which of the following laboratory findings would most likely prompt suspicion of an androgen-secreting tumor?
    A. Elevated SHBG, low DHEA-S
    B. Normal testosterone, slightly elevated LH
    C. Very high DHEA-S or total testosterone
    D. Decreased androstenedione with elevated FSH

Answers

1. B
2. B
3. B
4. C
5. A
6. B
7. B
8. C
9. C
10. C

References

1. Carter AE, Merriam S. Menopause. Med Clin North Am. 2023;107(2):199–212. https://doi.org/10.1016/j.mcna.2022.10.003.
2. Kamp E, Ashraf M, Musbahi E, DeGiovanni C. Menopause, skin and common dermatoses. Part 2: skin disorders. Clin Exp Dermatol. 2022;47(12):2117–22.
3. Lephart ED, Naftolin F. Menopause and the skin: old favorites and new innovations in cosmeceuticals for estrogen-deficient skin. Dermatol Ther (Heidelb). 2021;11(1):53–69. https://doi.org/10.1007/s13555-020-00468-7.

4. Thornton MJ. Estrogens and aging skin. Dermatoendocrinol. 2013;5(2):264–70. https://doi.org/10.4161/derm.23872.
5. Kanda N, Watanabe S. 17beta-estradiol stimulates the growth of human keratinocytes by inducing cyclin D2 expression. J Invest Dermatol. 2004;123:319–28.
6. Makrantonaki E, Vogel K, Fimmel S, Oeff M, Seltmann H, Zouboulis CC. Interplay of IGF-I and 17beta-estradiol at age-specific levels in human sebocytes and fibroblasts in vitro. Exp Gerontol. 2008;43(10):939–46. https://doi.org/10.1016/j.exger.2008.07.005.
7. Sobel H, Lee KD, Hewlett MJ. Effect of estrogen on acid glycosaminoglycans in skin of mice. Biochem Biophys Acta. 1965;101:225–9.
8. Maheux R, Naud F, Rioux M, Grenier R, Lemay A, Guy J, et al. A randomized, double-blind, placebo-controlled study on the effect of conjugated estrogens on skin thickness. Am J Obstet Gynecol. 1994;170:642–9.
9. Ashcroft GS, Ashworth JJ. Potential role of estrogens in wound healing. Am J Clin Dermatol. 2003;4:737–43.
10. Emmerson E, Hardman MJ. The role of estrogen deficiency in skin ageing and wound healing. Biogerontology. 2012;13:3–20.
11. Stevenson S, Thornton J. Effect of estrogens on skin aging and the potential role of SERMs. Clin Interv Aging. 2007;2(3):283–97.
12. Khunger N, Mehrotra K. Menopausal acne—challenges and solutions. Int J Women's Health. 2019;11:555–67.
13. Williams C, Layton AM. Persistent acne in women: implications for the patient and for therapy. Am J Clin Dermatol. 2006;7:281–90.
14. Grymowicz M, Rudnicka E, Podfigurna A, Napierala P, Smolarczyk R, Smolarczyk K, Meczekalski B. Hormonal effects on hair follicles. Int J Mol Sci. 2020;21(15):5342.
15. Ali I, Wojnarowska F. Physiological changes in scalp, facial and body hair after the menopause: a cross-sectional population-based study of subjective changes. Br J Dermatol. 2011;164(3):508–13.
16. Chaikittisilpa S, Rattanasirisin N, Panchaprateep R, Orprayoon N, Phutrakul P, Suwan A, Jaisamrarn U. Prevalence of female pattern hair loss in postmenopausal women: a cross-sectional study. Menopause. 2022;29(4):415–20.
17. Singal A, Sonthalia S, Verma P. Female pattern hair loss. Indian J Dermatol Venereol Leprol. 2013;79(5):626–40.
18. Martin KA, Anderson RR, Chang RJ, et al. Evaluation and treatment of hirsutism in premenopausal women: an Endocrine Society Clinical Practice Guideline. J Clin Endocrinol Metab. 2018;103(4):1233–5.
19. Zaman A, Rothman MS. Postmenopausal hyperandrogenism: evaluation and treatment strategies. Endocrinol Metab Clin N Am. 2021;50(1):97–111.
20. Angelou K, Grigoriadis T, Diakosavvas M, Zacharakis D, Athanasiou S. The genitourinary syndrome of menopause: an overview of the recent data. Cureus. 2020;12(4):e7586. https://doi.org/10.7759/cureus.7586.
21. Moral E, Delgado JL, Carmona F, Caballero B, Guillán C, González PM, Suárez-Almarza J, Velasco-Ortega S, Nieto C, as the writing group of the GENISSE study. Genitourinary syndrome of menopause. Prevalence and quality of life in Spanish postmenopausal women. The GENISSE study. Climacteric. 2018;21(2):167–17.
22. Gandhi J, Chen A, Dagur G, Suh Y, Smith N, Cali B, Khan SA. Genitourinary syndrome of menopause: an overview of clinical manifestations, pathophysiology, etiology, evaluation, and management. Am J Obstet Gynecol. 2016;215(6):704–11.

Mental Health in Menopause

13

Brijesh Saran

Abstract

Menopause signifies a crucial biological shift in a woman's life, generally occurring between the ages of 45 and 55, characterized by a reduction in estrogen and progesterone levels. These hormonal alterations significantly impact mental health, including mood control, cognition, and emotional stability. This chapter examines the mental aspects of menopause, emphasizing the heightened incidence of sadness, anxiety, bipolar disorder, cognitive deficits, and sleep difficulties during this phase. Disruptions in neurotransmitter systems, including serotonin, dopamine, and GABA, lead to mood instability, irritability, and cognitive impairments. Depression impacts over 50% of menopausal women, but anxiety problems affect up to 40%. Hormonal variations may exacerbate bipolar symptoms, complicating treatment approaches. Cognitive difficulties, such as memory deficits and "brain fog," are prevalent, while sleep disorders including insomnia and restless legs syndrome exacerbate emotional health. The interaction between neuroendocrine alterations and psychosocial stressors highlights the necessity for prompt identification and comprehensive care. Effective management encompasses psychotherapy, pharmaceutical treatments, lifestyle modifications, and, when applicable, hormone therapy. A complete understanding of these mental health effects is crucial for delivering effective care and enhancing the quality of life for women experiencing menopause.

Keywords

Menopause · Mental health · Depression · Anxiety · Bipolar Disorder · Cognitive Impairment · Sleep Disorders · Estrogen

B. Saran (✉)
Department of Psychiatry, Santosh Deemed to be University, Delhi NCR, India

R. Malik et al. (eds.), *Menopause Essentials*,
https://doi.org/10.1007/978-981-95-7498-8_13

13.1 Introduction to Menopause and Psychiatric Disorders

Menopause is a natural biological process that means a woman can no longer have children. It usually happens between the ages of 45 and 55. Menstrual periods stop for 12 months in a row, which is its defining feature. Perimenopause, the term for the period leading up to menopause, can persist for several years and is characterized by a number of symptoms, including mood swings, hot flashes, and nocturnal sweats. Recognizing the wider effects of menopause on women's health requires an understanding of these physiological changes. Menopause-related hormonal changes impair women's quality of life and emphasize socioeconomic gaps in symptom intensity by causing vasomotor symptoms, mood swings, cognitive problems, and genitourinary symptoms [1].

Psychiatric illnesses are more common around menopause; research suggests that up to 20% of women have severe depression symptoms during this time. About 10–15% of women going through menopause suffer from anxiety disorders, which are also prevalent. It is thought that these mental health problems are largely caused by changes in hormones, especially the drop in estrogen levels. These problems can also be made worse by the stress that comes with growing older and going through life changes [2].

Depression and anxiety are common during menopause, presenting as persistent sadness, loss of interest, and sleep changes. Anxiety includes excessive worry and physical symptoms like palpitations. Mood swings are also prevalent, affecting daily functioning [3].

Menopause-related hormonal fluctuations, particularly declines in estrogen and progesterone, have been linked to an increased risk of mental health conditions such as anxiety disorders, depressive symptoms, mood instability, insomnia, and cognitive impairments such as memory loss and decreased concentration. Symptoms might overlap and differ from woman to woman. Hormonal fluctuations, previous mental health conditions, and pressures in life are some of the contributing factors. For treatment to be effective, getting professional assistance is essential [4].

As women move out of their reproductive years, menopause can have serious psychological and emotional impacts, such as mood swings, impatience, and a sense of loss or mourning. This time is especially challenging because physical issues frequently exacerbate these emotional difficulties. The way society views menopause and aging can also have an effect on mental health outcomes. It is essential to comprehend these intricate and varied impacts in order to provide menopausal women with complete care. Menopausal patients' general health and quality of life can be enhanced by addressing both the emotional and physical aspects of the transition. Women who were early perimenopausal had the lowest psychosocial quality of life and the highest levels of stress, anxiety, and depression. The experiences of premenopausal and postmenopausal women were comparable. Regardless of age or menopausal stage, resilience and self-efficacy therapies may assist address psychological issues [5].

Improving quality of life during menopause requires addressing mental health issues. Relationships, everyday functioning, and physical health can all be significantly impacted by untreated mental health conditions. The required support is provided via early diagnosis and intervention. To support menopausal women, healthcare providers should evaluate for symptoms and give therapies such as medication, psychotherapy, and lifestyle modifications.

13.2 Pathophysiology

13.2.1 Hormonal Changes and Brain Function in Menopause

Menopause is characterized by a dramatic decrease in estrogen and progesterone levels, both of which are essential for brain function. These hormones control neurotransmitters like serotonin, dopamine, GABA, and acetylcholine, all of which affect mood, cognition, and emotional stability.

- Estrogen improves serotonin synthesis and receptor sensitivity, affects dopamine pathways (related to motivation and pleasure), and supports acetylcholine (essential for learning and memory).
- Progesterone decreases anxiety and neural excitability via influencing GABA, a neurotransmitter.

As these hormones deplete, serotonin levels decrease, increasing the risk of depression and irritability.

- Dopamine imbalance can cause mood swings and impaired motivation.
- GABA activity diminishes, leading to anxiety and sleep problems.
- Reduced acetylcholine levels can lead to memory and focus issues, commonly known as "brain fog."

13.2.2 Neuroendocrine Interactions and Cognitive Effects

The hypothalamic-pituitary-gonadal (HPG) and hypothalamic-pituitary-adrenal (HPA) axes are critical for hormonal control. During menopause, many systems are dysregulated.

- Estrogen withdrawal affects the hippocampus and prefrontal cortex, resulting in memory lapses and trouble concentrating.
- Hormonal imbalances can lead to increased cortisol (stress hormone), deplete serotonin levels, and worsen anxiety and depression.

Furthermore, vasomotor symptoms (VMS) such as hot flashes and night sweats, which are connected to hypothalamic neurons, are associated with poor sleep and cognitive impairment. These symptoms might last for years and vary by individual and ethnic group.

13.2.3 The Neuroprotective Role of Estrogen

Estrogen functions as a neuroprotective agent, protecting neurons from oxidative stress and inflammation. Its reduction during menopause reduces this barrier, potentially raising the risk of neurological illnesses like Alzheimer's.

13.3 Menopause and Psychiatric Disorders

An important stage of a woman's life, menopause is characterized by the cessation of menstrual cycles. Numerous physical and emotional changes are brought about by it. Hormonal fluctuations are one of the most important factors affecting mental health. Menopause-related drops in Estrogen and Progesterone levels can have a significant impact on a woman's mental health.

In addition to being reproductive hormones, Estrogen and Progesterone also have important effects on brain activity. In instance, Estrogen has neuroprotective qualities. It supports mood, cognitive function, and mental wellness in general. Depression, anxiety, and mood changes can result from a decrease in Estrogen levels during menopause. On the other hand, Progesterone calms the brain. Anxiety and irritation may be exacerbated by its reduction [6–8].

13.3.1 Impact of Menopause

- Mood Swings
- Depression
- Anxiety
- Cognitive Function
- Sleep Disturbances
- Reduced Energy Levels
- Stress Sensitivity
- Increased Risk of Mental Health Conditions
- Social Withdrawal
- Decreased Self-Esteem

These hormone shifts are caused by intricate neurological processes. Neurotransmitters that are essential for mood modulation, including serotonin, dopamine, and norepinephrine, interact with Estrogen. Mood disorders can result from these neurotransmitter systems being upset by a drop in Estrogen levels. Estrogen also possesses anti-inflammatory qualities that shield the brain from harm and stress. Insufficient Estrogen makes the brain more susceptible to stress, which can make mental health issues worse.

Additionally, Progesterone affects how the brain reacts to stress. It alters the action of the brain's main inhibitory neurotransmitter system, the gamma-aminobutyric acid (GABA) system. An elevated stress response and elevated

Table 13.1 Frequency of psychiatric disorders in menopausal women

Psychiatric disorder	Estimated prevalence	Clinical notes
Depressive mood disorders	30–50%	Often exacerbated by vasomotor symptoms and sleep disturbances
Anxiety disorders	25–40%	Includes generalized anxiety and panic symptoms; linked to hormonal fluctuations
Sleep disturbances	40–60%	Insomnia and fragmented sleep are common; often co-occur with mood symptoms
Somatoform symptoms	20–35%	Includes fatigue, muscle pain, and gastrointestinal complaints
Cognitive impairment	10–20%	Mild memory issues and concentration difficulties; often reversible
Sexual dysfunction	30–45%	Low libido, dyspareunia, and urogenital symptoms; may affect psychological health
Irritability & Mood Swings	35–50%	Often misdiagnosed; related to hormonal shifts and psychosocial stressors
Psychotic symptoms	<5%	Rare; may occur in severe cases or with comorbid conditions

anxiety might result from a decrease in Progesterone. Hormonal changes during menopause disrupt neurotransmitters like serotonin and dopamine, increasing mood disorders and stress vulnerability. Progesterone decline heightens anxiety by affecting the brain's GABA system [9].

These hormonal shifts can have a significant emotional impact. Women can feel a variety of emotions, such as anxiety, panic, and grief and irritation. These emotions can be debilitating and disrupt day-to-day activities. It is critical to recognize these feelings and get help when required. Confiding in a trusted friend or family member, joining a support group, or speaking with a healthcare professional can all have a big impact (Table 13.1).

13.4 Depression during Menopause

13.4.1 Risk and Prevalence Factors

Menopausal depression is a prevalent yet sometimes disregarded problem. During this time of transition, many women go through major mood swings. Compared to other life periods, menopausal women experience a significantly higher prevalence of depression. Hormonal changes, life pressures, and preexisting mental health disorders are all contributing factors to this increase. It is critical to understand that menopause is a significant emotional journey in addition to a physical shift [10, 11].

13.4.2 Summary of Risk Factors for Depression During Menopause [10, 11]

1. Hormonal Changes: Fluctuations and decline in Estrogen and Progesterone levels.
2. Life Stressors: Significant life events such as children leaving home, aging parents, and changes in marital status.
3. Preexisting Mental Health Conditions: History of depression or other mood disorders.
4. Neuroendocrine Disorders: Disorders involving the hormonal system getting worse.
5. Cardiovascular Disease: Links to serious health issues, like heart disease.
6. Metabolic Syndrome: Links to metabolic syndrome.
7. Osteoporosis: Connections with osteoporosis.
8. Reproductive Events: Increased depression around reproductive events like postpartum depression and premenstrual dysphoric disorder.
9. Sensitivity to Hormonal Shifts: Sensitivity to normal shifts in reproductive hormones.
10. History of Depression: Higher prevalence of depressive symptoms in women with a history of depression.

Depression during menopause is more likely to occur when a number of risk factors are present. Hormonal fluctuations are important, especially the drop in Estrogen levels. Depression and hopelessness can result from a decline in Estrogen, which has a major effect on mood regulation. Women who have experienced depression or other mood disorders in the past are also more vulnerable. Events in life like children moving out, parents becoming older, and marital status changes can also make depression worse.

13.4.3 Diagnostic Standards and Evaluation Instruments

Because menopausal and depressed symptoms sometimes overlap, diagnosing depression at menopause can be difficult. Persistent melancholy, loss of interest in activities, changes in eating and sleep patterns, exhaustion, and trouble focusing are typical signs of depression. These symptoms are easily confused with menopausal symptoms, which might result in an incorrect or undiagnosed.

13.5 ICD-10 Diagnostic Criteria for Depression [12]

13.5.1 Major Symptoms (At Least One Required for Diagnosis)

1. *Depressed Mood*: Persistent sadness or low mood most of the day, nearly every day.

2. *Loss of Interest or Pleasure*: Marked loss of interest or pleasure in all, or almost all, activities most of the day, nearly every day.
3. *Fatigue or Low Energy*: Persistent fatigue or loss of energy nearly every day.

13.5.2 Minor Symptoms (Additional Symptoms Required for Diagnosis)

4. *Disturbed Sleep*: Insomnia or hypersomnia nearly every day.
5. *Changes in Appetite or Weight*: Significant weight loss when not dieting, weight gain, or decrease/increase in appetite nearly every day.
6. *Psychomotor Agitation or Retardation*: Observable agitation or slowing down of physical movements nearly every day.
7. *Poor Concentration or Indecisiveness*: Diminished ability to think or concentrate, or indecisiveness, nearly every day.
8. *Low Self-Confidence*: Feelings of worthlessness or excessive/inappropriate guilt nearly every day.
9. *Suicidal Thoughts*: Recurrent thoughts of death, suicidal ideation without a specific plan, a suicide attempt, or a specific plan for committing suicide.

Medical professionals detect depression in menopausal women using a variety of evaluation instruments. One popular instrument for determining the degree of depression is the Patient Health Questionnaire (PHQ-9). It evaluates the frequency of depression symptoms during the previous 2 weeks using nine questions. The Beck Depression Inventory (BDI), which gauges the severity of depression, is another often used instrument. These resources aid in the precise diagnosis of menopausal depression when used in conjunction with a comprehensive clinical assessment (Table 13.2).

13.5.3 Impact on Emotions

Depression during menopause can have a significant emotional impact. The strength of women's emotions can overwhelm them. It can be quite distressing to experience both bodily and mental loss. Changes in identity and self-perception are equally as important as the cessation of menstrual cycles. Women may experience anxiety about aging and feelings of inadequacy, which can exacerbate symptoms of depression (Table 13.3).

13.6 Anxiety Disorder in Menopause

Anxiety disorder is a common mental illness marked by worrying and being afraid all the time.

Table 13.2 Depression rating scales [13]

Name of scale	No. of items	Scoring method	Score for diagnosis	Description
Hamilton Depression Rating Scale (HAM-D)	21	Administered by healthcare professionals	0–7 (Normal), 8–13 (Mild), 14–18 (Moderate), 19–22 (Severe), ≥23 (Very Severe)	Measures severity of depression; commonly used in clinical settings
Montgomery-Asberg Depression Rating Scale (MADRS)	10	Rated on a 7-point scale	0–6 (Normal), 7–19 (Mild), 20–34 (Moderate), ≥35 (Severe)	Measures severity of depression; sensitive to changes over time
Beck Depression Inventory (BDI)	21	Self-report	0–13 (Minimal), 14–19 (Mild), 20–28 (Moderate), 29–63 (Severe)	Assesses behavioral manifestations and severity of depression; widely used
Patient Health Questionnaire-9 (PHQ-9)	9	Self-report	0–4 (Minimal), 5–9 (Mild), 10–14 (Moderate), 15–19 (Moderately Severe), 20–27 (Severe)	Screens for depression and measures severity; commonly used in primary care
Center for Epidemiologic Studies Depression Scale (CES-D)	20	Self-report	≥16 (Indicates possible depression)	Measures major dimensions of depression experienced in the past week
Zung Self-Rating Depression Scale (SDS)	20	Self-report	20–44 (Normal), 45–59 (Mild), 60–69 (Moderate), 70–80 (Severe)	Measures affective, psychological, and somatic aspects of depression

During menopause, women often experience heightened anxiety due to hormonal changes, making it a critical period for mental health. Hormonal and thermoregulatory changes associated with ovarian aging cause menopausal hot flashes. Hormone therapy is helpful, but there is no scientific data on how to treat hot flashes, and the precise causes are unknown. Because the symptoms of anxiety and hot flashes coincide, anxiety is a contentious risk factor. It is uncertain if it is a precursor or a result. Women are more likely to suffer from anxiety disorders, which can lower their quality of life. There are many different types of anxiety, each with its own set of symptoms and causes, such as Panic disorder, Phobias, Generalized anxiety disorder (GAD), and anxiety-related disorders as Post-traumatic stress disorder [14].

Menopausal anxiety disorders can present in a variety of ways, each with distinct traits. The prevalent condition known as generalized anxiety disorder (GAD) is typified by excessive and uncontrollable worry over routine events. Women with generalized anxiety disorder (GAD) may experience chronic anxieties, be unable to

Table 13.3 The key themes identified

Key themes	Details
Loss of identity, womanhood, and control	Women reported feeling a loss of their previous identity and womanhood
	The transition led to feelings of invisibility and a loss of control over their lives
Negative self-appraisal	Participants described themselves using negative terms, indicating low self-esteem and confidence
	Body image concerns, particularly weight gain, were prevalent
Impact on quality of life	Menopause affected various aspects of life, including family, relationships, and work
	Some women resorted to isolation and alcohol as coping mechanisms
Emotional impact and overwhelm	Menopause can bring about significant emotional changes, including feelings of sadness, anxiety, and irritabilit
	These emotional shifts can be overwhelming and are often linked to hormonal fluctuations
Changes in identity and self-perception	The transition through menopause can challenge a woman's sense of identity and self-perception
	This period often coincides with other life changes, such as children leaving home or aging parents, impacting self-esteem and emotional well-being
Anxiety about aging and feelings of inadequacy	Menopause can trigger anxiety about aging and feelings of inadequacy
	These emotional responses are influenced by both the physical changes of menopause and societal attitudes towards aging and femininity

relax, and be on edge all the time. This might make day-to-day living feel tiresome and overwhelming.

Another type of anxiety issue that can develop or increase during menopause is panic disorder. It is distinguished by brief, intense bouts of fear, sometimes accompanied by physical symptoms such as sweating, shortness of breath, and palpitations. Women who have these severe panic episodes may feel helpless and unprotected.

Menopausal women are also prone to social anxiety disorder. This illness is characterized by a severe fear of social situations, which causes avoidance and social isolation. Women may be afraid of being judged or embarrassed, which can make them feel even more depressed and alone (Tables 13.4, 13.5 and 13.6).

Diagnosing anxiety during menopause involves a comprehensive approach to ensure accurate identification and appropriate treatment. The first step in the diagnostic process is to use the diagnostic criteria outlined in the ICD-10. Frequent, unprovoked panic attacks marked by abrupt spikes in extreme anxiety or distress are included in the ICD-10 Criteria for Panic Disorder (F41.0). Physical symptoms such a fast heartbeat, sweating, shaking, chest pain, shortness of breath, disorientation, and a feeling of impending doom or lack of control are frequently present

Table 13.4 Overview of various types of anxiety disorders

Anxiety disorder	Description
Generalized Anxiety Disorder (GAD)	Persistent and excessive anxiety about daily chores
Panic disorder	Panic episodes occur suddenly and repeatedly
Social anxiety disorder	Intense fear of social situations
Specific phobias	Irrational fear of specific objects or situations
Agoraphobia	Fear of places where escape might be difficult
Separation anxiety disorder	Excessive fear of being separated from loved ones
Selective mutism	Inability to speak in certain social situations

Table 13.5 Type of anxiety symptoms seen during menopause

Symptom type	Description
Physical symptoms	Palpitations, sweating, trembling, and hot flashes
Emotional symptoms	Irritability, restlessness, and feelings of dread
Behavioral symptoms	Avoidance of social situations and increased dependency on others
Cognitive symptoms	Difficulty concentrating, racing thoughts, and excessive worry

Table 13.6 The causes and risk factors contributing to anxiety during menopause

Cause/risk factor	Description
Genetic factors	Family history of anxiety disorders
Environmental factors	Stressful life events and lifestyle changes
Psychological factors	Pre-existing mental health conditions
Biological factors	Hormonal fluctuations, particularly the decline in estrogen levels

during these episodes. Other important characteristics include persistent concern about potential attacks in future and significant behavioral changes.

The Diagnostic and Statistical Manual of Mental Disorders, Fifth Edition (DSM-5) provides standardized criteria for diagnosing various anxiety disorders, including Generalized Anxiety Disorder (GAD), Panic Disorder, Social Anxiety Disorder, and Specific Phobias. These criteria help clinicians systematically evaluate the presence, duration, and severity of anxiety symptoms, ensuring a consistent and reliable diagnosis.

In addition to the DSM-5 criteria, Assessment Tools play a crucial role in the diagnostic process. These tools include standardized questionnaires and structured interviews designed to evaluate the severity and impact of anxiety symptoms. Commonly used questionnaires include the Generalized Anxiety Disorder 7 (GAD-7) scale, the Beck Anxiety Inventory (BAI), and the Zung Self-Rating Anxiety Scale. These tools help quantify the level of anxiety and provide a baseline for monitoring treatment progress. Structured interviews, such as the Mini International Neuropsychiatric Interview (MINI) or the Structured Clinical Interview for DSM-5 (SCID-5), allow clinicians to gather detailed information about the patient's symptoms, medical history, and psychosocial factors contributing to anxiety.

Differential Diagnosis is another critical component of the diagnostic process. This involves ruling out other medical conditions that may present with similar symptoms, such as hyperthyroidism, cardiovascular disorders, or other psychiatric conditions like depression or bipolar disorder. A thorough medical evaluation, including physical examinations and laboratory tests, is essential to exclude these conditions. Additionally, clinicians must consider the impact of hormonal fluctuations during menopause, as these can exacerbate anxiety symptoms. By carefully differentiating between anxiety disorders and other potential causes, clinicians can develop a more targeted and effective treatment plan.

Effective treatments for anxiety during menopause include Cognitive Behavioral Therapy (CBT), medications like antidepressants and benzodiazepines, lifestyle changes such as regular exercise and a healthy diet, and complementary therapies like yoga and meditation. Anxiety can impact daily life by decreasing productivity, straining relationships, and increasing health risks. Coping strategies involve stress management, relaxation techniques, and support groups. With proper treatment, many women see significant improvement, though some may need ongoing management. Current research focuses on new treatments and understanding hormonal roles in anxiety. Early intervention and professional help are crucial for managing symptoms effectively.

13.7 Cognitive Changes and Menopause

Cognitive performance is greatly impacted by menopause, which is characterized by a decrease in Estrogen and progesterone. Memory loss, concentration problems, and "brain fog" are common during this transition for women. Particularly in regions linked to memory and cognition, Estrogen is essential for brain function. Memory formation and retrieval may be impacted by reduced neuronal efficiency brought on by the decline in Estrogen levels after menopause. Subjective cognitive challenges during the menopausal transition are reported by about two-thirds of women. Developing solutions to promote mental clarity and brain health requires an understanding of these changes. To lessen the negative effects of hormone fluctuations on cognitive performance, effective strategies include hormone replacement treatment, lifestyle changes, and cognitive exercises.

Changes in memory during menopause is one of the most often observed cognitive abnormalities after menopause is memory loss. There is frequent talk about moments of forgetfulness, including losing things, skipping appointments, or having trouble remembering words and names. Studies show that the decrease in Estrogen levels, which are essential for brain function, is connected to this memory loss. The hippocampus, a part of the brain essential for memory formation and retrieval, is known to be influenced by Estrogen. Memory problems may result from a decline in the effectiveness of hippocampal neuronal connections caused by a drop in Estrogen levels.

Research has indicated that during menopause, up to two-thirds of women suffer from some form of cognitive impairment. These changes are not consistent; some women might have just minor disruptions, while others would experience major alterations in their day-to-day lives. Individual variations in hormone levels, hereditary variables, and general health can all be blamed for the heterogeneity in cognitive symptoms (Table 13.7).

Menopause can have an impact on verbal fluency, executive function, attention, and memory, among other areas of cognitive performance. Planning, problem-solving, and multitasking tasks all demand attention and executive function. Women may experience difficulties focusing, planning, or effectively switching between tasks during menopause. Conversations and verbal tasks can become more challenging as verbal fluency, or the capacity to locate and express words rapidly, deteriorates.

Hormonal changes are not the only cause of the loss in cognitive function that occurs with menopause. Cognitive decline is a natural by-product of aging, and menopause can make these changes worse. Cognitive function can also be further hampered by menopause-related symptoms such mood swings, hot flashes, and sleep problems. Because it impairs the brain's capacity to absorb information and build memories, poor sleep quality in particular has been connected to decreased cognitive function.

Table 13.7 The cognitive changes that can occur during menopause

Cognitive change	Description
Memory lapses	Forgetfulness, such as misplacing items or forgetting appointments
Difficulty concentrating	Challenges in maintaining focus and attention on tasks
Brain fog	A general sense of mental cloudiness or sluggish thinking
Reduced verbal fluency	Difficulty in finding and articulating words quickly
Decreased mental clarity	Feeling mentally fuzzy or having slower cognitive processing
Mood swings	Emotional fluctuations that can affect cognitive function
Sleep disturbances	Poor sleep quality, which can impair cognitive performance
Increased forgetfulness	More frequent episodes of forgetfulness and memory issues
Attention deficits	Problems with sustaining attention and multitasking
Executive function impairment	Difficulties with planning, problem-solving, and organizing activities

To support cognitive function during menopause, women can adopt a healthy diet, engage in regular exercise, participate in mentally stimulating activities, maintain good sleep hygiene, manage stress, stay socially active, and consider hormone replacement therapy (HRT) under medical supervision. These strategies help preserve mental clarity and promote brain health.

13.8 Sleep Disorders and Menopause

Menopause often leads to significant changes in sleep patterns, starting during perimenopause and continuing postmenopause. Insomnia, in which one has trouble going asleep, remaining asleep, or getting up at an inappropriate hour, is a common kind of sleep disruption. Night sweats, sudden episodes of intense heat and sweating, frequently cause awakenings. Sleep apnea, a condition where breathing repeatedly stops and starts during sleep, can be exacerbated by hormonal changes. Restless Legs Syndrome (RLS) is when you feel like moving your legs all the time, even when you're not trying to. This can make it hard to sleep. These disturbances can severely impact the quality of life, leading to daytime fatigue, irritability, and cognitive difficulties. Addressing these sleep issues is crucial for maintaining overall well-being during menopause. Effective management strategies may include lifestyle changes, medical treatments, and alternative therapies to improve sleep quality and mitigate the negative effects on daily functioning.

Managing sleep disturbances during menopause involves a combination of lifestyle changes, medical treatments, and alternative therapies. Hormone Replacement Therapy (HRT) can alleviate vasomotor symptoms like hot flashes and night sweats, which are major contributors to sleep disturbances, though it requires careful consideration of risks and benefits. Medications such as low-dose antidepressants, gabapentin, and clonidine can also help improve sleep quality. Good sleep hygiene practices is maintaining a regular sleep plan, making your bedroom comfortable, and setting up a relaxing bedtime routine are all important parts of good sleep hygiene.

Cognitive Behavioral Therapy for Insomnia (CBT-I) is effective in addressing sleep problems by changing negative thoughts and behaviors. Alternative therapies like acupuncture, yoga, and herbal supplements may provide relief, but should be discussed with a healthcare provider. Lifestyle modifications, including regular physical activity, stress management techniques, and a healthy diet, can further enhance sleep quality. Combining these strategies can help women manage sleep disturbances during menopause and improve their overall quality of life.

13.9 Bipolar Disorder and Menopause

Extreme mood fluctuations, including manic and depressive episodes, are a hallmark of bipolar disorder, a psychiatric illness. It has a major impact on everyday functioning and quality of life, affecting millions of people globally. Hormonal changes brought on by menopause, the natural end of menstruation, might have an impact on mental health issues including bipolar illness.

Hormonal changes during perimenopause and menopause can have a substantial effect on bipolar disorder. These modifications might make bipolar drugs less effective, which would exacerbate symptoms. Mood swings, sleeplessness, headaches, exhaustion, and sexual problems are common overlapping symptoms. The complex dynamic created by this symptom crossover makes managing both disorders more difficult and raises the risk of mood swings, sleep disturbances, and issues with sexual health.

Approximately 1% of people suffers with bipolar disorder. Women may have a more severe illness course, even if men and women are diagnosed with bipolar disorder at comparable rates. Panic disorder may be more prevalent among women. Rapid cycling and mixed and depressed episodes may also happen more frequently. Bipolar disease can affect people differently; some may struggle in many areas of life, while others may benefit from possibilities for social network expansion and professional advancement. In the context of living with bipolar disease, qualitative research emphasizes themes like "loss of control," "disruption, uncertainty, and instability," and "negative impact of symptoms across life."

Bipolar women may have higher mood swings throughout reproductive-cycle events like menstruation, pregnancy, the postpartum period, and menopause. Approximately 77% of women say their moods go worse during these periods. According to studies, 20% of women with bipolar disorder are more likely to have mood swings around menopause. Women with bipolar disorder scored higher on depression and mania rating measures throughout the late transition or early menopause phase than those in the early menopause phase. Compared to women with severe depression alone, those who experienced a symptomatic menopausal transition along with major depression were more likely to develop bipolar illness later on. In the general population, menopause can lead to mood instability; some women may experience anxiety, melancholy, and irritability. Hormone therapy and nonhormonal therapies like antidepressants are examples of medical treatments.

Menopausal symptoms can also be successfully treated with cognitive behavior therapy, health education, and psychoeducational programs. Since there is no concrete proof that depressive disorders are more prevalent during the menopause transition, it is crucial to avoid over abnormalize this period. Women's perceptions of psychological and physical changes, as well as social and cultural environment, all have an impact on the bio-psycho-socio-cultural shift that is menopause. Stressful life experiences, body mass index, and a history of depression and sexual abuse are associated with psychological suffering during the menopausal transition. Unpleasant perceptions of menopause might raise the risk of unpleasant psychological symptoms, and variations in Estradiol may increase emotional sensitivity to psychosocial stress.

A major life transition that can have a substantial influence on women with bipolar disorder is menopause. Bipolar illness symptoms might be made worse by the hormonal changes that take place after menopause, especially the drop in Estrogen and progesterone levels. It has been demonstrated that Estrogen stabilizes mood, and that its depletion can exacerbate mood instability. Because of this hormonal imbalance, women may have more frequent and severe mood swings, making it difficult for them to properly manage their bipolar symptoms.

The influence of menopause on mood regulation is one of the main ways that it impacts bipolar disorder. During this time, women may have more severe manic episodes or more frequent depression episodes. Because Estrogen and progesterone affect the brain's neurotransmitter systems, which include serotonin and dopamine and are essential for mood control, the relationship between hormonal changes and mood disorders is complicated. Women with bipolar disorder may experience mood disorders that are more severe as a result of these hormones fall, which might upset these systems.

Menopause can also have an impact on how well bipolar disorder drugs work. The metabolism and absorption of these drugs can be changed by hormonal fluctuations, which may lessen their efficacy. This calls for careful observation and potential modifications to treatment regimens by medical professionals. For women to adequately manage their menopausal symptoms, they may need various dosages or alternate drugs.

Bipolar illness management may become even more challenging when menopausal symptoms including hot flashes, night sweats, and sleep problems are accompanied by stress. In particular, poor sleep quality is a serious problem since it can lead to manic or depressed episodes. In order to create a thorough management plan that takes into account both menopausal and bipolar symptoms, it is imperative that women with bipolar disorder collaborate extensively with their medical professionals. For a well-rounded and successful course of treatment, this may involve lifestyle changes, hormone replacement therapy, and psychosocial support.

Menopause, marked by hormonal changes and reduced Estrogen levels, can significantly impact women with bipolar disorder by exacerbating mood swings and triggering episodes. The decline in Estrogen, crucial for mood regulation, increases vulnerability to depressive and manic states, leading to heightened irritability, anxiety, and more severe symptoms during menopause (Table 13.8).

Bipolar disorder symptoms include manic episodes (elevated mood, increased activity, reduced sleep, grandiosity, impulsivity), depressive episodes (persistent

Table 13.8 The types of bipolar disorder

Type of bipolar disorder	Description
Bipolar I Disorder	Manic episodes that last at least 7 days or having manic signs that are so bad that you need admission to the hospital right away. There are also episodes of depression, which usually last at least 2 weeks
Bipolar II Disorder	Characterized by a pattern of hypomanic and depressed episodes but not the full-blown manic episodes that are typical of bipolar I disorder
Cyclothymic Disorder	Periods of hypomanic and depressive symptoms that continue at least 2 years (1 year in children and adolescents), but do not match the diagnostic criteria for a hypomanic or depressive episode

sadness, fatigue, worthlessness, loss of interest), and mixed episodes (simultaneous mania and depression).

Bipolar disorder is influenced by genetic factors (family history), environmental factors (stressful life events, trauma), neurobiological factors (chemical imbalances in the brain), and psychological factors (preexisting mental health conditions). These elements interact to increase the risk of developing the disorder.

Diagnosing bipolar disorder involves using DSM-5 and ICD-10 criteria, employing assessment tools like questionnaires and structured interviews, and performing differential diagnosis to rule out other conditions. This comprehensive approach ensures accurate identification and effective management of bipolar disorder symptoms.

Menopausal symptoms like hot flashes, sleep disturbances, and mood swings can overlap with and intensify bipolar disorder symptoms, complicating diagnosis and treatment. Effective management requires a comprehensive approach, including medication adjustments to account for hormonal changes, cautious use of Hormone Replacement Therapy (HRT), and psychotherapy such as Cognitive Behavioral Therapy (CBT). Lifestyle modifications, including regular exercise, a balanced diet, and adequate sleep, are crucial. Building a strong support network of family, friends, and support groups can provide essential emotional and practical support, helping women navigate the challenges of managing both conditions concurrently.

Key Points

1. Menopause is a normal biological process that marks the end of a woman's reproductive years. It typically occurs between the ages of 45 and 55. Significant hormonal changes occur, which can have an impact on mental health.
2. Hormonal variations during menopause, especially the decrease in Estrogen and progesterone, can cause mood swings, sadness, anxiety, cognitive difficulties, and sleep disturbances.
3. Menopausal symptoms, including mood swings, depression, anxiety, and cognitive impairments, can have a major impact on everyday functioning, relationships, and quality of life.
4. Depression is widespread throughout menopause, with hormonal changes, life stressors, and preexisting mental health disorders playing key roles.
5. Anxiety disorders are common during menopause, and hormonal changes might exacerbate them. Symptoms include excessive worrying, panic attacks, and social anxiety.
6. Menopause might worsen bipolar disorder symptoms due to hormonal shifts. This can result in more frequent and severe mood swings, making management of both disorders difficult.
7. Menopause can cause cognitive abnormalities such as memory loss, attention issues, and "brain fog." Estrogen plays an important impact in brain function, notably memory and cognition.

8. Menopause is associated with sleep disorders such as insomnia, night sweats, sleep apnea, and restless legs syndrome. These difficulties can have a significant impact on quality of life and everyday functioning.

Long Answer Questions (LAQs)

1. Describe the hormonal mechanisms underlying psychiatric disorders during menopause. Include the roles of estrogen and progesterone and their effects on neurotransmitter systems.
2. Discuss the diagnostic challenges and tools used for identifying depression and anxiety in menopausal women. How do overlapping symptoms affect diagnosis?
3. Evaluate the bio-psycho-socio-cultural model in understanding the emotional impact of menopause. Support your answer with examples.
4. Compare and contrast the manifestations and management of depression, anxiety, and bipolar disorder in menopausal women. Address both pharmacological and non-pharmacological interventions.

Short Answer Questions (SAQs)

1. What are the most common psychiatric symptoms experienced during perimenopause?
2. Name two diagnostic tools used to assess depression severity in menopausal women.
3. Define "Brain Fog" and explain its clinical relevance during menopause.
4. List any three physical symptoms that can mimic anxiety during menopause.
5. What role does estrogen play in cognitive functioning?

Multiple Choice Questions (MCQs)

1. Which of the following neurotransmitters is most closely associated with mood regulation and is influenced by estrogen levels?

   A. Acetylcholine
   B. Serotonin
   C. GABA
   D. Glutamate

2. According to the ICD-10, which of the following is a major criterion for diagnosing depression?
   A. Appetite changes
   B. Loss of interest or pleasure
   C. Sleep disturbances
   D. Weight gain
3. Which of the following is a primary factor contributing to depression during menopause?
   A. Increased testosterone levels
   B. Elevated dopamine activity
   C. Decline in estrogen and progesterone
   D. High melatonin levels
4. Which anxiety disorder is marked by intense fear of social judgment and avoidance of social settings?
   A. Panic Disorder
   B. Generalized Anxiety Disorder
   C. Social Anxiety Disorder
   D. Agoraphobia
5. Decline in which hormone is most commonly associated with increased anxiety sensitivity in menopausal women?
   A. Testosterone
   B. Melatonin
   C. Estrogen
   D. Oxytocin
6. The most commonly used self-report tool to assess severity of anxiety is:
   A. MADRS
   B. PHQ-9
   C. BAI
   D. HAM-D
7. What is the impact of poor sleep on cognitive functioning in menopausal women?
   A. Improved stress tolerance
   B. Reduced estrogen production
   C. Impaired memory and attention
   D. Lower serotonin metabolism
8. Which of the following is not a commonly reported emotional impact of menopause?
   A. Loss of self-esteem
   B. Increased libido

C. Anxiety about aging
D. Feelings of invisibility

9. Cognitive Behavioral Therapy is especially effective in managing:

   A. Hormonal imbalances
   B. Sleep disturbances and anxiety
   C. Osteoporosis
   D. Hot flashes

10. Which of the following is a minor symptom for depression according to ICD-10?

   A. Persistent sadness
   B. Suicidal thoughts
   C. Poor concentration
   D. Loss of pleasure

Answers

1. B
2. B
3. C
4. C
5. C
6. C
7. C
8. B
9. B
10. C

References

1. Santoro N, Roeca C, Peters BA, Neal-Perry G. The menopause transition: signs, symptoms, and management options. J Clin Endocrinol Metabol. 2021;106:1–15. https://doi.org/10.1210/clinem/dgaa764.
2. Zhang Y, Hu T-T, Cheng Y-R, Zhang Z-F, Su J. Global, regional, and national burden of anxiety disorders during the perimenopause (1990–2021) and projections to 2035. BMC Womens Health. 2025;25:11. https://doi.org/10.1186/s12905-025-03547-z.
3. Bromberger JT, Kravitz HM, Chang Y, Randolph JFJ, Avis NE, Gold EB, et al. Does risk for anxiety increase during the menopausal transition? Study of Women's Health Across the Nation. Menopause. 2013;20:488. https://doi.org/10.1097/gme.0b013e3182730599.
4. Freeman EW, Sammel MD, Liu L, Gracia CR, Nelson DB, Hollander L. Hormones and menopausal status as predictors of depression in womenin transition to menopause. Arch Gen Psychiatry. 2004;61:62–70.

5. Kuck MJ, Hogervorst E. Stress, depression, and anxiety: psychological complaints across menopausal stages. Front Psych. 2024;15:1323743. https://doi.org/10.3389/fpsyt.2024.1323743.
6. Jones HJ, Minarik PA, Gilliss CL, Lee KA. Depressive symptoms associated with physical health problems in midlife women: a longitudinal study. J Affect Disord. 2020;263:301–9. https://doi.org/10.1016/j.jad.2019.11.166.
7. Newhouse PA, Dumas J, Wilkins H, Coderre E, Sites CK, Naylor M, et al. Estrogen treatment impairs cognitive performance after psychosocial stress and monoamine depletion in postmenopausal women. Menopause. 2010;17:860. https://doi.org/10.1097/gme.0b013e3181e15df4.
8. Nair B. Obstetrics and Gynecology patients: menstrual cycle, pregnancy, and postpartum-related psychiatric disorders. In: Leigh H, Streltzer J, editors. Handbook of consultation-liaison psychiatry. Cham: Springer International Publishing; 2015. p. 465–96. https://doi.org/10.1007/978-3-319-11005-9_31.
9. Bendis PC, Zimmerman S, Onisiforou A, Zanos P, Georgiou P. The impact of estradiol on serotonin, glutamate, and dopamine systems. Front Neurosci. 2024:18. https://doi.org/10.3389/fnins.2024.1348551.
10. Bromberger JT, di Scalea TL. Longitudinal associations between depression and functioning in midlife women. Maturitas. 2009;64:145–59.
11. Cizza G, Primma S, Csako G. Depression as a risk factor for osteoporosis. Trends Endocrinol Metab. 2009;20:367–73.
12. World Health Organization WH. The ICD-10 classification of mental and behavioural disorders: diagnostic criteria for research. World Health Organization; 1993.
13. Bech P. Rating scales in depression: limitations and pitfalls. Dialogues Clin Neurosci. 2006;8:207–15.
14. Freeman EW, Sammel MD. Anxiety as a risk factor for menopausal hot flashes: evidence from the Penn Ovarian Aging cohort. Menopause. 2016;23:942–9. https://doi.org/10.1097/GME.0000000000000662.

Menopause and Sexuality

14

Padmini Prasad and Anuradha Singh

Abstract

Menopause is a complex transition that affects various aspects of a woman's life, including biological, psychological, relational, and sociocultural factors. This chapter looks at how hormonal changes, especially decreases in estrogen and androgens, relate to sexual health. It highlights how common and often overlooked female sexual dysfunction (FSD) is. The genitourinary syndrome of menopause (GSM), which includes symptoms like vaginal dryness, pain during intercourse, and urinary issues, significantly contributes to sexual discomfort. Psychological factors such as anxiety, depression, and concerns about body image, along with relationship dynamics and cultural stigma, also make sexual challenges worse. The chapter recommends a biopsychosocial approach to diagnosis and treatment, using tools like the FSFI and DSDS, hormonal assessments, and pelvic exams. Treatment options include local and systemic hormone therapies, psychosexual counseling, pelvic floor physiotherapy, and new methods such as PRP and laser therapy. It stresses the importance of communication models like the PLISSIT framework to encourage open discussions and partner involvement. By using a multidisciplinary, patient-focused approach, healthcare providers can help menopausal women regain their sexual health, dignity, and quality of life. The chapter emphasizes that addressing sexuality is essential for effective menopausal care.

P. Prasad (✉)
Institute of Sexual Medicine, Ramamani Nursing and Maternity Home, Bangalore, India

A. Singh
Department of Obstetrics and Gynaecology, Lady Hardinge Medical College, New Delhi, India

R. Malik et al. (eds.), *Menopause Essentials*,
https://doi.org/10.1007/978-981-95-7498-8_14

Keywords

Female sexual dysfunction (FSD) · Genitourinary syndrome of menopause (GSM) · Biopsychosocial approach · Hormone therapy · Psychosexual counseling

14.1 Introduction

Menopause marks the permanent end of menstruation due to reduced ovarian follicular activity, leading to significant hormonal changes—especially in estrogen, progesterone, and testosterone levels. These shifts affect multiple organ systems, resulting in symptoms like hot flashes, sleep disturbances, and metabolic changes. Of particular relevance to sexual health is the genitourinary syndrome of menopause (GSM), which includes vaginal dryness, dyspareunia, urinary urgency, and recurrent infections. Neuroendocrine changes also impact mood, cognition, and sexual arousability, with declining androgens and altered estrogen metabolism influencing neurotransmitter activity, libido, and emotional regulation.

Beyond biological symptoms, menopause is a biopsychosocial transition involving emotional and social changes [1].

The women may face psychological challenges such as low self-esteem, body image concerns, and mood fluctuations, especially in cultures that equate youth with femininity. Social factors—like caregiving roles, relationship shifts, and societal stigma around aging and sexuality—further shape the menopausal experience. For gynecologists, recognizing these layers is essential. A patient-centered approach that includes empathetic communication, sexual history-taking, and individualized care plans—incorporating counseling, partner involvement, hormonal therapy, and lifestyle support—can help women navigate menopause with dignity and improved quality of life.

This chapter explores how menopause affects sexual function, the emotional and relational aspects of sexuality, and practical approaches to counseling and treatment that support women in maintaining a fulfilling sexual life during and after this transition.

14.2 Midlife and Menopausal Sexual Health: Definitions, Expectations, and Facts

For midlife women, sexual health is an essential but frequently most neglected aspect of total well-being. According to the World Association for Sexual Health (WAS), sexual health is more than just the absence of illness or dysfunction; it is a condition of physical, emotional, mental, and social well-being in connection to sexuality. Regardless of age or reproductive status, this inclusive definition highlights the significance of autonomy, respect, safety, and enjoyment in sexual experiences.

Sexual desire, arousal, lubrication, and orgasmic response are all impacted by the physiological changes that women experience throughout the perimenopause and postmenopause. The changes are mainly attributed to the decrease in estrogen and androgens. Sexual discomfort is frequently caused by genitourinary syndrome of menopause (GSM), vaginal dryness, dyspareunia, and urinary symptoms. GSM is still underdiagnosed and undertreated despite its prevalence, frequently as a result of patient and healthcare professional embarrassment or ignorance [2–4].

14.3 Epidemiology

A significant percentage of menopausal women suffer from FSD. According to the PRESIDE study, low sexual desire with distress was experienced by 7.4% of women over 65 and 12.3% of women between the ages of 45 and 64. According to research conducted worldwide, the prevalence of FSD ranges from 25% to 43%, with greater rates among women who have undergone surgery to menopause because of the sudden drop in hormones.

Even though it's common, almost 50% of women who experience symptoms don't tell medical professionals about their worries. Cultural taboos, humiliation, and the belief that sexual dysfunction is a natural aspect of aging are some of the obstacles. Healthcare professionals may also encounter difficulties like a lack of training, time limits, and awkwardness when talking about sexual matters.

Menopausal women's FSD is a complicated and common illness that needs medical care. Accurate diagnosis and successful treatment depend on a biopsychosocial approach that takes into account relational, psychological, and medical aspects. Gynecologists need to be prepared to identify and treat FSD to improve midlife women's sexual health and general quality of life.

14.4 Factors affecting Sexual Health in Menopause

Various factors affecting sexual function in menopause are listed below.

- Physical health—changes in skin, hair, muscles, and urogenital region
- Mental health—anxiety, depression, low self-esteem, feeling of decreased attractiveness
- Relationship factors—partner's health, sociocultural factors
- Surgery
- Illness and medication effects on the nerves, blood vessels, hormones, muscles, and erectile tissue can affect the sexual function and sexual response.

- Psychosocial factors: Misconceptions about sex, perception of menopause changes, loss of sexual confidence, personal, emotional, and occupational distress
- Partner's general health or sexual problem
- Sociocultural factors: Cultural, religious expectations and restrictions, life stressors like divorce, death, and economic hardships.

Regardless of age and menopausal status, sexual interest continues for many women. Seventy-six percent of middle-aged women in the SWAN (Study of Women's Health Across the Nation) reported that sex was moderately or extremely important to them. In the Women's Healthy Ageing Project (WHAP) cohort, as an extension of the Melbourne women's midlife health project, a significant decline from 74% to 56% in sexual activity was reported between early postmenopausal women and late postmenopausal women. The decline may be multifactorial. Emotional issues such as anxiety, depression, and low self-esteem, often linked with body image concerns and fear of aging, can lower sexual desire and satisfaction. Relationship dynamics, like poor communication, emotional disconnect, or a partner's health problems, also play a major role in sexual well-being. In many cultures, older women's sexuality is ignored or stigmatized, leading to shame and reluctance to seek help. Healthcare providers must break these myths through education and open dialogue. By routinely asking about sexual health, listening empathetically, and offering evidence-based guidance, clinicians can help women maintain fulfilling sexual lives well into midlife and beyond.

14.4.1 FSD in Menopause

A complex disorder, female sexual dysfunction (FSD) includes recurring or ongoing issues with sexual responsiveness, desire, arousal, orgasm, or pain during sexual activity that lead to severe suffering or interpersonal problems. Hormonal fluctuations, aging-related physiological changes, and psychosocial factors make FSD more common in menopausal women. FSD is nevertheless underdiagnosed and undertreated despite its significant prevalence, frequently as a result of stigma, ignorance, and a lack of clinical expertise.

14.5 Classification of Sexual Dysfunction

A classification system for sexual dysfunctions is given by the Diagnostic and Statistical Manual of Mental Disorders (DSM-5) (Table 14.1). The following are the main categories for women:

For a diagnosis to be made, symptoms must be present in at least 75% of sexual interactions, last for at least 6 months, and cause discomfort.

Table 14.1 Diagnostic and statistical manual of mental disorders

Category	Description	DSM-IV equivalents
Female sexual interest/arousal disorder (FSIAD)	Persistent/recurrent lack of sexual interest, erotic thoughts, initiation, and receptivity to sexual cues	Combined: Hypoactive sexual desire disorder + sexual arousal disorder
Female orgasmic disorder	Difficulty or inability to achieve orgasm despite adequate stimulation and arousal	Female orgasmic disorder
Genito-pelvic pain/penetration disorder	Pain during intercourse, fear/anxiety about penetration, involuntary pelvic muscle tightening	Combined: Dyspareunia + vaginismus
Substance/medication-induced sexual Dysfunction	Sexual dysfunction due to medications or substances (e.g., SSRIs, antihypertensives, hormones)	New category in DSM-5

14.6 Pathophysiology

Hormones, neurotransmitters, and physiological systems interact intimately to govern sexual function in women. Emerging research emphasizes the larger hormonal landscape—including androgens, progesterone, and neurosteroids—that regulates sexual desire, arousal, and satisfaction, even though estrogen insufficiency is a well-known cause of sexual dysfunction in menopausal women. Developing thorough and customized treatment plans requires an understanding of these variables [5].

Menopausal hormonal changes and sexual behavior: Beyond estrogen deficiency

During menopause, hormonal changes—especially the drop in estrogen and androgens—significantly affect a woman's sexual health. Estrogen plays a key role in maintaining vaginal health, lubrication, and blood flow, and its decline leads to symptoms like vaginal dryness, pain during sex (dyspareunia), and increased risk of infections, known collectively as genitourinary syndrome of menopause (GSM). Estrogen also influences brain pathways that regulate mood and sexual arousal. However, estrogen deficiency alone doesn't explain all sexual dysfunctions [6]. Androgens like testosterone, though present in lower levels in women, are crucial for sexual desire and arousal. Their gradual decline with age—especially after surgical menopause—can lead to hypoactive sexual desire disorder (HSDD). Testosterone therapy may help some women, but concerns about safety and side effects limit its widespread use.

Sexual dysfunction in menopausal women is also influenced by aging-related changes like pelvic floor weakening, chronic illnesses (e.g., diabetes, hypertension, depression), and medications such as SSRIs and cardiovascular drugs. These factors can reduce sexual desire, energy, and self-image. Neurosteroids like DHEA, which convert into estrogen and testosterone, also play a role in sexual function by affecting brain regions involved in emotion and arousal. Intravaginal DHEA has shown benefits in improving vaginal health and sexual satisfaction. Overall, sexual well-being in menopause is shaped by a complex interplay of hormones, brain function, physical health, and psychological factors—highlighting the need for personalized, holistic treatment approaches [5].

Psychological factors such as mood swings, anxiety, poor sleep, and body image concerns can lower sexual confidence and desire. Past trauma or mental health issues may resurface during menopause, making sexual health more complex. Relationship quality also plays a major role—emotional closeness, communication, and partner support are essential, but may be disrupted during this phase.

Cultural and social beliefs strongly influence women's views and expression of their sexuality in midlife. In many cultures, older women are discouraged from discussing or seeking help for sexual concerns due to shame or stigma. Religious views, life stressors like caregiving or financial strain, and lack of education or access to care can further limit sexual well-being [7]. Women with higher education and economic independence are more likely to seek help. Gynecologists must create a safe, respectful space for open discussion and be trained in sexual history-taking and counseling.

Addressing psychological, relational, and cultural factors is key to restoring sexual health and improving quality of life for menopausal women.

14.7 Diagnosis

A detailed history is extremely important to make an accurate diagnosis of FSD. Important elements consist of: Inquiry into the frequency of sexual activity, desire, arousal, orgasm, and pain is part of the detailed sexual history. Relationship dynamics and partner health should also be investigated.

The Important Medical and Surgical History: Hormonal state, pelvic surgeries, cancer therapies, and chronic conditions (e.g., diabetes, hypertension) are essential to assist in making a diagnosis.

Sexual dysfunction can be a multifactorial issue, often influenced by various medications across therapeutic domains. Several psychotropic agents are implicated, including antidepressants and mood stabilizers such as selective serotonin reuptake inhibitors (SSRIs), tricyclic antidepressants (TCAs), monoamine oxidase inhibitors (MAOIs), benzodiazepines, lithium, and antipsychotics. These may interfere with neurotransmitter pathways critical to sexual desire and arousal. Cardiovascular medications also contribute, notably beta blockers, digoxin, antilipid agents, and spironolactone, which can impair vascular flow and hormonal balance. Hormonal preparations like oral contraceptives, GnRH agonists, and antiandrogens may suppress endogenous sex hormone production, further dampening libido and sexual responsiveness. Additional contributors include neuroleptics, steroids, antiepileptics, antihistamines, and anticholinergics, each affecting sexual function through diverse mechanisms such as sedation, hormonal disruption, or altered nerve conduction.

Psychosocial assessment is also the key assessment area, which includes the study of interpersonal connections, cultural beliefs, body image, and mental health.

Use of Validated Questionnaires: Instruments like the Decreased Sexual Desire Screener (DSDS) and the Female Sexual Function Index (FSFI) help measure dysfunction and direct treatment.

General and pelvic examinations should be included in the physical examination, with special care paid to pelvic floor integrity, vulvovaginal atrophy, and indications of infection or dermatological disorders. Additionally, quantitative sensory testing in the vulval region can help detect altered sensation or pain, offering insight into potential neurogenic or localized causes of sexual discomfort or dysfunction.

To evaluate underlying physiological contributors, a hormonal profile including estradiol, follicle-stimulating hormone (FSH), luteinizing hormone (LH), prolactin, and thyroid-stimulating hormone (TSH) is essential to identify endocrine imbalances. A lipid panel is also relevant, as dyslipidemia may lead to arterial changes and hypertension, compromising genital blood flow. Genital ultrasonography may also be recommended [8].

14.8 Management: Standardizing Care Through Clinical Guidelines

Comprehensive guidelines for treating sexual dysfunction in midlife women have been given by the European Menopause and Andropause Society (EMAS), the International Society for the Study of Women's Sexual Health (ISSWSH), and the North American Menopause Society (NAMS) [9]. These guidelines highlight regular sexual health screenings throughout menopausal consultations, use of proven instruments like the Decreased Sexual Desire Screener (DSDS) and the Female Sexual Function Index (FSFI), customized treatment programs according to patient preferences, contraindications, and the intensity of symptoms.

These guidelines promote a proactive, patient-centered approach.

14.8.1 Multidisciplinary Management: An Approach Based on Collaboration

First-line treatment for genitourinary syndrome of menopause (GSM) is with local estrogen therapy. When mood or vasomotor symptoms mix with sexual dysfunction, systemic hormone therapy may be considered. Clinicians can tailor treatments beyond traditional estrogen replacement by having an understanding of hormonal impacts. Estrogen, progesterone, and testosterone combination treatments may have complementary effects. Tibolone, a synthetic steroid with estrogenic and androgenic qualities, selective estrogen receptor modulators (SERMs), and more recent medications like bremelanotide and flibanserin increase sexual desire by targeting brain neurotransmitter pathways. Relationship support and psychosexual counseling are incorporated into holistic care.

A multidisciplinary team approach to treatment is the most successful because sexual dysfunction is a complex condition. To address the biological, psychological, and relational aspects of sexual health, specialists from various fields of medicine are required. Gynecologists are in charge of care coordination, hormonal management, and evaluation.

The psychologists and sex therapists use methods including mindfulness, cognitive behavioral therapy (CBT), and psychodynamic counseling to help clients overcome emotional and cognitive obstacles. Targeted exercises and biofeedback are offered by pelvic floor physiotherapists to increase sexual function, decrease pain, and improve muscle tone.

Urologists treat incontinence and other urinary problems that may accompany GSM. Skin disorders that impact sexual comfort and vulvar dermatoses are treated by dermatologists.

Endocrinologists help with complicated hormonal assessments, particularly for women who have many medical conditions.

14.9 Communication and Education

Open communication and education are the first steps toward empowering women. Because of cultural taboos, shame, or fear of rejection, many women are reluctant to talk about sexual difficulties. Using frameworks such as the PLISSIT model (Permission, Limited Information, Specific Suggestions, Intensive Therapy) to direct discussions and interventions, clinicians must provide a secure, nonjudgmental environment for communication. Partners should also get education, which should promote supportive intimacy and assist them in comprehending the mental and physical changes brought on by menopause.

14.10 Comprehensive Treatment Modalities

1. Psychotherapy and Psychosocial Interventions
   - Psychodynamic Therapy: Addresses unconscious conflicts and resistance to change
   - Cognitive Behavioral Therapy (CBT): Identifies and modifies irrational beliefs and dysfunctional thoughts
   - Mindfulness & Relaxation Techniques: Reduces anxiety and enhances body awareness
   - Basic Sexual Counseling:
     - Education on sexuality and human sexual behavior
     - Dispelling myths and misconceptions
     - Partner communication

- Psychosexual Interventions:
  - Sensate focus exercises (Masters & Johnson)
  - Behavior therapy
  - Relaxation exercises

2. Lifestyle Modifications
   - Diet, exercise, sleep hygiene
   - Avoid alcohol, smoking, and medications that impair sexual function
   - Weight reduction and bariatric surgery for obesity-related dysfunction
   - Screening for medications and illnesses affecting sexual function
3. Complementary Therapies
   - Yoga and acupuncture: modest benefits in sexual function and mood
   - Nutraceuticals: L-Arginine, Ginkgo, Maca, Ginseng, Tribulus terrestris, Ashwagandha
     - Mechanism: Improve nitric oxide pathways and blood flow
     - Evidence: Limited; better results when combined with sex therapy
   - Improving Body Image and Self-Esteem
     - Body awareness education
     - Enhancing stimulation through changes in sexual techniques
     - Distraction techniques to reduce anxiety
4. Pelvic Floor Physiotherapy
   - Kegel exercises
   - Biofeedback
   - Targeted muscle training to improve tone and reduce pain
5. Pharmacotherapy

   Hormonal Treatments:
   - Estrogen (local/systemic)
   - Estrogen + Progesterone
   - Tibolone
   - Testosterone
   - DHEA

   Nonhormonal Treatments:
   - Flibanserin
   - Wilysee
   - Sildenafil
   - Buspirone
   - Bupropion
   - Nutraceuticals
6. Surgical and Cosmetic Procedures
   - Pelvic floor repair (PFR)
   - Hymenoplasty
   - Prolapse correction
   - Vaginal rejuvenation
   - Laser treatments
   - Cosmetic injections (G-shot, O-shot)

14.10.1 Role of Communication and Education

14.10.1.1 The PLISSIT Model

An incremental approach to office-based counseling could be a useful approach for practitioners. Women are given:

- Permission (P) to discuss their problems and emotions and to explore solutions
- Then, the practitioner provides limited information (LI), which includes basic sexual function education and/ or resources (e.g., literature, videos, and erotica), and
- Specific suggestions (SS) for addressing the problem in the form of directives and advice
- If the individual needs more intensive treatment (IT) for HSDD, then the practitioner can refer her for individual or couple's therapy
- Creating a nonjudgmental, culturally sensitive environment
- Addressing shame, taboos, and fear of rejection

Partners should also get education, which should promote supportive intimacy and assist them comprehend the mental and physical changes brought on by menopause

14.10.2 Management of GSM

14.10.2.1 Vaginal Moisturizers and Lubricants

Indications

- First-line for mild to moderate vaginal dryness
- Useful when estrogen therapy is contraindicated

Type of Lubricants used for GSM are given below

Type	Features	Examples
Water-based	Gentle, easy to clean, short-lasting	KY Jelly
pH-balanced	Maintains vaginal Ph	–
Silicone-based	Long-lasting, suitable for water play	Astroglide, Silk-n-Slide
Glycerin-based	Sticky texture, plant-derived	KY Jelly

Moisturizers

- Mimic natural secretions
- Hydrate vaginal epithelium
- Effects last 2–3 days

14.10.2.2 Hormonal Therapies

The Various options for hormonal therapy

Type	Indication
Estrogen alone	Women posthysterectomy
Estrogen + Progesterone	Women with intact uterus
Estrogen + Progesterone + Testosterone	GSM with HSDD
Tibolone	Mixed estrogenic, androgenic, progestogenic effects

Mechanism

- Enhances blood flow via nitric oxide and VIP pathways
- Improves lubrication, arousal, clitoral sensitivity, and orgasm
- Modulates sensory thresholds via central nervous system

The various forms of local estrogen therapy for GSM are given in Table 14.2.

Systemic Estrogen Risks

- Venous thromboembolism
- Stroke

Table 14.2 The Various forms of Local Estrogen Therapy for GSM

Delivery route	Medication	Brand name	Dose	FDA-approved dosage regimens	Typical serum estradiol levels
Vaginal creams	17-β estradiol vaginal cream	Estrace vaginal cream	0.1 mg per gram of cream	2–4 g/day for 1–2 weeks and then reduce to 1 g 1–3 times per week	Variable
	Conjugated estrogens vaginal cream	Premarin vaginal cream	0.625 mg per gram of cream	0.5–2 g/day for 21 days and then drug holiday for 7 days OR 0.5 g twice weekly	Variable
Vaginal rings	17-β estradiol	Estring	2 mg	7.5 μg/d for 90 days	7.8 pg/ml
	Estradiol acetate	Femring	12.4 mg	50 mcg/d for 90 days	40.6 pg/ml
		Femring	24.8 mg	100 mcg/day for 90 days	76 pg/ml
Tablet	Estradiol hemihydrate	Vagifem	10 mcg	1 tablet/d for 2 weeks then 1 tablet twice weekly	4.5 pg/ml

14.10.2.3 Selective Estrogen Receptor Modulators (SERMs)

Mechanism

- Tissue-specific agonist/antagonist effects on estrogen receptors

Agents

- Ospemiphene: 60 mg/day for women contraindicated for estrogen
- Bazedoxifene + Conjugated Estrogens (CEE/BZA): Improves Vasomotor Symptoms (VMS), Vulvovaginal Atrophy (VVA), and Bone Health

14.10.2.4 Tibolone

- Estrogenic, androgenic, and progestogenic properties
- Improves sexual function and climacteric symptoms
- Dose: 1.25–2.5 mg/day

14.10.2.5 Androgen Therapy

Testosterone

- Enhances libido and sexual desire
- Especially useful in surgically menopausal women with HSDD
- Safety concerns: Virilization, lipid profile changes, cardiovascular and cognitive risks

Formulations

- 300 mcg/24 h patch
- 1% cream (10 mg/mL)
- 2% gel

Note: Blood levels do not correlate well with clinical outcomes

Dehydroepiandrosterone (DHEA): Moderate to severe dyspareunia can be treated with intravaginal DHEA. It has no systemic hormonal effects and works locally to increase lubrication and regenerate vaginal epithelium [10].

Mechanism

- Prohormone converted to active steroids
- Intravaginal DHEA (Prasterone):
  - Approved for moderate to severe dyspareunia
  - Improves vaginal pH, epithelial thickness, and sexual function

14.10.2.6 Neurotransmitter-Based Therapies

Flibanserin

- 5HT1A agonist and 5HT2A antagonist
- Normalizes serotonin, dopamine, and norepinephrine
- Dose: 100 mg at bedtime
- Approved for HSDD in premenopausal women

Bremelanotide
- Melanocortin receptor agonist
- Subcutaneous injection (1.75 mg) before sexual activity
- Approved for acquired, generalized HSDD

Bupropion
- Norepinephrine and dopamine reuptake inhibitor
- Off-label use for HSDD

Buspirone
- Serotonin and dopamine receptor modulator

Combination Therapies
- Sublingual Testosterone + Sildenafil: Enhances arousal and desire
- Sublingual Testosterone + Buspirone: Targets HSDD

Phosphodiesterate inhibitors: e.g., Sildenafil citrate (Viagra)

Not FDA approved. It can improve genital blood flow through vasodilatation. It can improve arousal.

14.10.2.7 Combination Therapy

(a) Sublingual testosterone and sildenafil in women with HSDD and arousal disorder
(b) Sublingual testosterone with buspirone in HSDD

14.11 New and Developing Treatments: Regenerative Medicine and Cosmetic Gynecology

The subject of menopausal sexual health has recently included creative and regenerative methods in addition to more conventional hormone and psychosexual therapy. These new approaches, which range from physiologically active therapies to cosmetic gynecology, present encouraging options for women who want to improve genital appearance, regain sexual function, and generally improve their quality of life both during and after menopause.

14.11.1 Cosmetic Gynecology

A range of operations targeted at enhancing the vulvovaginal region's beauty and functionality is included in cosmetic gynecology. Many of these treatments, which were once created for aesthetic reasons, have shown promise in treating sexual dysfunction, particularly in postmenopausal women. Procedures such as labiaplasty, clitoral hood reduction, and mons pubis fat reduction can enhance sexual confidence and genital self-image, but they must be performed with ethical awareness and transparent patient counseling.

Laser therapy (CO_2 and Er: YAG lasers) for vaginal rejuvenation increases collagen synthesis, improves tissue suppleness, and increases vaginal wetness. Women with genitourinary syndrome of menopause (GSM), including cancer survivors who are unable to utilize hormonal therapies, benefit most from it [11].

By boosting vascularity and nerve sensitivity, G-Shot and O-Shot (platelet-rich plasma injections into the Grafenberg spot or clitoral region) are intended to improve sexual enjoyment. Despite encouraging anecdotal accounts, thorough clinical trials are still required to confirm efficacy.

14.12 Regenerative Medicine: Cellular Function Restoration

The goal of regenerative therapies is to use biological processes to restore tissue health and function. These consist of Growth factors found in platelet-rich plasma (PRP) that aid in tissue regeneration and repair. When paired with hyaluronic acid, it effectively alleviates vaginal dryness and dyspareunia in breast cancer survivors. PRP may also improve sexual responsiveness and aid in pelvic floor rehabilitation.

Although they are still in the experimental stage and are not yet a standard component of clinical practice, stem cell therapy and tissue engineering are being studied for their potential to rejuvenate pelvic and vaginal tissues.

14.13 Role of Complementary Therapy and Lifestyle Modification

Complementary therapies, including yoga, acupuncture, and nutraceuticals (such as maca, ginseng, and L-arginine), are becoming more and more popular. Although there is little data, these treatments may improve sexual function by promoting hormonal balance, lowering stress, and increasing circulation. Any treatment method must start with lifestyle changes like quitting smoking, managing weight, and pelvic floor physical therapy.

14.14 Conclusion

Sexual health is a key part of a woman's identity and happiness. Especially after menopause, when many women face issues like low desire, vaginal dryness, and pain during sex. These problems can affect their confidence, relationships, and emotional well-being, but are often overlooked. Gynecologists play a key role in starting open conversations, explaining the changes that happen during menopause, and offering help through hormone therapy, lubricants, and counseling. By working with psychologists and other experts, and following clear medical guidelines with compassion, healthcare providers can support women in improving their sexual health and overall quality of life.

Key Points

- Sexual changes during menopause arise from hormonal, psychological, relational, and sociocultural factors—requiring a nuanced, interdisciplinary approach.
- GSM significantly impacts sexual function and quality of life. Routine screening and proactive management—especially with local estrogen therapy—are essential.
- Gynecologists should ensure safe, empathetic spaces for discussing sexual concerns, challenging stigma, and validating diverse experiences of aging and intimacy.
- Treatment should be tailored to each woman's symptoms, preferences, and risk profile balancing hormonal, nonhormonal, and psychosexual interventions.
- Addressing sexuality is central to comprehensive menopausal care and reflects a commitment to patient-centered, dignified practice.

Conflicts of Interest None

Long Answer Questions (LAQs)

1. Describe the role of hormones in menopausal sexual dysfunction?
2. How do you evaluate a case of hypoactive sexual desire disorder in a perimenopausal woman?
3. What are the commonly used sexual functionary questionnaires that can be utilized by a practitioner?
4. Describe hormonal treatment of menopausal sexual dysfunction?

Short Answer Questions (SAQs)

1. What is DSM -5 classification of sexual dysfunction?
2. Describe the a) biopsychosocial model. b) PLISSIT Model?
3. Vaginal moisturizers and lubricants?
4. Write briefly about Flibanserin, the Female Viagra?

Multiple Choice Questions (MCQs)

1. Sexual Health is for?

   A. Procreation
   B. Recreation
   C. Relation
   D. All of the above

2. Menopause is the end of sex life?
   - A. True
   - B. False
3. Sexual problems in menopausal women are due?
   - A. Oestrogen decline
   - B. Testosterone decline
   - C. Cortisol deficiency
   - D. All of the above
4. Present classification of sexual dysfunction is as per?
   - A. DSM – 3
   - B. DSM – 4
   - C. DSM-5
   - D. DSM-6

   (DSM – Diagnostic and Statistical Manual of American Psychiatric Association)
5. What Is Female Viagra?
   - A. Flibanserin
   - B. Bremelanotide
   - C. Buspirone
   - D. Buspirone
6. The treatment of choice for Genitourinary Syndrome of Menopause (GSM)?
   - A. Local oestrogen therapy
   - B. Systemic oestrogen therapy
   - C. Testosterone
7. Masters & Johnsons sex therapy is known?
   - A. Sensate focus exercises
   - B. Counselling
   - C. PLISSIT
8. Hypoactive sexual desire disorder due to surgical menopause responds well to?
   - A. Testosterone,
   - B. Estrogen
   - C. Flibanserine,
   - D. All of the above

Answers

1. A
2. B
3. D
4. C
5. A
6. A
7. A
8. D

References

1. Roeca C, Al-Safi Z, Santoro N. The postmenopausal women. In: Feingold KR, Ahmed SF, Anawalt B, Blackman MR, Boyce A, Chrousos G, et al., editors. Endotext [Internet]. South Dartmouth: MDText.com, Inc.; 2000. [cited 2025 Aug 15].
2. Scavello I, Maseroli E, Di Stasi V, Vignozzi L. Sexual health in menopause. Medicina (Kaunas). 2019;55(9):559.
3. Shifren JL. Genitourinary syndrome of menopause. Clin Obstet Gynecol. 2018;61(3):508–16.
4. Wasnik VB, Acharya N, Mohammad S. Genitourinary syndrome of menopause: a narrative review focusing on its effects on the sexual health and quality of life of women. Cureus. 15(11):e48143.
5. Cameron JL. Hormonal mediation of physiological and behavioral processes that influence fertility. In: Offspring: human fertility behavior in biodemographic perspective [Internet]. National Academies Press; 2003. [cited 2025 Aug 15].
6. Thornton K, Chervenak J, Neal-Perry G. Menopause and sexuality. Endocrinol Metab Clin N Am. 2015;44(3):649–61.
7. Namazi M, Sadeghi R, Behboodi Moghadam Z. Social determinants of health in menopause: an integrative review. Int J Women's Health. 2019;11:637–47.
8. Parish SJ, Hahn SR, Goldstein SW, Giraldi A, Kingsberg SA, Larkin L, et al. The International Society for the Study of women's sexual health process of care for the identification of sexual concerns and problems in women. Mayo Clin Proc. 2019;94(5):842–56.
9. Krakowsky Y, Grober ED. A practical guide to female sexual dysfunction: an evidence-based review for physicians in Canada. Can Urol Assoc J. 2018;12(6):211–6.
10. Berndt S, Vischer S, Turzi A, Dällenbach P. Optimizing the regenerative potential of vaginal fibroblasts. the role of autologous platelet-rich plasma and hyaluronic acid in vitro. Maturitas. 2025;194:108196.
11. Capito L, Antsaklis A, Gupte S, The FIGO Committee on Ethical Aspects of Human Reproduction and Women's Health. FIGO statement: cosmetic genital surgery. Int J Gynecol Obstet. 2025;170(1):11–4.

Dental Hygiene in Menopause

15

Mrinalini Ahuja

Abstract

Menopause is marked by reduction in estrogen and progesterone levels. This influences systemic and oral health. The hormonal decline significantly affects the dental tissues, as there are estrogen receptors present in oral mucosa, salivary glands, gingiva, and jawbones. Postmenopausal women are commonly faced with xerostomia, burning mouth syndrome, altered taste perception, periodontal disease, and osteoporosis-related bone loss leading to tooth mobility or loss. These changes compromise quality of life and increase susceptibility to dental caries, mucosal discomfort, and oral infections. These conditions are exacerbated by factors such as medications, nutritional deficiencies, systemic illnesses, and lifestyle habits.

Preventive and management strategies include meticulous oral hygiene, topical fluoride use, dietary modifications with adequate calcium and vitamin D, and regular dental visits for early detection of periodontal and mucosal conditions. Hormone replacement therapy although beneficial for oral symptoms, individualized risk–benefit evaluation is essential. Importantly, comprehensive care can be provided only by collaboration between dental professionals and gynecologists. By recognizing the oral implications of menopause, healthcare providers can enhance both systemic and oral health outcomes in midlife women.

Keywords

Dental hygiene · Postmenopausal women · Xerostomia · Burning mouth syndrome

M. Ahuja (✉)
Santosh Dental College, Ghaziabad, Uttar Pradesh, India

R. Malik et al. (eds.), *Menopause Essentials*,
https://doi.org/10.1007/978-981-95-7498-8_15

15.1 Introduction

Menopause is the permanent cessation of menstruation for 12 consecutive months. This typically occurs between 45 and 55 years of age. The transition is marked by a sharp reduction in production of estrogen and progesterone levels, bringing systemic changes, and ends up affecting nearly every organ system [1]. These hormonal changes impact the quality of life and have important implications for overall health. Menopause may lead to changes in the oral cavity that mirror systemic effects as oral and dental tissues are also hormone-sensitive. Estrogen receptors are present in oral mucosa, salivary glands, bone, and gingival tissues [2]. With estrogen deficiency, the oral cavity may undergo adaptive changes:

- Gums—more susceptible to plaque and inflammation.
- Saliva—composition or flow can alter.
- Bone density in the jaws—may decrease [3].

As a result, menopausal women often face unique oral health challenges [4]. This chapter provides an overview of menopause-related oral health concerns and dental hygiene considerations.

15.2 Oral Health Concerns in Menopause

15.2.1 Impact of Estrogen Deficiency on Oral Health

During menopause, the hormonal milieu—which is characterized by low estrogen and progesterone—has a direct impact on oral tissues.

Normally, the estrogen helps maintain the integrity of the oral mucosa, salivary gland function, and the skeletal system (which includes the maxilla and mandible, as well as the periodontium). Estrogen plays a role in maintaining the integrity of oral mucosa, salivary gland function, and the skeletal system (including the jawbones and the periodontium). With estrogen deficiency, several physiological changes occur in the oral cavity:

1. The oral mucosal epithelium may become thinner and less keratinized, salivary gland secretions can be altered, and during bone turnover, resorption is more rapid than deposition [3].
2. In gingival tissue, periodontal ligament cells, and jaw bone osteoblasts, all have been identified with estrogen receptors [2], and so, the drop in estrogen during menopause can make the gums and oral mucosa more susceptible to inflammation and injury. The gingiva may appear dry or shiny and can bleed more easily, which is referred to as menopausal gingivostomatitis. The gingival tissues become pale or erythematous and easily bleed causing discomfort [5]. These changes possibly happen because of reduced local estrogenic effect, which leads to decreased collagen content and reduced microvascular supply in oral tissues.

3. Increased osteoclastic activity happens during menopause throughout the skeleton. This consequently leads to accelerated bone loss in the alveolar bone that supports the teeth. Higher levels of bone resorption activity are observed in postmenopausal women due to the absence of estrogen's protective effect [6]. If systemic osteoporosis develops, density of jaw bones reduces, potentially reducing the bony support for teeth. This can manifest as greater alveolar resorption, and in severe cases, it may also cause tooth loss. Studies show that women with osteoporosis may have more enhanced jawbone loss and an increased risk of tooth loss [5]. However, this may also be due to other factors—age, genetics, and oral hygiene practices—as they may influence periodontal health. It is clear that maintaining hormonal and bone health is an important component of preserving oral health in menopause.

15.3 Common Oral Manifestations of Menopause

15.3.1 Xerostomia (Dry Mouth)

Xerostomia is one of the most common complaints in postmenopausal women [4]. Patients often complain of a dry, sticky feeling in the mouth or throat, difficulty swallowing dry foods or needing frequent sips of water. This can be either due to hyposalivation or saliva composition alteration, which is associated with hormonal shifts.

Estrogen receptors present in salivary gland tissue suggest that menopause could influence the salivary production [2]. Some studies have found reduction in the salivary flow rates in menopausal women along with the changes in saliva electrolytes and proteins. For example, one study noted a decrease in the production of saliva, with increased salivary immunoglobulin A (IgA) and total protein in menopausal participants [7]. Clinically, approximately 25% of menopausal women report dry mouth symptoms [4]. However, roughly only 33% of symptomatic women show true glandular hypofunction on testing. In healthy women, some studies (e.g., Ship et al.) have found no significant difference in unstimulated salivary flow between premenopausal and postmenopausal women [7]. This is suggestive of factors like medications, stress or other health conditions may also contribute to xerostomia.

No matter what the etiology is, xerostomia can have multiple oral consequences. Saliva is protective in nature as it helps with oral cleansing, buffering acids and antimicrobial defense. Reduced saliva leads to a dry oral mucosa, making it more vulnerable to ulceration, sensitivity and infection. Patients with dry mouth often develop increased incidence of dental caries (especially root caries). Due to lack of salivary lubrication they may also have trouble wearing dentures. Fungal infections such as oral candidiasis thrive in a dry environment and are seen often in these conditions [5].

When there is severe dry mouth accompanied by salivary gland enlargement or systemic dryness (eyes, etc.) in a postmenopausal woman, Sjögren's syndrome (an autoimmune exocrinopathy) should be considered as a differential diagnosis. Serologic tests and salivary gland biopsy are required for final diagnosis.

Xerostomia (dry mouth): The tongue and oral mucosa appear dry with a cracked, dehydrated surface due to reduced salivary flow. Postmenopausal women commonly report dry mouth, which can increase the risk of dental caries and oral infections.

Management of Xerostomia

- This requires symptomatic relief and prevention of complications. The aim is to keep the mouth moist, which can be done by increasing frequency of water intake and sugar-free chewing gum or lozenges (which will stimulate the salivary glands).
- For temporary moisture, over-the-counter saliva substitutes or gels (biomimetic lubricants) can be used.
- However, in more severe cases, sialogogues like Pilocarpine or Cevimeline may be prescribed [2].
- As the caries risk increases, patients should be advised on meticulous oral hygiene and regular dental visits. Using fluoride toothpaste or fluoride mouthwashes can help reduce the incidence of dental caries. Interestingly, humidifier at night is helpful to reduce oral dryness during sleep [4].
- With hormone replacement therapy (HRT), some women noted an alleviation of symptoms. Up to 45% of women on HRT have reported reduced oral discomfort as well as increased salivary flow [7]. Even though this is not completely correctible, systemic estrogen therapy may partially improve xerostomic symptoms in certain individuals [3].

Overall, managing dry mouth in menopause is about keeping the mouth well hydrated, preventing dental disease, and addressing any underlying causes.

15.3.2 Burning Mouth Syndrome (BMS)

Burning mouth syndrome is another common oral complaint during menopause and is often seen with xerostomia. BMS is defined as a chronic burning, scalding, or tingling sensation in the oral mucosa, typically in the absence of any visible lesions or abnormalities on examination. Areas commonly affected include the tongue (especially the tip and lateral borders) but can also involve the lips, palate, or widespread areas of the mouth.

This is commonly seen in females. The female-to-male ratio is as high as 7:1 [3]. This may be due to hormonal changes as most BMS patients are menopausal middle-aged women. The distinguishing symptom is bilateral burning pain that can range from moderate to severe, often worsening as the day progresses. Individuals with this condition often describe a scorching or burning sensation in the mouth, similar to the feeling of having consumed a hot liquid. Associated symptoms can include disruptions in taste, such as experiencing bitter or metallic flavors, or a reduction in the ability to taste, along with a sensation of dryness in the mouth [4]. A notable characteristic that distinguishes this condition from other oral issues is that a clinical examination typically shows no visible abnormalities or pathology in the oral tissues, such as ulcers or redness.

The etiology of primary BMS is not fully understood, but menopause is considered a significant risk factor. One of the theories suggests hormonal changes (especially estrogen deficiency) can alter the pain perception or neurosensory function in the oral mucosa.

Most patients of BMS have anxiety and depression, suggesting that psychological factors may have an impact, though it's often unclear if they are causes or results of the chronic pain. Interestingly, many women with BMS have nutritional deficiencies (low B vitamins, iron, folate) or underlying conditions like hypothyroidism or diabetes, so a thorough systemic workup is important to identify secondary causes. If an underlying cause is found (e.g., candidiasis, Vitamin B12 deficiency, lichen planus, etc.) and this condition is treated, the patient is relived of their burning mouth symptoms. In such cases, it is called secondary burning mouth syndrome. The true etiology of BMS is unidentifiable and it is usually a diagnosis of exclusion [3].

Management of BMS: Managing BMS can be challenging and typically focuses on symptom relief. First, all local aggravating factors (sharp teeth, oral habits, vitamin deficiencies, dry mouth, etc.) should be treated. Topical therapies such as mouthrinses containing anesthetics (e.g., viscous lidocaine) or capsaicin rinse which may desensitize nerve endings provide temporary relief. Surprisingly, low dose clonazepam, when dissolved in the mouth without swallowing, has been helpful for many patients. Systemic clonazepam or tricyclic antidepressants (like amitriptyline or nortriptyline in low doses) are also used in managing BMS pain, by altering the neuropathic pain pathways.

Women with atrophic mucosa are greatly benefitted by using HRTs to improve BMS. Patients undergoing HRT complain less of oral burning and taste complaints, though this is not a universal effect. For a holistic management, we should be aware that unexplained oral burning in a menopausal patient may be BMS and a multidisciplinary approach (involving dental specialists, pain specialists, and possibly psychologists) [3].

15.3.3 Periodontitis and Gum Changes

With decline in estrogen in menopausal women, there is a negative impact on the gingiva and periodontal tissue. This is commonly associated with gingivitis, receding gums and rarely tooth mobility. As estrogen leads to an exaggerated inflammatory response, the oral tissue has a higher reaction to plaque and calculus, meanwhile reducing the healing capacity of the periodontal tissues [6].

In the menopausal age group, women have gums that appear dry, pale, or reddened and bleed easily on probing. This condition is termed menopausal gingivostomatitis [5].

There is a significant link in periodontitis and menopause. However, this may be attributed to age as well. So disentangling age effects from hormonal effects is challenging [6]. Some studies have reported that postmenopausal women on HRT have better periodontal health than those who aren't. It was reported that women not on HRT had deeper periodontal pockets, clinical loss of attachment of gingiva and even fewer teeth (due to loosening of gingiva). In contrast, postmenopausal women on hormone replacement therapy (HRT) often show periodontal health more comparable to premenopausal women.

Estrogen helps regulate the immune response and maintains bone density. Estrogen deficiency can contribute to periodontal bone loss. HRT might be associated with preservation of periodontal bone. The Women's Health Initiative and other large studies found that current HRT users had a much lower risk of tooth loss than nonusers (one analysis showed a 24% reduction in risk of tooth loss). Moreover, cross-sectional studies in populations have noted that postmenopausal women on estrogen therapy tend to have more teeth present than those not on therapy. However, not all researchers agree—other factors like oral hygiene practices, smoking, and calcium/vitamin D intake also play major roles in periodontal outcomes [5].

Menopausal women should be counseled on observing persistent gingival bleeding, gum recession or loosening of teeth, they must visit a professional due to rapid rate of progression of inflammation.

15.3.4 Osteoporosis-Related Tooth Loss

Due to estrogen deficiency, osteoporosis is commonly observed in postmenopausal women, this unfortunately affects the maxilla and mandible as well. The bone mineral density reduces, making the resorption rates much faster, especially in when chronic periodontal inflammation is present too [6]. This can result in tooth instability or tooth loss over time.

In edentulous women, as there is an acceleration of the resorption rate of the residual ridge, a lot of women are left with ill-fitting dentures. It's important to clarify that osteoporosis itself does not cause cavities or gum disease, but it creates a bone environment that is vulnerable to inflammation and stress. Studies have shown that women with more fractures due to osteoporosis tend to have fewer teeth, showing a direct link between bone mineral density and oral health [5]. Therefore, effective management of osteoporosis may positively influence oral outcomes.

Another factor to consider: the pharmacological treatment of osteoporosis, antiresorptive medications (like bisphosphonates or denosumab) can rarely lead to a condition called medication-related osteonecrosis of the jaw (MRONJ). MRONJ is an uncommon but serious adverse effect where an area of jawbone is exposed and fails to heal, often after a dental extraction or trauma, in a patient on these medications. Therefore, postmenopausal women receiving treatment for osteoporosis should maintain meticulous dental hygiene and get any dental work involving bone healing done (like dental implants) before starting therapy to minimize risks [6]. Gynecologists should coordinate with dentists in such cases—for a dental examination and address any active dental infections or extractions prior to therapy. While the incidence of MRONJ in osteoporosis patients is very low, it is still valuable to make the patient aware.

Prevention can be done easily by optimizing bone health (with diet and medications as appropriate) and preventing periodontal disease. For the patient, maintaining a diet rich in calcium and vitamin D is imperative [6]. Regular dental examinations can catch early signs of bone changes in the jaw—dentists may even notice thinning of jawbone in dental X-rays as an early indicator of low bone density [5].

15.3.5 Other Oral and Dental Issues

During menopause, women may encounter various oral health issues, not all of which are universally experienced. Some women report unexplained oral discomfort or pain, potentially linked to mucosal changes or minor neuropathic alterations. Others experience changes in taste perception, such as a persistent metallic or bitter taste, known as dysgeusia. This condition may be associated with dry mouth, burning mouth syndrome (BMS), or zinc deficiency, and often resolves with time or targeted treatment of underlying causes, such as ulcers or redness.

There is also a higher incidence of certain oral mucosal disorders around this time. Even conditions like oral lichen planus often have an onset in the 40 s–50 s and have a female predominance [5]. Even though it is not caused by menopause, the stress and immune changes around this age might trigger lichen planus. Lichen planus is a condition in which the patient presents with white lacy patches or erosive lesions in the mouth, commonly associated with burning sensations. Similarly, aphthous ulcers (canker sores) could be triggered by stress or nutritional deficiencies common in menopausal women (like B12 or folate deficiency). If a patient presents with such lesions, they should be properly evaluated. Management includes topical steroids or other immunomodulatory medications if needed [3].

High stress can result in parafunctional habits like bruxism or teeth grinding, leading to tooth wear and/or temporomandibular joint (TMJ) pain. Additionally, some women may neglect oral care when dealing with significant menopausal symptoms or mood disorders. Clinicians should take a holistic view—addressing mental health and stress can have positive effects on oral health behaviors.

15.3.6 Risk Factors for Poor Dental Hygiene during Menopause

Recognizing these risk factors is important for both prevention and management:

- Inadequate Oral Hygiene Practices: These habits need to be adjusted with age. The inflammatory response increases with estrogen and so do periodontal diseases. Effective oral hygiene practices include brushing as well as flossing. The plaque build-up in this age group can very aggressively harm the gingival and periodontal tissue. As this age group is also associated with tooth loss, meticulous cleaning of the prosthesis/denture is recommended on the daily [2].

- Diet and Nutrition: Dietary changes during menopause can impact oral health. Women experiencing mood swings or sleep disturbances might "midnight snack" on foods high in sugar. With already low secretion of saliva, the caries index can massively increase. Others may have reduced appetite and lower intake of vitamins—both calcium and vitamin D intake is crucial in midlife to support bone health. If there is a deficiency, it can worsen osteoporotic changes and by extension, affect jawbone density [6]. Deficiency of B-complex vitamins, iron, or zinc can lead to glossitis, mouth soreness, or delayed oral tissue healing.
- Medications: Menopausal women may be on various medications for chronic conditions (e.g., antihypertensives, antidepressants, anxiolytics). A common side effect associated with these drugs is dry mouth. Anticholinergic drugs reduce salivary flow. Diuretics and beta-blockers or SSRIs and other antidepressants frequently cause xerostomia as well. This further adds to the dryness that might already be present due to menopause. Some medications, like calcium channel blockers can cause gingival hyperplasia and even alter taste.
- Smoking and Alcohol Use: In menopausal women, smoking can further reduce salivary flow, impair healing of gum tissue, exacerbate bone loss and even affect bone density, causing loss of teeth. Similarly, excessive alcohol intake causes dehydration, which in turn may accentuate the dry mouth, as well as increase the risk for oral cancers when combined with tobacco [8].
- Low Awareness and Dental Care Utilization: Unfortunately, oral health is sometimes neglected by patients and even healthcare providers during menopause. Attention is often focused on managing systemic complications, while dental check-ups might be overlooked. According to the National Oral Health Programme in India, low awareness among the population and care providers has led to neglect of dental care, especially in adults [8]. One survey indicated that a majority of women over 40 do not stick to twice-yearly dental visits as recommended [9]. This lack of awareness is a risk factor in itself, as women may not report oral symptoms to their doctors or seek care in a timely manner.
- Psychosocial Factors: Menopause can be a stressful period due to physical symptoms and life changes. Stress and anxiety can lead to oral habits like bruxism (teeth grinding) or clenching, which cause tooth wear, jaw pain, and contribute to TMJ disorders. High stress can also influence immune function and eventually triggering conditions like recurrent oral ulcers or lichen planus as mentioned. Moreover, depression or low motivation might lead some women to be less diligent with self-care, including oral hygiene.
- Systemic Conditions: Around the age of menopause, incidence of systemic conditions like type 2 diabetes increases. Diabetes, especially if uncontrolled, is a major risk factor for periodontal disease and oral infections. Autoimmune conditions (rheumatoid arthritis, Sjögren's syndrome, thyroid disorders) often manifest in midlife women and can affect oral health (e.g., Sjögren's causes severe dry mouth; rheumatoid arthritis in the hands can make brushing/flossing difficult).

15.4 General Dental Hygiene Measures for Menopausal Women

15.4.1 Routine Oral Hygiene Practices

Adhering to a consistent and thorough oral hygiene routine is the first line of defense against dental problems. Menopausal women should be encouraged to:

- Brush Effectively: Brush teeth at least twice a day with a fluoride toothpaste. Use a soft-bristled toothbrush to avoid gum abrasion, especially if gums are fragile or receding. Electric toothbrushes can be helpful for those with limited manual dexterity or arthritis. This is necessary to counter the reduction in the salivary flow and its cleansing action [2].
- Floss Daily: Flossing (or use of interdental cleaners like water flossers or interdental brushes) once a day helps clean between teeth and under the gumline where toothbrush bristles can't reach. This is vital for preventing interdental cavities and periodontal pockets. These areas are most prone to decay due to dry mouth [2].
- Manage Dry Mouth in Hygiene Routine: In case the patient has xerostomia, some small adjustments improve comfort during oral care. For instance, rinsing the mouth with water or a moisturizing mouthrinse before brushing can help lubricate tissues. Using toothpaste for sensitive mouths, without sodium lauryl sulfate (surfactant), may reduce irritation. Also, a fluoride mouthwash or high-fluoride prescription toothpaste (5000 ppm fluoride) can be used daily to remineralize enamel against caries in the context of dry mouth [4]. The Indian Dental Association recommends supplemental topical fluoride and even custom trays for applying fluoride gel at home or in the dental office in patients with high caries risk due to hyposalivation [2].
- Dentures: If the patient wears any removable dentures, strict hygiene for those is necessary. Removable dentures, if not cleaned can cause fungal infections like denture stomatitis. Menopausal dry mouth can cause more friction and sore spots under dentures, so keeping them clean and well-fitting (with periodic dentist checks for adjustments or reline) is important. Additionally, the adjacent teeth on which the partial denture rests will be more prone to caries. The small gap between the tooth and the denture acting as a pocket for food to get stuck and along with hyposalivation its a recipe for dental caries.
- Regular Dental Check-ups and Cleanings: Professional dental visits at least twice per year are advised. Dental professionals can perform thorough cleanings to remove tartar (calculus) that contributes to gum disease. They also conduct oral exams to monitor for any signs of cavities, gum detachment, or oral lesions. Early detection of problems means simpler and more successful treatment [1].

15.4.2 Dietary and Lifestyle Recommendations

During menopause, nutrition and lifestyle play a vital role in oral health. Some dietary adjustments not only improve general health (bone health, cardiovascular health) but also directly benefit the teeth and gums:

1. Ensure Adequate Calcium and Vitamin D: Supports alveolar bone maintenance and overall tooth retention [6].
2. Limit Sugary and Acidic Foods: Emphasis on a diet that's low in fermentable carbs and high in fiber [3].
3. Balanced Diet Rich in Nutrients: Adequate protein intake is important for tissue repair and immune function. Vitamins A and C are needed for mucosal and collagen health. Additionally, fruits and vegetables mechanically help clean teeth when chewed. Crunchy fruits and veggies can stimulate saliva and naturally scrub tooth surfaces. Folic acid and B-vitamin rich foods may help in maintaining healthy gums. Conversely, extremely spicy or salty foods might aggravate oral burning in susceptible women and might be moderated if a patient has BMS [3].
4. Avoid Tobacco and Moderate Alcohol [8].
5. Phytoestrogens and Diet: Some have speculated that phytoestrogens might help alleviate menopausal symptoms. Stay Hydrated and Use Sugar-Free Chewing Aids: For those with dry mouth, sipping water often and sucking on sugar-free mints or xylitol-sweetened candies can provide relief and also reduce cavity risk [3].
6. Exercise and Health Maintenance [6].

Key Points Summary

1. Menopause and Oral Health: Menopause is associated with estrogen deficiency that can adversely affect the oral cavity. Common oral manifestations include dry mouth (xerostomia), burning mouth syndrome (BMS), altered taste sensation, and a higher risk of gum disease and tooth loss due to bone loss. Gynecologists should be aware that oral discomfort (burning, pain, dryness) can be part of menopausal symptoms.
2. Estrogen Deficiency Effects: Estrogen receptors in oral tissues mean menopause can lead to thinner oral mucosa, reduced salivary secretion, and accelerated alveolar bone resorption. Consequently, postmenopausal women may experience menopausal gingivostomatitis (dry, easily bleeding gums) and have an increased prevalence of periodontitis unless mitigated by good oral care or hormone therapy.
3. Importance of Oral Hygiene and Diet: Diligent oral hygiene (brushing twice daily with fluoride toothpaste, daily flossing) and a noncariogenic diet (low sugar, adequate calcium/Vitamin D) are crucial in menopause. These measures counteract the higher caries risk from dry mouth and support bone and gum

health. Regular dental check-ups (every 6 months) and professional cleanings should be maintained or increased in frequency if periodontal issues exist.

4. Collaborative Care: Gynecologists should incorporate oral health screening questions during menopause evaluations and encourage patients to seek dental care for any issues. Referral to a dentist for persistent dry mouth, oral lesions, or periodontal concerns is recommended. Likewise, gynecologists should inform dentists if a patient is on therapies like bisphosphonates or HRT. A team approach (physician + dentist) ensures comprehensive care—for example, treating periodontal disease and optimizing calcium/Vitamin D and osteoporosis management together help preserve teeth.
5. Therapeutic Considerations: Hormone replacement therapy can improve some oral parameters (like reducing tooth loss risk and possibly alleviating burning mouth symptoms), but it is prescribed based on overall indications. Saliva substitutes, sialogogues (pilocarpine), topical fluoride, and antifungals are useful dental treatments for managing xerostomia and its complications.

Long Answer Questions (LAQs)

1. Discuss the oral manifestations associated with menopause. Explain the role of estrogen in maintaining oral health and describe how its deficiency impacts the periodontium, salivary glands, and oral mucosa.
2. What is burning mouth syndrome (BMS)? Elaborate on its etiology, clinical features, diagnostic approach, and the multidisciplinary management strategies for menopausal women.
3. Describe xerostomia in postmenopausal women. Include its causes, associated complications, differential diagnoses, and current management protocols.
4. Explain the relationship between postmenopausal osteoporosis and oral health. How do bisphosphonates affect dental treatment planning in these patients?

Short Answer Questions (SAQs)

1. What is menopausal gingivostomatitis? Describe its signs, symptoms, and possible underlying pathophysiology.
2. List and explain the modifiable risk factors for poor oral health during menopause. What precautions should be taken before initiating antiresorptive therapy (like bisphosphonates) in menopausal women from a dental perspective?
3. How can hormonal replacement therapy influence oral health in postmenopausal women?
4. Explain how psychological changes during menopause can indirectly affect oral health.

Multiple Choice Questions (MCQs)

1. Which of the following oral symptoms is most commonly reported by post-menopausal women?
   A. Halitosis
   B. Xerostomia
   C. Herpes labialis
   D. Glossopharyngeal neuralgia
2. Burning mouth syndrome (BMS) is best characterized by:
   A. Burning sensation with visible ulcers
   B. Unilateral oral burning with viral cause
   C. Bilateral burning pain with normal oral examination
   D. Pain only when eating spicy food
3. Estrogen receptors are NOT found in which of the following oral tissues?
   A. Gingival tissues
   B. Enamel
   C. Salivary glands
   D. Alveolar bone
4. Menopausal gingivostomatitis is typically associated with:
   A. Blue discoloration of gums
   B. Pale or erythematous gums with easy bleeding
   C. Excessive gingival hyperplasia
   D. Spontaneous gum regeneration
5. Which of the following medications is most likely to cause medication-related osteonecrosis of the jaw (MRONJ)?
   A. Calcium carbonate
   B. Pilocarpine
   C. Bisphosphonates
   D. Ibuprofen
6. Which of the following is a common oral fungal infection seen in menopausal women with dry mouth?
   A. Herpangina
   B. Oral candidiasis
   C. Hairy leukoplakia
   D. Actinomycosis
7. Which hormone's deficiency is primarily responsible for oral mucosal thinning during menopause?
   A. Progesterone

   B. Cortisol
   C. Estrogen
   D. Testosterone

8. Which lifestyle habit worsens both xerostomia and periodontal bone loss in menopausal women?

   A. Vegan diet
   B. Yoga practice
   C. Smoking
   D. Intermittent fasting

9. In the management of xerostomia, which of the following is used as a sialogogue?

   A. Metronidazole
   B. Chlorhexidine
   C. Pilocarpine
   D. Fluconazole

10. A 54-year-old woman presents with tooth mobility and alveolar bone loss. She is postmenopausal and has a history of hip fracture. What underlying systemic condition should be suspected?

   A. Diabetes mellitus
   B. Sjögren's syndrome
   C. Osteoporosis
   D. Thyroid carcinoma

Answers

1. B
2. C
3. B
4. B
5. C
6. B
7. C
8. C
9. C
10. C

References

1. Mehta M, Haldiya KR, Bhatia P, et al. Clinical Practice Guidelines on Menopause (IMS 2020–21): an executive summary and recommendations. J Midlife Health. 2021;12(1):9–26.
2. Sen S, Mandal A, Dutta A. Oral manifestation and its management in postmenopausal women: an integrated review. J Int Soc Prev Community Dent. 2020;10(4):431–8.
3. Friedlander AH. The physiology, medical management and oral implications of menopause. J Am Dent Assoc. 2002;133(1):73–81.
4. Dutt P, Chaudhary K, Kumar P. Oral health and menopause: a comprehensive review on current knowledge and associated dental management. Ann Med Health Sci Res. 2013;3(3):320–3.
5. López-Marcos JF. Menopause and oral health. Med Oral Patol Oral Cir Bucal. 2005;10(2):130–5.
6. Jafri Z, Bhardwaj A, Sawai M, Sultan N. Influence of female sex hormones on periodontium: A case series. J Midlife Health. 2015;6(1):41–4.
7. Ship JA, et al. Salivary function and menopause. J Gerontol. 1991.
8. World Health Organization. Oral health. WHO Fact Sheet [Internet]. 2022 [cited 2025 Mar 9].
9. Sharma N, Bhat A. Oral health considerations in postmenopausal women. J Obstet Gynaecol India. 2016;66(4):246–51.

Hormone Therapy at Menopause

16

Meeta Meeta, Tanvir Tanvir, and Akanshi Madan

Abstract

Menopausal hormone therapy (MHT) is an established first-line therapy for moderate to severe vasomotor symptoms and genitourinary syndrome of menopause (GSM), and it helps maintain bone density to prevent osteoporosis. MHT typically consists of estrogen (e.g., 17β-estradiol or conjugated equine estrogens) with addition of a progestogen for women with a uterus. It can be administered orally or transdermally for systemic relief, or via low-dose vaginal estrogen for isolated GSM symptoms. Therapy should be individualized in terms of patient selection, timing, dose, and route: initiating MHT within 10 years of menopause onset or before age 60 optimizes benefits and minimizes risks. MHT effectively alleviates hot flashes (~90% reduction) and urogenital atrophy, prevents bone loss and fractures, and may confer metabolic and mood benefits, thereby improving quality of life. Adverse effects include nausea, bloating, and mood swings; prolonged or late-initiated therapy can increase risks of breast cancer, venous thromboembolism, and stroke. Absolute contraindications include estrogen-dependent malignancies, unexplained vaginal bleeding, and active thromboembolic or cardiovascular disease. Newer alternatives such as tibolone (a synthetic steroid) and estetrol (a novel estrogen) are being explored to expand therapeutic options. Overall, when used judiciously in appropriate candidates, MHT safely improves menopausal symptom control and quality of life.

Keywords

Menopausal hormone therapy · Vasomotor symptoms · Osteoporosis

M. Meeta (✉) · T. Tanvir · A. Madan
Tanvir Hospital, Hyderabad, Telangana, India

R. Malik et al. (eds.), *Menopause Essentials*,
https://doi.org/10.1007/978-981-95-7498-8_16

16.1 Introduction

Menopause is a natural and an inevitable event, with similar physiological changes, yet in some women, the immediate effects and sequelae of estrogen deficiency are profound and may need pharmacological intervention. The role of menopause hormone therapy (MHT) at menopause transition and post menopause as a safe treatment option for women with vasomotor symptoms (VMS) and without contraindications is established. MHT also maintains bone and urogenital health by reducing fracture risk and prevents the atrophic changes of genitourinary syndrome (GSM) of menopause [1].

It needs to be understood that there is biological variability in the response of women to endogenous estrogen and exogenous estrogen therapy. It has been shown that the physiological and pharmacological response to estrogen varies at different phases of a women's life and is modulated by her health status, presence of comorbidities, genetics, and lifestyle [2]. The challenge lies in choosing the right woman, right combination, right dose, right route, and the right regime. Prescribing MHT is an art based on science, needs to be individualized by offering the low, effective and adjustive dose to the woman and has to be monitored.

The prescription of MHT showed a precipitous decline of use of MHT from 8.6% before WHI to 1.9% after the Women's Health Initiative (WHI), due to the hasty release of the inappropriately analyzed data from the WHI study in 2002. Despite the proven efficacy and safety of MHT from the results of the reanalyzed data of WHI, the underutilization of MHT persists as shown in the study by Yang and Toriola. The study has important messages regarding improving health care professional education and public awareness, reducing disparities in health care access, and advancing menopause research to optimize appropriate MHT use and enhance quality of life for postmenopausal women [3].

16.2 Pharmacotherapy

16.2.1 Nomenclature and Types of Hormone Therapy (HT)

The estrogen deficiency at menopause may lead to somatic symptoms (VMS, psychological disorders), organic changes (skin changes, urogenital changes, weight changes), and metabolic effects (lipid changes, atherosclerosis, osteoporosis). Correction of the deficient estrogen at an age-appropriate menopause is termed MHT, and replacing estrogen in women with premature ovarian insufficiency (POI) is called hormone replacement therapy (HRT). The term HT covers therapies including estrogens, progesterone, combined estrogen and progestogen, selective estrogen receptor modulator (SERM), and gonadomimetics, such as tibolone, which contain estrogen, progestogen, and an androgen.

The estrogens generally used in MHT are micronized 17 beta estradiol (estradiol hemihydrate E2), conjugated equine estrogen (CEE), and estriol. CEE is a mixture of conjugated estrogens, including estrone sulfate, estradiol sulfate, and equilin sulfate. E2 is bioidentical to the estradiol produced from the ovaries. Less commonly used is estradiol valerate (EV). EV is an esterified form of estradiol, while E2 is the nonesterified form, EV 1 mg is equal to E2 0.76 mg. Estetrol is under investigation to be used as MHT. The effectiveness between E2 and CEE in treating VMS is comparable according to a meta-analysis, and the adverse events outcomes were inconsistent. E2 was more effective as an anxiolytic and antidepressant indicating differences in cognitive outcomes between types of estrogen and the brain serotonergic system. Ethinyl estradiol (EE) is the component of the oral contraceptive pill (OCP) with high potency and is restricted to be used for younger women with POI and for contraception.

The role of progesterones in MHT is to protect the endometrium from hyperplasia and cancer caused by the use of unopposed estrogen. The natural progesterones, micronized progesterone (MP) and dydrogesterone are preferred in MHT as they have an effective antiproliferative effect on the endometrium and are devoid of action on the metabolic receptors unlike progestins. Natural progesterones needs to be adequately dosed for endometrial protection. Moreover, observational studies have indicated that the risk of breast cancer may be less with the use of MP and dydrogesterone compared with synthetic progestogens. Natural progesterones needs to be adequately dosed for endometrial protection. Various progestins have been used in MHT, but the common ones are medroxyprogesterone (MPA), norethisterone, and levonorgesterol (LNG). The most common progestogen derivatives studied in the WHI was MPA which exerts good antiestrogenic effect at the endometrium, but has an undesirable effect on lipids. Progesterone can help with sleep disturbances and mood instability and is given before bedtime.

The role of androgen therapy in MHT is limited, formulations for use in women are not available in India.

16.3 Accepted Indications for MHT

MHT is the first line of treatment for VMS and GSM of menopause as per most menopause societies' guidelines. At menopause transition and early postmenopause, it has shown to reduce fractures in unselected population in the Women's Health Initiative (WHI) trial. Some of the guidelines advocate the use of HT as first line in the protection of bone health and prevention of features in women with POI, early menopause and in the early post menopause period.

16.3.1 Vasomotor Symptoms

In a study by Gartoulla et al., VMS was found to begin as early as 11 years before the final menstrual period (FMP) and persisted for 11–12 years after the FMP. VMS affects the quality of life (QOL) by decreasing the day-to-day functioning and restless nights [4]. This leads to decreased output at home and workplace leading to a feeling of worthlessness. VMS may indicate a higher risk for cardiovascular disease, cognitive functions, bone loss due to the common effects of deficient estrogen. MHT is the most effective treatment for VMS. MHT use reduces VMS by nearly 90%, usually within 1 month of initiation as seen in the WHI. The therapy, dose, route, and duration of therapy is individualized.

16.3.2 The Genitourinary Syndrome of Menopause

Estrogen deficiency leading to urogenital atrophy may lead to unspoken distress and decreased QOL due to vaginal dryness, dyspareunia, vulvar itching and burning, and dysuria, urinary frequency, urgency, and recurrent lower urinary tract infections. The discomfort leads to dyspareunia and reduced sexual desire and in some with a reduced hormone-driven sexual desire may result in discordance in relationships [5]. Both topical and systemic estrogens have been shown to improve the symptoms of GSM. Low-dose vaginal estrogen is adequate when estrogen is considered only for GSM and progesterone therapy in not needed. Long-term therapy is required to maintain the beneficial effects or symptoms generally recur after stopping HT and the safety data for continuous use for up to 1 year is available. For women with breast cancer, low-dose vaginal estrogen may be prescribed in consultation with their oncologists, when all other treatments fail.

Transdermal estrogen improves sexual functioning by not affecting the circulating testosterones levels as seen with oral preparations and systemic estrogen has local physiological effects like increase lubrication, blood flow, and sensation of vaginal tissues. Oral estrogens increase the sex hormone-binding globulin (SHBG) and decrease the circulating testosterone levels [6]. It's is prudent to understand that the effects of estrogen on sexual functioning is seen only in the presence of menopausal symptoms. Tibolone is a good option and has an androgenic effect.

16.3.3 Osteoporosis

Osteoporosis is common affecting one out of three postmenopausal women and estrogen deficiency is one of the important risk factors. At menopause, the bone loss is maximum (1–5%) within the first 2–3 years and sensibly can be prevented by MHT and reduces the risk of fracture at all bone sites by 20–40%. Absolute risks based on results from the WHI trial indicated that 5 years of combined hormone therapy reduced the incidence of hip fractures by about 1 case per 1000 women younger than 70 years and by about 8 cases per 1000 women aged 70–79 years even in unselected population. Data suggests that estrogen is beneficial for bone protection at all ages, more so when started within the first 5 years of menopause. Women who have a decreased bone mineral density and those with a known history of osteoporotic fractures benefit from HT. Women with premature menopause also benefit from the bone-protective benefit of HT. The consensus regarding MHT as the first line in bone protection is divided, Indian Menopause Society, International

Menopause Society advocates MHT as first-line therapy in the early post menopause in healthy woman [1].

16.4 Possible Benefits of MHT

16.4.1 Joint Pain

Women in the WHI and other studies have shown less joint pain or stiffness compared with those on placebo.

16.4.2 Diabetes

Metabolic changes associated with menopausal transition increases the risk of developing to type 2 diabetes mellitus (T2DM) and a meta-analysis suggest that MHT use reduces the prevalence of diabetes by 30%. Oral estrogens are beneficial in women with diabetes and low cardiovascular disease CVD risk, while transdermal administration is preferred in those with moderate CVD risk and or in obese women, as the risk of stroke and venous thromboembolism (VTE) is increased with oral administration. The preferred progesterone are MP and dydrogesterone. Interestingly a Korean study, including 58,060 postmenopausal women, showed that MHT is not associated with CVD or T2DM development [7].

CVD—Refer Timing hypothesis.
Central Nervous System (CNS)—Refer Timing hypothesis.

16.4.3 Other Effects of MHT

The other effects of MHT are prevention of senile macular degeneration and geriatric blindness, maintain oral health and prevent tooth loss, and reduce the risk of osteoarthritis as seen in the WHI. The risk of colorectal cancer was reduced with combined CEE and MPA use and no significant difference found with CEE alone therapy.

16.4.4 QOL and MHT

MHT improved the health related QOL in women with menopausal symptoms and no change in when without symptoms at baseline.

16.5 Absolute Contraindications of MHT

Undiagnosed abnormal vaginal bleeding—Needs to be investigated before starting MHT.

Breast carcinoma—Known, suspected, or current invasive breast carcinoma, premalignant changes of breast (atypical ductal hyperplasia, lobular neoplasia), and a ductal carcinoma in situ (intraductal carcinoma) and at high risk for breast cancer.

Estrogen-dependent cancers—Known, suspected, or history of estrogen-dependent cancers, i.e., endometrial, endometrial stromal, leiomyosarcoma, granulosa cell tumors, low-grade serous, and nongynecological estrogen and/or progesterone receptor positive cancers like the meningioma, glioma, lung, gastric, bladder cancer, and advanced malignant melanoma.

CVD—Active or history of CVD and at severe increased risk of CVD, untreated hypertension, active or history of venous thromboembolism (VTE), active or history of stroke. History of blood clotting disorder, the most common being Factor V Leiden mutation carriers (may consider transdermal estrogen).

Age ≥60 years or menopause onset >10 years—Prior with moderate risk for CVD, moderate risk for breast cancer.

Severe or active liver disease.

Diabetes with end organ failure.

Known or suspected pregnancy.

Known intolerance to a certain constituent of the preparation.

16.6 HT to Be Given with Caution

Age and Time since Menopause—Initiating treatment after 60 years of age or after 10 years postmenopause and moderate risk for CVD, history of deep vein thrombosis, varicose veins, superficial thrombophlebitis, and at moderate risk for breast cancer.

High triglycerides—In women with triglyceride levels between 250 and 500 mg/dL, estrogen should be provided with great caution, and a transdermal route of administration is preferred. A level >500 mg/dL may precipitates acute pancreatitis.

After start of HT, the triglyceride response is rapid, and a repeat level should be obtained in 2–4 weeks. If increased, hormone therapy must be discontinued.

Active gallbladder disease, obesity, and fibroids.

Smoking enhances the thromobogenic potential of estrogen.

Migraine with aura is a risk factor for ischemic stroke. Estrogen may potentiate the thrombogenic state seen in women with migraines. Transdermal routes and the lowest dose should be prescribed to control VMS. It is important to monitor the increase in the migraine attacks.

Autoimmune Disorders: The impact of HT use on risk and severity of autoimmune conditions such as systemic lupus erythematosus (SLE) or rheumatoid arthritis (RA) are few, but those with antiphospholipid syndrome, a hypercoagulable state associated with SLE, should avoid HT. [8]

16.7 Timing Hypothesis—Concept of Early Initiation of MHT

16.7.1 CVD

The timing hypothesis in the use of MHT is appropriate for its effect on the outcome of CVD. At menopause transition, lipid profiles tend to become atherogenic with a significant increase in total cholesterol, low-density lipoprotein (LDL) cholesterol, and apolipoprotein B (ApoB), independent of ethnicity, age, or weight. Moreover, blood pressure levels tend to rise in postmenopause. Estrogen deficiency induces the production of pro inflammatory markers and accelerates the atherosclerosis process. The effects of MHT on CVD outcomes depends on chronological age and menopausal age, individual health status, route of delivery of estrogens, and type of progestogen. Long term use of transdermal E2 has been shown to reduce ambulatory blood pressure in normotensive postmenopausal women. Oral MHT had a largely neutral effect on blood pressure in normotensive women. Use of transdermal E2 may therefore be preferable to oral CEE/E2 in hypertensive postmenopausal women. HT initiated within 10 years of menopause onset and less than 60 years, there may be a cardioprotective effect and risks are not increased, hence beneficial to women in low and moderate risk for CVD.

16.7.2 Type 2 Diabetes

Early initiation of MHT may offer benefits related to cardiovascular health and glucose metabolism and later initiation, especially in women with established T2DM and atherosclerosis, can be associated with increased risks. HT significantly reduced diabetes risk in those with a BMI of up to 30, but not in those with a BMI of 30 kg/m^2 or higher.

16.7.3 CNS

Clinical data is controversial regarding effects on the brain. Association of HT use and risk of Alzheimer disease (AD) may depend on timing of use. Similarly, the effect on CVD outcomes, HT use if taken during a critical window near menopause is possibly beneficial, initiated in later life may be associated with increased risk. Moreover, early use of HT might reduce risk of AD by lowering cardiovascular risk factors. Data on the effect on cognition with CEE do not seem to convey long-term benefit or adverse consequences.

16.8 Adverse Effects

Nausea—Prescribe oral estrogen with meals or before bed, switch to another oral estrogen, switch to transdermal estrogen or lower the estrogen or progestogen dose.

Bloating, weight gain, fluid retention—Switch to low-dose transdermal estrogen; lower the progestogen dose a level that still protects the uterus; switch to another progestin or to MP.

Mood swings—May be associated with use of relatively androgenic progestogens. Lower the progestogen dose, switch progestogen, switch from systemic progestin to the progestin IUS or tibolone. Change to a continuous-combined (CC) EPT regimen, ensure adequate water intake, restrict intake of salt, caffeine, and alcohol.

Breast tenderness—Lower the estrogen dose, switch to another estrogen, restrict salt intake; switch to another progestin, cut down on caffeine and chocolate.

Chloasma—Use sun screen lotion.

16.8.1 Vaginal Bleeding

Unscheduled bleeding is the most common problem for women on MHT. Some bleeding for up to 6 months after beginning MHT is acceptable. If bleeding is heavy or frequent, investigations should be carried out sooner. Investigations should include history, physical examination, vulvar and vaginal, rectal inspection, Pap smear, and bimanual examination. Pelvic ultrasound to check for endometrial thickness and an endometrial thickness ≤4 mm is reassuring. If bleeding recurs, endometrial biopsy, diagnostic hysteroscopy, or sonohysterogram should be performed. Therapeutic options are to switch from continuous progestogen use to cyclical progestogen, to reduce the dose of estrogen or the route of administration.

Tension headache will frequently respond to lifestyle modifications, stress management, and use of nonnarcotic analgesics.

16.8.2 CVD

In women at high risk for CVD as seen in the WHI and established CVD, estrogen may increase the CVD events in the first year of treatment as seen in the Heart and Estrogen/progestin Replacement Study (HERS) [9]. The WHI clinical trials found an excess CHD risk among women with a baseline LDL-C ≥130 mg/dL taking CEE with or without MPA. Moreover, in the WHI trials, statin use did not lower the event rate in women on EP Oral HT use increases triglycerides, transdermal HT decreases triglyceride levels by 5–30%; hence, it's advised to use transdermal HT in women with dyslipidemia.

16.8.3 Venous Thromboembolism

Oral estrogen (CEE more than E2) and synthetic progestogens, may increase risk of VTE, more so in women with obesity and transdermal mitigates this risk. Progesterone and pregnane derivatives, such as dydrogesterone and chlormadinone acetate, were found to be neutral on the risk of VTE unlike other progesterones [10].

16.8.4 Stroke

The risk for stroke is increased in women who initiate treatment after age 60 years and the risk of stroke is greatest for high-dose oral >0.625 mg CEE, >2 mg E2 formulations. Stroke risk was not found to increase with increasing doses of transdermal estrogens. No association was found with the use of progesterone and duphaston while a positive association has been reported for formulations containing norpregnane derivatives [11].

16.8.5 Gall Bladder

Risk of gallstones, cholecystitis, and cholecystectomy is increased with oral estrogen-alone and combination oral MHT. Observational studies report lower risk with transdermal MHT than with oral estradiol compared with CEE, but neither observation is confirmed in RCTs.

16.9 Risk of Cancer with HT

Breast Cancer: The WHI trial showed that the use of CEE and MPA resulted in 29% increased risk of breast cancer. After about 19 years of follow-up, CEE alone resulted in a significant 23% reduction in breast cancer incidence. Mortality from breast cancer was 45% increase with CEE + MPA and a significant 44% reduction with CEE alone. Conclusions drawn from the WHI and European studies indicate a decreased risk with estrogen alone, progesterone and dydrogesterone compared with MPA. The safety in prescribing HT also depends on the baseline risk of breast cancer in the woman [12].

Endometrial cancer: Unopposed estrogen therapy increased risk of endometrial cancer, sequential combined (SC) HT >5 years may be associated with small increase in risk of endometrial cancer, with risk inversely proportional to number of days progestogen is given. CC estrogen and progestogen has a neutral effect on risk of endometrial cancer compared to placebo. WHI showed significant reduction in endometrial cancer risk in the post intervention phase.

Ovarian cancer: Epidemiological studies indicate an increase in risk of serious and endometrioid ovarian cancer with HT, while WHI data did not show an increased risk.

Colorectal cancer: WHI results showed reduced risk of colorectal cancer with oral combined HT. The risk reduction reduced after stopping HT over 13 years cumulative follow-up. No effect in the estrogen alone group.

Lung Cancer: In nonsmokers, MHT may reduce or have no effect on lung cancer risk. In the EPT arm of WHI, current and former smokers over age 60 were shown to have a small increase in the risk of death from nonsmall cell lung cancer (4/10,000 per year).

16.10 Safety of HT After Cancer Diagnosis

HT may be advantageous in endometrial cancer type I, cervical adenocarcinoma, hematological malignancies, local cutaneous malignant melanoma, colorectal cancer, and hepatocellular cancer [13].

HRT is neutral in BRCA 1/2 mutation carriers without cancer, endometrial cancer type II, uterine carcinosarcoma and adenosarcoma, most types of ovarian cancer, cervical, vaginal, and vulvar squamous cell carcinoma, prolactinoma, kidney cancer, pancreatic cancer, and thyroid cancer.

HT is contraindicated in ER/PR positive breast cancer, leiomyosarcoma, endometrial stromal sarcoma, endometroid types of ovarian tumors, low-grade serous, sertoli leydig, estrogen-dependent granulosa cell tumors, meningioma, glioma, advanced metastatic malignant melanoma, lung cancer, and gastric and bladder cancer.

16.11 Doses, Route, Regimes, Monitoring, and Tapering

It is good practice to start with a low effective dose and increase as needed. The estrogen doses used are ultra-low dose (CEE 0.3 mg/day, E2 0.25 mg/day, transdermal E2 0.014 mg/day), low dose (CEE 0.45 mg/day, E2 0.5 mg/day, transdermal E2 0.025 mg/day), and standard dose (CEE 0.625 mg/day, E2 1 mg/day, transdermal E2 0.0375–0.05 mg/day).

The transformation dose of MP and dydrogesterone used in MHT depends on the dose of estrogen and the regime. With a standard dose of 1 mg E2 daily, 100 mg of daily MP or 5–10 mg of dydrogesterone protects the endometrium in a CC regime and 200–300 mg of MP and 10–20 mg of dydrogesterone in SC regime. The levonorgestrel intrauterine device (LNG-IUD) contains 52 mg and delivers 20 μg of LNG is an alternative to systemic progestogen therapy and may be used for 5 years.

In an SC MHT regime, estrogen is used every day, with progesterone added cyclically for 10–14 days during each month. Uterine bleeding occurs in about 80% of women when progestogen is withdrawn, although bleeding can begin 1–2 days earlier, depending on the type and dose of progestogen use. This is the regime for the perimenopausal woman. In a CC MHT, fixed doses of estrogen and progesterone are administered every day. Approximately 40% incidence of irregular spotting or bleeding in the first 6 months and prescribed for women after 1 year of menopause. CC regimens should not be used in perimenopausal women because of the high risk of irregular bleeding.

Estrogen given by transdermal route by passes the hepatic metabolism that produces activated protein-C resistance, negating the risk of blood clotting seen with oral formulations. The indications for transdermal therapy are triglyceridemia, hyperlipidemia, migraine, diabetes with mild to moderate CVD risk, hypertension, obesity, smoking, previous VTE, varicose veins, bowel disorders, e.g., irritable bowel syndrome, gall bladder disease, and sexual dysfunction. Transdermal estrogen is available as gel and spray.

Vaginal estrogens may be used alone, or they may be added at standard doses to systemic treatment when it does not fully treat GSM. Low-dose vaginal estrogen therapy may be administered as long as it is needed because of the low systemic impact.

Women on systemic HT should have a review at 1 and 3 months to assess symptom relief and adverse effects. Long-term follow-up should be annual, including a medical examination, updated history, and breast assessment. Any unscheduled or prolonged bleeding after 3–6 months requires investigation. Generally, after 3–5 years of menopause hormone therapy, there should be an attempt to taper and eventually discontinue treatment. Tapering of systemic therapy does not seem to offer greater benefits in the long term compared to stopping abruptly. If symptoms persist, lower doses or transdermal therapy could be offered, with periodic reevaluation of the risks and benefits.

16.12 Prescribing MHT

16.12.1 Asses the Profile of the Woman to Individualize Treatment

1. Counseling: A patient-centered approach is vital, with individualized treatment plans that consider each woman's risk factors to create a benefit risk profile and tailor HT to each woman seeking relief for menopausal symptoms. The Importance of shared decision-making in menopause care to increase compliance include discussion on indications, benefits, risks & side effects of MHT, pre-HT work up, economic considerations, monitoring and follow up.
2. Detailed history, clinical examination, and relevant investigations, risk assessment for comorbidities.
3. Evaluation of women's individual benefits and risks

   This allows you to classify women into two major groups.

   Group 1—Women with no menopausal symptoms (VMS).

   Group 2—Women with menopausal symptoms (VMS).

   In practice, charting out an individualized long-term management plan becomes simple.
4. Prescribing therapy depending on type and stage of menopause.

A. Surgical menopause—estrogen only/tibolone.
B. Menopause transition—cyclical progesterone/OCP/ MHT cyclical.
C. Early menopause—estrogen and progesterone SC regime (more estrogen).
D. Late menopause >12 months—estrogen and progesterone CC regime/ Tibolone.
E. POI—MHT SC regime full dose, OCP.
F. GSM—Local estrogens.

16.13 Long-Term Management of HT

The guidelines after 20 years of WHI study indicate that HT does not need to be routinely discontinued at the age of 60 years but requires continued monitoring for new health concerns, periodic trials of tapered HT doses, and attempts at HT discontinuation should be made for women nearing the age of 60–65 years old [14].

A study looked at 13 different outcomes using 40 different hormonal therapies that were started or continued in women older than 65. They found that the use of estrogen-only HRT for those older than 65 was linked to significant reductions in mortality (19%) and risks for several conditions, including breast, lung, and colorectal cancer, congestive heart failure, VTE, atrial fibrillation, myocardial infarction, and dementia [15].

16.14 MHT in the Elderly

There can be three situations in the elderly:

- On MHT and wants to continue, this may be considered in healthy women at low risk of CVD and breast cancer with persistent VMS or at elevated risk of fracture for whom other therapies are not appropriate.
- Was on MHT, stopped and wants to restart. Initiation of HT in this group requires careful consideration of individual benefits and risks.
- MHT for the first time—Commencing MHT de novo is not conventionally recommended. If MHT is to be initiated, it is important that very low doses are prescribed and ideally with transdermal estrogen [16].

16.15 Tibolone

Tibolone is a progestogen with selective tissue estrogenic activity (STEAR) and exhibits weak estrogenic, progestogenic, and androgenic activity. The recommended dose is 2.5 mg/day to treat menopausal symptoms and it improves vaginal atrophy without affect the endometrium. It has a protective effect on bone mass, even in a dose of 1.25 mg/day. In young healthy postmenopausal women, it reduces proliferation of breast epithelial cells, does not increase mammographic density, and reduces cyst diameter of fibrocystic mastopathy and does not increase the risk of breast cancer development compared with placebo. Tibolone does not cause an increased VTE risk or increase of CHD events. Tibolone should only be used in women >12 months since menopause as it may cause irregular bleeding in younger women. In younger women, tibolone has place in POI with sexual dysfunction and mood swings and long-term add-back therapy of agonists gonadotropin-releasing hormone [17].

In the elderly with risk factors for CVD and established CVD, risk of stroke rises exponentially with age, tibolone should generally be avoided. There is also evidence that tibolone could slightly increase the risk of recurrence in breast cancer patients.

16.16 Selective Estrogen Receptor Modulators

Bazedoxifene (BZA) is a new SERM that verifiably reduces bone mass loss in postmenopausal women and reduces the risk of vertebral and nonvertebral (in the high-risk group) fractures without stimulating breast tissue or endometrium. This is not available in India [18].

16.17 Estetrol

It is produced exclusively by fetal liver and has a very good oral bioavailability. It binds to estrogen receptor (ER) alpha 4–5 times stronger than to ER beta. Although VMS frequency seems to be reduced with as low as 2 mg E4, a minimum dose of 15 mg was needed to reduce VMS severity [19]. The potential of E4 when used as hormone replacement in women after breast cancer surgery, in women treated by aromatase inhibitors or tamoxifen, has been indicated by initial observation within a clinical study.

16.18 Compounded "Bioidentical" Hormone Therapy (cBHT)

"Bioidentical" hormones are defined as substances that have exactly the same chemical and molecular structure as hormones that are produced in the human body. Any hormone can be made to be "bioidentical," and there are many FDA-approved hormone preparations that are "bioidentical."

CBHT particularly estrogen and progesterone, have been promoted by some as safer and more effective alternatives to manufactured FDA-approved hormone therapies (HT) for relief of symptoms of the menopause. They are not accepted by the medical societies, since the formulation have not gone through the vigor of clinical safety and efficacy studies.

Key Message

1. MHT initiated in early postmenopausal period in healthy women is safe.
2. Like all medicines, MHT needs to be used appropriately, but it is essential that women in early menopause who are suffering menopausal symptoms should have the option of using MHT.
3. A complete evaluation of risks and benefits has to be done objectively.
4. Informed choices.
5. Right woman, right age, right MHT, right dose, and right route.

Long Answer Questions (LAQs)

1. What are the main indications for initiating hormone therapy during menopause, and how should the decision to start treatment be individualized?
2. What are the different types and routes of hormone therapy available for menopausal women, and how are they selected based on patient needs?
3. What are the potential benefits and risks associated with hormone therapy at menopause, and how should these influence ongoing management?
4. What are the current recommendations regarding the duration of hormone therapy at menopause, and what considerations should guide the discontinuation of therapy?

Short Answer Questions (SAQs)

1. How does hormone therapy specifically alleviate hot flashes and night sweats during menopause?
2. What are the long-term health risks associated with prolonged hormone therapy at menopause?
3. In what ways can hormone therapy impact bone health and prevent osteoporosis in menopausal women?
4. How is the MHT regimen selected and individualized?
5. When is topical estrogen preferred over systemic MHT?

Multiple Choice Questions (MCQs)

1. Which of the following is an approved indication for menopausal hormone therapy (MHT)?
   A. Prevention of cognitive decline
   B. Vasomotor symptoms
   C. Prevention of breast cancer
   D. Treatment of hypertension
2. What is the main risk associated with using estrogen-only therapy in women with an intact uterus?
   A. Ovarian cancer
   B. Endometrial cancer
   C. Colon cancer
   D. Macular degeneration
3. Which form of estrogen delivery is associated with a lower risk of venous thromboembolism (VTE)?
   A. Oral estrogen
   B. Transdermal estrogen
   C. Vaginal estrogen
   D. Intramuscular estrogen
4. Which of the following is a common symptom that hormone therapy can effectively relieve during menopause?
   A. Hypertension
   B. Hyperlipidemia
   C. Hot flashes
   D. Diabetes
5. Which of the following is a contraindication for hormone replacement therapy (HRT)?
   A. Osteoporosis
   B. Unexplained vaginal bleeding
   C. Insomnia
   D. Vaginal dryness
6. For women with premature ovarian insufficiency, what is the recommended approach regarding MHT?
   A. Avoid MHT
   B. Use only nonhormonal therapies
   C. Standard dose MHT until the average age of natural menopause
   D. Use only phytoestrogens

7. What is the recommended minimum duration of HT to minimize risks?
   A. As long as possible
   B. Shortest time and lowest dose necessary
   C. Indefinitely
   D. At least 10 years
8. Which symptom is NOT typically improved by hormone therapy at menopause?
   A. Vaginal dryness
   B. Osteoporosis prevention
   C. Cognitive decline
   D. Hot flashes
9. What should be added to estrogen therapy in women with an intact uterus to reduce the risk of endometrial cancer?
   A. Testosterone
   B. Progestogen
   C. Calcium
   D. Vitamin D
10. Which of the following is a benefit of hormone therapy in postmenopausal women?
    A. Reduced risk of colon cancer
    B. Increased risk of stroke
    C. Increased risk of hypertension
    D. Reduced risk of diabetes

Answers

1. B
2. B
3. B
4. C
5. B
6. C
7. B
8. C
9. B
10. A

References

1. Meeta M, Digumarti L, Agarwal N, Vaze N, Shah R, Malik S. Clinical practice guidelines on menopause: Indian Menopause Society, 2020.
2. Bardakjian T, Gonzalez-Alegre P. Towards precision medicine. Handb Clin Neurol. 2018;147:93–102.
3. Yang L, Toriola AT. Menopausal hormone therapy use among postmenopausal women. JAMA Health Forum. 2024;5(9):e243128.
4. Gartoulla P, Worsley R, Bell RJ, Davis SR. Moderate to severe vasomotor and sexual symptoms remain problematic for women aged 60 to 65 years. Menopause. 2018;25:1331–8.
5. Nappi RE, Palacios S, Bruyniks N, Particco M, Panay N, EVES Study investigators. The burden of vulvovaginal atrophy on women's daily living: implications on quality of life from a face-to-face real-life survey. Menopause. 2019;26:485–91.
6. Taylor HS, Tal A, Pal L, Li F, Black DM, Brinton EA, Budoff MJ, Cedars MI, Du W, Hodis HN, et al. Effects of oral vs. transdermal estrogen therapy on sexual function in early postmenopause: ancillary study of the Kronos Early Estrogen Prevention Study (KEEPS). JAMA Intern Med. 2017;177:1471–9.
7. Kim J-E, Choi J, Park J, Shin A. Effects of menopausal hormone therapy on cardiovascular diseases and type 2 diabetes in middle-aged postmenopausal women: analysis of the Korea National Health Insurance Service Database. Menopause. 2021;28:1225–32.
8. Grygiel-Gorniak B, Limphaibool N, Puszczewicz M. Clinical implications of systemic lupus erythematosus without and with antiphospholipid syndrome in peri- and postmenopausal age. Prz Menopausal. 2018;17(2):86–90.
9. Herrington DM. The HERS trial results: paradigms lost? Heart and Estrogen/progestin Replacement Study. Ann Intern Med. 1999;131(6):463–6.
10. Vinogradova Y, Coupland C, Hippisley-Cox J. Use of hormone replacement therapy and risk of venous thromboembolism: nested case-control studies using the QResearch and CPRD databases. BMJ. 2019;364:k4810.
11. Canonico M, Carcaillon L, Plu-Bureau G. Postmenopausal hormone therapy and risk of stroke: impact of the route of estrogen administration and type of progestogen. Stroke. 2016;47:1734–41.
12. Asi N, Mohammed K, Haydour Q, et al. Progesterone vs. synthetic progestins and the risk of breast cancer: a systematic review and meta-analysis. Syst Rev. 2016;5(1):121.
13. Deli T. Hormone replacement therapy in cancer survivors—review of the literature. Pathol Oncol Res. 2020;26(1):63–78.
14. The NAMS 2022 Hormone Therapy Position Statement Advisory Panel. The 2022 hormone therapy position statement of the North American Menopause Society. Menopause. 2022;29(7):767–94.
15. Baik SH, Baye F, McDonald CJ. Use of menopausal hormone therapy beyond age 65 years and its effects on women's health outcomes by types, routes, and doses. Menopause. 2024;31(5):363–71.
16. Panay N, Ang SB, Cheshire R, Goldstein SR, Maki P, Nappi RE, on behalf of the international menopause society board. Menopause and MHT in 2024: addressing the key controversies—an International Menopause Society White Paper. Climacteric. 2024.
17. Kenemans P. Speroff Tibolone: clinical recommendations and practical guidelines. Maturitas. 2005;51:21–8.
18. Archer DF, Pinkerton JV, Utian WH, et al. Bazedoxifene, a SERM: effects on the endometrium, ovarium, and breast from a randomized controlled trial in osteoporotic postmenopausal women. Menopause. 2009;16:1109–15.
19. Coelingh Bennink HJ, Verhoeven C, Zimmerman Y, Visser M, Foidart JM, Gemzell-Danielsson K. Clinical effects of the fetal estrogen estetrol in a multiple-rising-dose study in postmenopausal women. Maturitas. 2016;91:93–100.

Nonhormonal Management of Menopausal Symptoms

17

A. G. Radhika and Sana Ahmed

Abstract

As a natural phase of life, menopause is characterized by symptoms such as hot flashes, vaginal dryness, sleep disturbances, and concerns regarding bone health. Although hormone replacement therapy (HRT) is effective, its potential risks make nonhormonal alternatives more attractive. The article discusses nonhormonal methods for managing menopausal symptoms. SSRIs and serotonin-norepinephrine reuptake inhibitors (SNRIs) are effective medications for treating vasomotor symptoms, along with cognitive behavioral therapy (CBT) and hypnosis. The use of lifestyle modifications, such as weight reduction and cooling techniques, can also help to alleviate insomnia. As a first-line treatment, CBT for insomnia (CBT-I) is an effective method for treating insomnia. A short-term use of benzodiazepines and Z-class drugs may also be an option. Lubricants, moisturizers, and hyaluronic acid may alleviate symptoms associated with the genitourinary system. In addition to improving vaginal health, ospemifene, a nonsteroidal agent, can improve bone health with exercise, calcium, and vitamin D supplementation. The use of bisphosphonates and denosumab is effective in managing osteoporosis. Long-term safety and efficacy of these alternatives require further research.

Menopausal symptoms can be effectively managed with nonhormonal therapies, thus allowing for individualized treatment. The importance of patient education and the education of healthcare professionals cannot be overstated.

A. G. Radhika (✉) · S. Ahmed
Department of Obstetrics and Gynaecology, UCMS & GTB Hospital, Delhi, India

R. Malik et al. (eds.), *Menopause Essentials*,
https://doi.org/10.1007/978-981-95-7498-8_17

Keywords

Menopause · Nonhormonal management · Menopausal symptoms · Alternative therapies · Women's health

Menopausal symptoms are reported not only in menopause but also in the transition phase and are of varying severity, decreasing the quality of life. Menopause produces varying symptoms ranging from hot flushes (vasomotor), psychological (mood changes, irritability, sleep disturbances) and genitourinary discomfort, and vaginal dryness, leading to pruritus and dyspareunia and loss of libido.

17.1 Why the Need for Nonhormonal Treatment Options?

Menopause hormone therapy (MHT) is the most effective in managing menopausal symptoms. The associated side effects and contraindications of hormone therapy (history of breast cancer, severe liver disease, porphyria, thromboembolic disease, and undiagnosed vaginal bleeding) necessitate the use of nonhormonal methods to relieve postmenopausal symptoms. Another problem with hormone therapy is reappearance of symptoms following cessation of treatment. Management of symptoms therefore requires detailed evaluation and provides individualized treatment [1].

A landmark study, Women's Health Initiative (WHI study), which was terminated prematurely in 2002, reported stroke, breast cancer and cardiovascular risks associated with MHT, thus necessitating the exploration of nonhormonal methods.

The nonhormonal management of menopausal symptoms is discussed symptom wise as follows.

17.2 Vasomotor Symptoms

17.2.1 Pharmacological Treatment

Selective serotonin reuptake inhibitors (SSRI) and selective norepinephrine reuptake inhibitors (SNRI) have shown to be effective for vasomotor symptoms in healthy women (Table 17.1).

Clinicians should be aware of potential drug interactions with Paroxetine. In patients with bipolar disease, uncontrolled seizures, liver or kidney insufficiency, uncontrolled hyponatremia or poorly controlled hypertension, concurrent use of other SSRIs or SNRIs. SSRI, specially, paroxetine and fluoxetine, in women with breast cancer on tamoxifen may lead to inhibition of CYP2D6 (the enzyme that converts tamoxifen to its most active metabolite, endoxifen). These patients can be prescribed venlafaxine or desvenlafaxine (SNRIs) or escitalopram or citalopram (SSRIs).

Table 17.1 Medical management of vasomotor symptoms [3]

Type of drug and dose	Efficacy	Side effects
Selective serotonin reuptake inhibitors (SSRIs)[a]		
1. Paroxetine mesylate 7.5/day 2. Paroxetine HCl 10–25 mg/d (the only nonhormonal FDA-approved drug)	Improves sleep, reduces hot flashes [2]	Dose-related nausea Contraindicated in tamoxifen users as it inhibits CYP2D6 enzyme
3. Fluoxetine 10–30 mg/day	Relieves hot flashes in 24% [3]	Nausea
4. Sertraline 25–100 mg/day	Moderate reduction in hot flashes [3]	Nausea Decreased libido Compliance—90%
5. Citalopram 10–20 mg/day	Significant relief seen in 49–55% in hot flashes [3] Alternative option to paroxetine Can be given to those on tamoxifen	80% compliance rate
6. Escitalopram 10–20 mg/day	Relief in hot flashes—seen in 24% [3] Best tolerated option	Nausea Drowsiness Weakness
Selective norepinephrine reuptake inhibitors (SNRIs)[a]		
1. Duloxetine 30–120 mg/day	Relief in symptoms—seen in 62%	Nausea Difficulty sleeping Xerostomia Constipation
2. Venlafaxine[b] 37.5–150 mg/day	Immediately effective (30–58%) Better sleep [4]	Nausea Headache Xerostomia Sleeping difficulties Reduced appetite
3. Desvenlafaxine[b] 100–150 mg/day	24–29% relief in hot flashes Safest in breast cancer patients	At treatment initiation—Dizziness, nausea, and headache
Gabapentin and pregabalin		
Gabapentin 300–900 mg/day, 8–12 weeks	Nearly 45% decrease in intensity and frequency of hot flashes [5]	Day time sleepiness 13% rate of withdrawal Suicidal tendencies
Pregabalin 75–150 mg/day	64–75% reduced frequency of hot flashes [6]	Somnolence Dizziness 12–17% rate of withdrawal Suicidal thoughts

(continued)

Table 17.1 (continued)

Type of drug and dose	Efficacy	Side effects
Clonidine		
0.1 mg/day for 12 weeks	26% reduction in hot flashes	Xerostomia Constipation Hypotension Chance of sudden hypertension (if abruptly stopped)
Oxybutynin		
2.5–5 mg twice a day	Reduced frequency of hot flushes [6, 7]	Xerostomia Dryness of eyes Urinary retention Pain abdomen
Fezolinetant[b]		
Neurokinin receptor 3 antagonist—3 mg/kg/day approved by FDA and European Union (EU) for management of hot flushes, in 2023	Better control of hot flash frequency and intensity [8]	Elevated liver enzymes, diarrhea, head ache, back pain, insomnia [8]

[a]Start at lowest effective dose, increase dosage if needed. When withdrawing, decrease to minimal dose for 2 weeks and then stop completely

[b]Not available in India

17.2.2 Nonpharmacological

(a) *Cognitive Behavioral Therapy (CBT)*:

CBT fits perfectly with how we see menopause—not just hormones, but a woman's mindset, expectations, how she makes sense of symptoms, her mood, social life, and past experiences. Many "menopausal" issues beyond hot flushes have other roots or mix with things like midlife stress or anxiety from life changes and finances. In sessions, CBT shares information and practical tools to help women handle hot flushes, stress, and sleep on their own, cutting down symptom triggers. Low estrogen can aggravate stress and negative thoughts can make it worse, but staying calm with deep breaths and shifting focus, eases the distress [9].

The program runs over 4–6 weekly sessions, totaling about 8 h. It covers menopause basics and why hot flushes happen, plus a simple cognitive behavioral approach.

- *Sessions*: 4–6 weekly meetings, about 8 h total.
- *Information*: Learn basics of menopause and hot flushes, with a simple explanation of why they happen and the cognitive behavioral approach.
- *Track Triggers*: Monitor and adjust things that spark hot flushes.
- *Relax & De-stress*: Practice breathing exercises and CBT techniques to cut stress.

- *Challenge Thoughts*: Explore and reframe unhelpful beliefs about menopause and symptoms.
- *Helpful Habits*: Build behaviors like less avoidance, pacing your day.
- *Night Sweats & Sleep*: Get tips for managing them better.
- *Personal Goals*: Set your own at the start, with tailored homework between sessions.
- *Key Skills*: Gain knowledge to handle symptoms.
- *Wrap-Up*: Final review and plan to keep using what works for you.

(b) *Hypnosis*: Effective reduction in hot flashes was seen with sessions lasting 1 h taken over 5 weeks. Cases showed 80% and 85% improvement in frequency and severity of symptoms when compared with controls receiving gabapentin. The mechanism by which hypnosis provides relief is not known but theories have been proposed whereby it acts on the medial preoptic hypothalamic area, which has been shown to be the thermoregulatory center [10].

(c) *Weight Reduction*: The severity of menopausal symptoms is worsened with increasing weight gain. The following strategies can be used to manage weight:

1. Dietary modifications and portion control—Eating a balanced diet that is rich in fruits, vegetable, lean protein, and whole grain promotes fullness for longer periods, thus reducing craving and binge eating. Portion control (having smaller, more frequent meals throughout the day) can help in managing intake.
2. Exercise—The recommended exercises include strength training for at least 2 days a week or 150 min of moderate intensity exercise per week or yoga and Pilates to improve joint strength and balance [11].

(d) *Lifestyle Modifications:* Measures like environmental cooling, avoiding triggers and exercising can also help, although studies are still underway to establish their efficacy [12].

1. Environmental cooling: These measures aim to decrease core body temperature. Loose layered clothing, wearing breathable materials like cotton, using handheld fans, air conditioners and drinking cold fluids can help avoid triggering an episode of hot flash.
2. Avoiding triggers: Smoking cessation, decreasing alcohol intake and avoiding spicy food may help in reducing frequency of hot flashes.
3. Regular exercise: studies have not reported a direct benefit of exercise but it may help by reducing weight, allaying anxiety, improved muscle tone and better sleep pattern [13].

(e) *Yoga:* Although limited evidence exists on its effectiveness, yoga has shown to improve psychological symptoms like anxiety, mood disorders and sleep problems. It effectively reduced vasomotor symptoms in perimenopausal and postmenopausal women at 8 and 12 weeks respectively. The recommended frequency is three times per week for 4, 8, 12, 16, and 20 weeks with the longer the duration, the better the results [14].

(f) *Acupuncture*: It has been proposed that endorphins secreted during acupuncture therapy may have a role in improving vasomotor symptoms. [15]
(g) *Stellate Ganglion Block*: It involves injecting local anesthetic into the stellate ganglion in the neck. The proposed mechanism is that menopause results in increased nerve growth factor concentration, which causes raised norepinephrine levels. Stellate ganglion block has been shown to reduce nerve growth factor levels and decreases the intensity of hot flashes. Its use is precluded by its invasive nature and cost [16].
(h) *Phytoestrogens and Herbal Remedies*: Alternative estrogen sources—soybeans and soy protein—have high level of isoflavones which have biological activity same as that of estrogens, and their safety and efficacy profile is still under research [17, 18].

17.3 Insomnia

1. *Sleep Hygiene*: Avoidance of caffeine, mobile use, television watching and bright lights in the bed room, promote sleep.
2. *Cognitive Behavioral Therapy for Insomnia (CBT-I)*: CBT has been found to be an effective substitute for medication. The American Academy of Sleep Medicine and the European Sleep Research recommend it as first-line therapy, particularly in patients with chronic insomnia [18]. CBT-I therapy targets and modifies patients' sleep beliefs and attitudes. It educates them on sleep hygiene to improve sleep patterns, restrictions, stimulus control, and relaxation therapy. Correcting dysfunctional ideas about sleep is achieved with cognitive therapy. [19] CBT in conjunction with pharmacological methods show better results.in both peri and postmenopausal patients, CBT-I reported better sleep habits as soon as 8 week. Barriers to its usage as standard therapy include time-intensive sessions, cost, transportation and scheduling difficulties. These can be addressed via telephone-based education control [20].
3. *Benzodiazepines and Z-Class Drugs*: These drugs treat insomnia by acting on the $GABA_A$ receptor complexes. They decrease sleep latency and night time awakenings and increase total sleep time while ameliorating sleep quality. Z-class drugs (Zolpidem, Zopiclone, and Zaleplon) selectively bind to the type 1 $GABA_A$ receptor, thus minimizing side effects. Usage should be limited to ≤4 weeks at the lowest possible dose due to data paucity about their long-term effects, tolerance, dependency potential, and abuse risk. Adverse effects reported are dizziness, somnolence, headaches, confusion and increased risk of falls and fractures because of muscle relaxation [21].
4. *Antidepressants (SSRIs and SNRIs)*: Coexisting depression and insomnia is seen commonly and is treated with SSRIs and SNRIs. The US-FDA approves Doxepin (3–6 mg/day) for insomnia management. Trazodone (25–50 mg) used in sleep maintenance has minimal side effects of dependence or substance abuse [20].
5. *Melatonin*: Ramelteon is a melatonin receptor agonist, proven to have beneficial effects on insomnia and is US-FDA approved. Prolonged release preparations

(2 mg) are also under study [22]. The advantage of melatonin is that it is well tolerated and not habit forming.

6. *Orexin Antagonist and Gabapentin*: Orexins are hypothalamic neuropeptides involved in varied functions including control of feeding behavior, sleep–wake rhythm, and neuroendocrine homeostasis. The estrogenic disinhibition of orexins may have a role in insomnia seen in menopause. Further evaluation is needed to recommend use of orexin receptor antagonists in treating menopause associated insomnia [23]. Gabapentin in a dose of 300 mg can reduce nighttime awakenings and help improve sleep.

17.4 Genitourinary Symptoms

(a) *Lubricants*: Vaginal dryness and dyspareunia are relieved by using oil-based or water and silicon-based lubricants. Using locally applied estrogen cream can also help. Caution must be exercised when using oil-based formulations in conjunction with latex condoms (due to risk of condom breakdown) and counsel regarding risk of sexually transmitted infections. [24, 25]

(b) *Moisturizers*: Their hydrophobic and bio-adhesive properties (adhering to superficial cells of vagina) help in absorption into skin and moisture retention, thus alleviating symptoms of pruritus and dyspareunia [24, 25].

(c) *Hyaluronic Acid*: It is a naturally occurring hydrophilic polysaccharide. Relieves vaginal atrophy by retaining water with good tolerability and almost no side effects.

(d) *Laser*: Lasers are becoming increasingly popular for menopausal vaginal symptoms. Examples include Erbium and CO_2 lasers. [24] They act by raising the local temperature which promotes vasodilation, neovascularization, and collagen synthesis and remodeling. Side effects include risks of burning, bladder injury, scarring and further dyspareunia. The US-FDA cautions against its routine use.

(e) *Ospemifene*: It is a synthetic, nonsteroidal drug for improving genitourinary symptoms of menopause (GSM). It acts by increasing the vaginal superficial epithelial cell count and helps to normalize pH like in the premenopausal state. The effects are seen after a month to 1 year of regular use. It has also been implicated in improving other associated symptoms like bladder and sexual problems. Ospemifene is postulated to be even more efficacious than vaginal estrogen in a dose of 60 mg/day. Adverse effects include abnormal vaginal discharge, muscular spasms, vaginal candida infection and vaginal bleeding. Absolute contraindications include vaginal bleeding of unknown etiology- and estrogen-dependent neoplasia.

17.5 Bone Health [26]

(a) *Bisphosphonates*: In women over 60 years of age, they have been found to be beneficial in bone remodeling and reducing the risk of fractures with a good tolerance profile. Poor compliance is linked to adverse effects like gastric irritation and use of effervescent forms or risedronate can help overcome this. They may also adversely affect renal function and decrease serum vitamin D levels; thus, they should be monitored. Rare complications include osteonecrosis of the jaw. There is no study on the optimum duration of use for effectiveness but are usually given for up to 5 years (limited RCT evidence).

Continuing treatment beyond 5 years is of unproven benefit and stopping therapy is not associated with increased risk of fractures.

(b) *Denosumab*: It is a monoclonal antibody that binds to the nuclear factor-kb ligand and decreases the osteoclast activation and bone resorption. It can also be used in patients with a compromised renal function. Rare but serious side effects include femur fractures and osteonecrosis of the jaw.

(c) *Teriparatide*: Although not routinely used due to the need for daily injections and high cost, it effectively decreases rate of vertebral fractures by up to 65% and nonvertebral fractures by up to 35%. Prolonged use poses the additional risk of osteosarcomas and so usage must be restricted to a maximum of 2 years.

(d) *Selective Estrogen Receptor Modulators (SERM)*: They help to improve bone mineral density, decrease bone resorption, and prevent vertebral fractures by 40%. Options include raloxifene and bazedoxifene. They have estrogenic action on the bone, increasing the bone mineral density and reducing bone resorption. Raloxifene hydrochloride 60 mg tablets given daily have been found to be effective.

(e) *Exercise*: Regular exercises improve muscle tone, thus decreasing the propensity to falls and trauma and include options like tai-chi, yoga, and resistance training.

(f) *Calcium and Vitamin D Supplementation*: The daily recommended calcium and vitamin D necessary for bone health is 1000–1500 mg/day and 600–800 IU/day respectively.

17.6 Sarcopenia and Muscle Health

High protein diet, weight bearing and resistance training exercise can help in sarcopenia management to prevent falls and fracture in menopausal women [27]. There is no role of hormonal treatment for sarcopenia at present.

17.7 Libido and Sexual Function

1. *Education and correcting modifiable factors*: Educating women on sexual dysfunction, sexual stimulation and involving partners in correcting sexual behaviors and demands for sex and partner pressure may help. Pelvic floor muscle training and use of vibrators may also be beneficial.
2. *Cognitive behavioral therapy and mindfulness*: May be effective in orgasmic dysfunction, hypoactive sexual disorder and problems in arousal.
3. *Ospemifene*: It can help treat moderate to severe dyspareunia when used at a dose of 60 mg/day. It has no adverse effects on the endometrium, bone or breast tissue.
4. *Vaginal moisturizers and lubricants*: Moisturizers are an option for women with mild to moderate symptoms, although eventually require hormonal therapies. There are similar improvements for the outcomes of vaginal dryness and pH compared with local vaginal estrogens application.
5. *Lasers therapies*: Laser can help in re-epithelization and better vaginal elasticity. However, it is not approved by FDA.
6. *Flibanserin* is a novel multifunctional serotonin agonist and antagonist. It has been recently approved for postmenopausal hypoactive sexual disorder in women less than 65 years of age. The dose is 100 mg prior to sleep [28].

17.8 Conclusion

Nonhormonal management of menopausal symptoms is preferred by some women, especially older women more than 65 years and those with contraindications to MHT like breast cancer or deep vein thrombosis.

Key Points

1. Nonhormonal treatment can be given to symptomatic menopausal who have contraindication to MHT or those unwilling to take hormonal treatment.
2. Breast cancer patients suffering from hot flashes can benefit from nonhormonal treatment like desvenlafaxine and venlafaxine.
3. SSRIs like paroxetine and fluoxetine are not to be given with tamoxifen in breast cancer patients.
4. CBT is very effective in relief of hot flushes.
5. Lubricants and moisturizers are effective in GSM for relief of vaginal dryness, itching, and dyspareunia.

Long Answer Questions (LAQs)

1. What is the nonhormonal treatment for vasomotor symptoms?
2. What is the nonhormonal treatment for GSM?

Short Answer Questions (SAQs)

1. Neurokinin receptor 3 antagonists.
2. Cognitive behavioral therapy in menopause.
3. Ospemifene in genitourinary syndrome of menopause.
4. Bisphosphonates in bone health during menopause.

Multiple Choice Questions (MCQs)

1. Following are the SSRIs used in the treatment of vasomotor symptoms except:

   A. Paroxetine
   B. Sertraline
   C. Citalopram
   D. Duloxetine

2. Following are the benzodiazepines used in the treatment of insomnia during menopause except:

   A. Zolpidem
   B. Zopiclone
   C. Mirtazapine
   D. Zaleplon

3. Mechanism of action of ramelteon is:

   A. Melatonin receptor agonist
   B. Melatonin receptor antagonist
   C. SSRI
   D. SNRI

4. Mechanism of action of suvorexant is:

   A. Orexin receptor antagonist
   B. Orexin receptor agonist
   C. Benzodiazepine
   D. SSRI

5. Following are the drugs used in the treatment of osteoporosis during menopause except:

   A. Denosumab
   B. Teriparatide
   C. Zolpidem
   D. Risedronate

6. Fracture Risk Assessment Tool (FRAX) is used to calculate:

   A. 7-year risk of fractures
   B. 5-year risk of fractures
   C. 10-year risk of fractures
   D. 15-year risk of fractures

7. Mechanism of action of ospemifene is:

   A. Synthetic, nonsteroidal agent
   B. Synthetic, steroidal agent
   C. SSRI
   D. SNRI

8. Dose of ospemifene is:

   A. 20 mg once a day
   B. 40 mg once a day
   C. 60 mg once a day
   D. 80 mg once a day

9. All the following appear to decrease hot flushes in menopausal women except:

   A. Androgens
   B. Raloxifene
   C. Isoflavones
   D. Tibolone

10. Most common menopausal symptom is:

    A. Sleep disorders
    B. Vasomotor symptoms
    C. Sexual complaints
    D. Cognitive decline

Answers

1. D
2. C
3. A
4. A
5. C
6. C
7. A
8. C
9. B
10. B

References

1. Hickey M, Szabo RA, Hunter MS. Non-hormonal treatments for menopausal symptoms. BMJ. 2017;359:j5101.
2. Simon JA, Portman DJ, Kaunitz AM, Mekonnen H, Kazempour K, Bhaskar S, et al. Low-dose paroxetine 7.5 mg for menopausal vasomotor symptoms: two randomized controlled trials. Menopause. 2013;20(10):1027–35.
3. Sahni S, Lobo-Romero A, Smith T. Contemporary non-hormonal therapies for the management of vasomotor symptoms associated with menopause: a literature review. touchREV Endocrinol. 2021;17(2):133–7.
4. Ensrud KE, Guthrie KA, Hohensee C, Caan B, Carpenter JS, Freeman EW, et al. Effects of estradiol and venlafaxine on insomnia symptoms and sleep quality in women with hot flashes. Sleep. 2015;38(1):97–108.
5. Yoon SH, Lee JY, Lee C, Lee H, Kim SN. Gabapentin for the treatment of hot flushes in menopause: a meta-analysis. Menopause. 2020;27(4):485–93.
6. Nguyen ML. The use of pregabalin in the treatment of hot flashes. Can Pharm J (Ott). 2013;146(4):193–6.
7. Leon-Ferre RA, Novotny PJ, Wolfe EG, et al. Oxybutynin vs placebo for hot flashes in women with or without breast cancer: a randomized, double-blind clinical trial (ACCRU SC-1603). JNCI Cancer Spectr. 2020;4(1):pkz088.
8. Prague JK, Roberts RE, Comninos AN, Clarke S, Jayasena CN, Nash Z, et al. Neurokinin 3 receptor antagonism as a novel treatment for menopausal hot flushes: a phase 2, randomised, double-blind, placebo-controlled trial. Lancet. 2017;389(10081):1809–20.
9. Hunter MS. Cognitive behavioral therapy for menopausal symptoms. Climacteric J Int Menopause Soc. 2021;24(1):51–6.
10. Muñiz V, Padilla VJ, Alldredge CT, Elkins G. Clinical hypnosis and cognitive behavioral therapy for hot flashes: a scoping review. Womens Health Rep. 2025;6(1):1–20.
11. Swift DL, Johannsen NM, Lavie CJ, Earnest CP, Church TS. The role of exercise and physical activity in weight loss and maintenance. Prog Cardiovasc Dis. 2014;56(4):441–7.
12. Australian Menopause Society. Lifestyle and behavioural modifications for menopausal symptoms: Australian Menopause Society; [cited 2024 Aug 13].
13. Kapoor E, Collazo-Clavell ML, Faubion SS. Weight gain in women at midlife: a concise review of the pathophysiology and strategies for management. Mayo Clin Proc. 2017;92(10):1552–8.

14. Susanti HD, Sonko I, Chang P, Chuang Y, Chung M. Effects of yoga on menopausal symptoms and sleep quality across menopause statuses: a randomized controlled trial. Nurs Health Sci. 2022;24(2):368–79.
15. Chien TJ, Hsu CH, Liu CY, Fang CJ. Effect of acupuncture on hot flush and menopause symptoms in breast cancer – a systematic review and meta-analysis. PLoS One. 2017;12(8):e0180918.
16. Kirkpatrick K, Khan MH, Deng Y, Shah KB. A review of stellate ganglion block as an adjunctive treatment modality. Cureus. 2023;15(2):e35174.
17. Hall E, Frey BN, Soares CN. Non-hormonal treatment strategies for vasomotor symptoms: a critical review. Drugs. 2011;71(3):287–304.
18. ACOG Practice Bulletin No. 141: management of menopausal symptoms. Obstet Gynecol. 2014;123(1):202–216.
19. Jeon GH. Insomnia in postmenopausal women: how to approach and treat it? J Clin Med. 2024;13(2):428.
20. McCurry SM, Guthrie KA, Morin CM, Woods NF, Landis CA, Ensrud KE, et al. Telephone-based cognitive behavioral therapy for insomnia in perimenopausal and postmenopausal women with vasomotor symptoms: a MsFLASH randomized clinical trial. JAMA Intern Med. 2016;176(7):913–20.
21. Baker FC, Lampio L, Saaresranta T, Polo-Kantola P. Sleep and sleep disorders in the menopausal transition. Sleep Med Clin. 2018;13(3):443–56.
22. Proserpio P, Marra S, Campana C, Agostoni EC, Palagini L, Nobili L, et al. Insomnia and menopause: a narrative review on mechanisms and treatments. Climacteric. 2020;23(6):539–49.
23. Messina G, Viggiano A, De Luca V, Messina A, Chieffi S, Monda M. Hormonal changes in menopause and orexin-a action. Obstet Gynecol Int. 2013;2013:1–5.
24. Silva ASD, Baines G, Araklitis G, Robinson D, Cardozo L. Modern management of genitourinary syndrome of menopause. Fac Rev. [Internet] 2021 [cited 2024 Aug 15];10. Available from: https://www.ncbi.nlm.nih.gov/pmc/articles/PMC7946389/.
25. Danan ER, Sowerby C, Ullman KE, Ensrud K, Forte ML, Zerzan N, et al. Hormonal treatments and vaginal moisturizers for genitourinary syndrome of menopause: a systematic review. Ann Intern Med. 2024;177(10):1400–14.
26. Eastell R, Rosen CJ, Black DM, et al. Pharmacological management of osteoporosis in postmenopausal women: an Endocrine Society clinical practice guideline. J Clin Endocrinol Metab. 2019;104(5):1595–622.
27. Najm A, Niculescu AG, Grumezescu AM, Beuran M. Emerging therapeutic strategies in sarcopenia: an updated review on pathogenesis and treatment advances. Int J Mol Sci. 2024;25(8):4300.
28. Vallejos X, Wu C. Flibanserin: a novel, nonhormonal agent for the treatment of hypoactive sexual desire disorder in premenopausal women. J Pharm Pract. 2017;30(2):256–60.

Postmenopausal Bleeding in Menopause 18

Sudhaa Sharma and Asna Beg Ashraf

Abstract

Postmenopausal bleeding (PMB), defined as any bleeding that occurs more than 12 months after the final menstrual period in women not on menopause hormone therapy, is a common clinical condition with significant implications. Although more than 90% of women with endometrial cancer (EC) present with PMB, over 90% of PMB cases are due to benign conditions such as endometrial or cervical polyps, vaginal atrophy, and endometrial hyperplasia. A thorough evaluation is essential, as up to 10% of women with PMB may harbor EC or premalignant lesions. Risk factors such as age, obesity, unopposed estrogen exposure, diabetes, and tamoxifen use must be carefully considered. Diagnostic modalities like transvaginal sonography (TVS), office hysteroscopy, and targeted endometrial sampling have now replaced blind dilatation and curettage (D&C), offering higher accuracy and safety. Management strategy is guided by the underlying etiology—ranging from local estrogen therapy for atrophy, hysteroscopic removal for polyps and submucous myomas, to hysterectomy for atypical hyperplasia and carcinoma. A structured, risk-based evaluation and individualized management remain essential to optimize outcomes and reduce morbidity.

S. Sharma (✉)
Department of Obstetrics and Gynaecology, GMC Jammu, Jammu, India

Indian Menopause Society (IMS), Mumbai, India

A. B. Ashraf
Ujala Medical Center, Lucknow, India

Lucknow Menopause Society, Lucknow, India

Stillbirth Society of India, Lucknow, India

R. Malik et al. (eds.), *Menopause Essentials*,
https://doi.org/10.1007/978-981-95-7498-8_18

Keywords

Postmenopausal bleeding · Endometrial cancer · Transvaginal sonography · Endometrial hyperplasia · Hysteroscopy · Menopausal hormone therapy · Endometrial sampling

18.1 Introduction

One of the most common gynecological concerns in menopausal women is postmenopausal bleeding [1]. Any bleeding occurring after 1 year of permanent cessation of menses in women who are not on menopause hormone therapy (MHT) is considered postmenopausal bleeding (PMB) [2]. Up to 10% of cases of PMB can be due to endometrial cancer (EC) or premalignant conditions depending on age and risk factors [1, 3]. Many other conditions, such as endometrial or cervical polyps, vaginal atrophy, or nongynecologic conditions, may also cause PMB [1]. Women with PMB should always be evaluated thoroughly and promptly to find the cause of bleeding because PMB is the most common symptom of EC and other serious conditions like atypical hyperplasia or endometrial intraepithelial neoplasia (EIN) [4]. In the past, dilatation and curettage (D&C) used to be the mainstay of investigating PMB, but now newer approaches like transvaginal sonography (TVS) and office hysteroscopy have revolutionized the diagnosis of PMB by offering safer, more accurate, and less invasive alternatives to the traditional D&C [1].

18.2 Associations or Risk Factors for PMB

All clinical risk factors for endometrial cancer should be taken into consideration when evaluating a woman for PMB. A comprehensive list of risk factors includes increasing age, obesity, reproductive factors, medical comorbidities, genetic factors, lifestyle and iatrogenic factors [3, 4] (Table 18.1).

18.3 Causes of PMB

More than 90% of women with endometrial cancer (EC) present with PMB, but over 90% of women with PMB have a benign underlying cause for their symptoms [3] (Table 18.2).

1. *Atrophy* is the most common cause of bleeding in postmenopausal patients. It is usually due to vaginal atrophy resulting from the changes occurring in the vulvovaginal tissues due to estrogen deficiency, known as genitourinary syndrome of menopause (GSM). Postcoital spotting or bleeding is also a common symptom of GSM. Endometrial atrophy may also cause PMB in some cases [1].
2. *Polyps* (endocervical and/or endometrial) are also very common in postmenopausal women [1]. Endometrial polyps are a common cause of PMB, and while

Table 18.1 Risk factors for PMB [3, 4]

Advancing age
Obesity
Reproductive Early menarche Late menopause Nulliparity
Medical comorbidities Polycystic ovary syndrome Type 1 and 2 diabetes mellitus Hypertension Atypical glandular cells on screening cervical cytology
Genetic Lynch syndrome, Cowden syndrome Family history of endometrial or colorectal cancers
Lifestyle Physical inactivity Diet
Iatrogenic Use of unopposed estrogen therapy Tamoxifen therapy

Table 18.2 Causes of PMB [3]

Malignant Endometrial cancer Cervical cancer Vulval cancer Vaginal cancer Ovarian or fallopian tube cancer Choriocarcinoma Cancer in adjacent organs (e.g., urethra, bladder, bowel)
Premalignant Endometrial hyperplasia
Benign Endometrial polyps Atrophy of the vaginal mucosa or endometrium Endometritis
Iatrogenic Unscheduled bleeding in women using hormone replacement therapy Anticoagulant therapy Post radiation therapy
No cause identified

most are benign, the risk of malignancy ranges from 1.5% to 12.9%. The risk of endometrial hyperplasia and cancer in polyps is 4.4 times higher in postmenopausal women with PMB compared to asymptomatic women [1].

3. *Myomas* may rarely present as PMB. Myomas and adenomyosis should not cause PMB in the absence of postmenopausal hormone therapy. If a submucous myoma causes PMB, it should be evaluated for sarcomatous change [5].

4. *Endometrial hyperplasia (EH)*—According to the World Health Organization, the EH classification system has only two categories: hyperplasia without atypia (nonneoplastic) and atypical hyperplasia (endometrial intraepithelial neoplasm, EIN) [6]. Hyperplasia without atypia is benign and often regresses with hormonal correction. The chances of coexisting invasive cancer at diagnosis are 1%, and the risk of progression to cancer is 1–3% if estrogen excess persists. Atypical hyperplasia is a precursor to endometrioid endometrial cancer. Up to 60% have coexisting invasive cancer or are at high risk of developing it [6].
5. *Endometrial cancer*—PMB is the most common symptom of EC; therefore, the complaint of PMB should always be taken very seriously and never ignored, no matter how inconsequential it may appear.
6. *Vaginal, vulval, and cervical cancers* are also considered, in the differential diagnosis for women presenting with PMB [7].
7. *Urological (urethra/bladder) and gastrointestinal (anal/rectal/bowel) cancers* are also considered in women presenting with bleeding that is thought to be coming from the genital tract [7].
8. *Iatrogenic causes* can be unscheduled bleeding in women using MHT, anticoagulant therapy, tamoxifen, or following radiation therapy [3].
9. *Other causes* could be foreign bodies like forgotten IUCD or forgotten pessary for prolapse, and nonprescription medications—herbals/phytoestrogens.
10. *Chronic tubercular endometritis* can be a rare cause of PMB in the developing world.
11. *Coagulopathies* including thrombocytopenia, leukemia, liver disease, pancytopenia, and dengue hemorrhagic fever are also rare causes of PMB.

18.4 Evaluation of PMB

18.4.1 History

A detailed history including general medical history, menstrual and obstetric history, duration since menopause, and characteristics of PMB (severity, frequency, duration, pattern, and amount) should be elicited. History of associated symptoms (pain, discharge, weight loss), gynecologic surgeries, and cervical smears are also important [1, 2]. Drug history includes the use of MHT, current or past tamoxifen, and use of anticoagulants such as warfarin, heparin, and clopidogrel which many women with cardiac problems take. Clinical risk factors for endometrial cancer, including but not limited to age, obesity, use of unopposed estrogen, comorbidities (e.g., polycystic ovary syndrome, type 2 diabetes mellitus, atypical glandular cells on screening cervical cytology), and family history of gynecologic malignancy should be considered when evaluating PMB [4]. Assessments should aim to identify and monitor the multiple identifiable risk factors associated with endometrial cancer [7]. History of any known coagulopathy is important.

18.4.2 Examination [1, 2]

A thorough general and systemic examination should include general appearance, signs of coagulopathy, body mass index (BMI), blood pressure, and breast examination. Abdominal palpation should be done to rule out any abdominal or pelvic masses. Local examination should be done to check for visual signs of bleeding and any lesions/growth. A speculum examination is done to inspect the vulva, vagina and urethra for atrophy, suspicious lesions, trauma, foreign body, atrophic vaginitis, cervical polyps, and cancer. Uterine size, mobility, and the adnexa are evaluated by bimanual vaginal examination. Per rectal examination is done to rule out anal fissures or bleeding hemorrhoids.

18.4.3 Investigations

There is no universal consensus on the ideal approach for diagnosing PMB. The order of investigations for patients presenting with PMB may vary depending on several factors, including clinical judgment, available resources, and patient preference [1]. Ultimately, the choice of diagnostic approach should be tailored to the individual patient's circumstances.

1. Transvaginal ultrasound (TVS).
2. Endometrial sampling/biopsy.
3. Saline infusion sonohysterography (SIS).
4. Hysteroscopy.
5. Advances in diagnostic techniques.

18.4.3.1 Transvaginal Sonography (TVS)

TVS is a valuable, noninvasive tool and is now accepted as the first-line investigation for evaluating a postmenopausal woman with first episode of bleeding [4]. All women with PMB or abnormal uterine bleeding on MHT should undergo a TVS to assess the thickness and features of the endometrium [7]. The thickness of the double-layer endometrium helps guide clinical decisions on whether further investigations, such as endometrial biopsy or hysteroscopy are required [3]. Endometrial thickness (ET) is measured as the maximum anterior-posterior thickness of the endometrial echo on the long-axis transvaginal view of the uterus [4]. The adnexal region should also be covered in the ultrasound to exclude extrauterine pelvic masses. Transabdominal ultrasound should complement TVS if there is an enlarged uterus or pelvic mass [7].

Interpretation of TVS

- A uniform, thin, distinct endometrial echo will accurately identify the 40% of women in whom atrophy is the cause of the bleeding. If the echo is visualized in its entirety and is 4 mm, no further investigations are necessary in the average-risk woman [2]. An ET of 4 mm or less has a greater than 99% negative predictive value (NPV) for endometrial cancer [4].

- TVS can help assess malignancy risk based on endometrial characteristics. A heterogeneous endometrium with cystic changes is highly suspicious of underlying disease [3]. A thickened endometrial echo does not diagnose any particular pathology and is an indication for further investigation which can be hysteroscopy with directed biopsy, sonohysterography or endometrial sampling [4]. In low-resource settings, if these investigations are not routinely available, blind endometrial sampling may be undertaken. It is important to recognize the limitations of this approach.

Limitations of TVS

- An axial uterus, obesity, coexisting myomas, polyps, adenomyosis, and previous scars do not allow proper assessment of ET [4].
- Endometrial fluid when present, should not be included in measuring endometrial thickness [4].
- TVS evaluation depends on the experience of the examiner, the equipment and the quality of visualization.

18.4.3.2 Endometrial Sampling

Dilatation and Curettage (D&C) was once the standard for evaluating PMB. However, isolated D&C is no longer the first-line method because it can miss focal pathology (>50% of the cavity) due to blind sampling [7]. Later on, in-office endometrial sampling devices (e.g., Pipelle and Vabra) became available [1]. An endometrial biopsy (EB) is indicated if a woman with PMB has a thickened endometrium (ET >4 mm) on TVS. Although it is easy and quick to perform in an outpatient setting, endometrial biopsy is an invasive procedure with many disadvantages and risks. There can be a failure to obtain a tissue sample (11%), inadequate sample (31%), pain, bleeding, infection, and rarely perforation. Since it is a blind procedure, small, localized cancers can be missed by endometrial sampling [1, 3].

Endometrial sampling in the form of office-based biopsy, is now used in combination with TVS with or without hysteroscopy for evaluating women with PMB [7]. Endometrial sampling is conclusive only if hyperplasia, or malignancy, is found. If it is negative but bleeding persists, further evaluation by hysteroscopy is needed to detect missed abnormalities. The likely findings will be endometrial polyps or undetected histological abnormalities missed on blind biopsy [2]. Women with benign or inconclusive histology but persistent symptoms or suspicious ultrasound findings should be offered hysteroscopy.

18.4.3.3 Saline Infusion Sonography (SIS)

In SIS, visualization of intracavitary lesions is enhanced by infusing saline into the uterine cavity. The diagnostic accuracy for endometrial pathology in PMB varies from 85% to 95% sensitivity and 84% to 91% specificity. SIS helps stratify women for further hysteroscopic evaluation. The diagnostic success was found to be lower in postmenopausal women (87%) vs. premenopausal women ($p < 0.01$). SIS is a valuable tool for assessing abnormal uterine bleeding but may be less effective in postmenopausal women [1].

18.4.3.4 Hysteroscopy

Hysteroscopy is the direct visualization of the uterine cavity to identify pathology, take directed biopsies, and carry out therapeutic procedures, such as polypectomy. Hysteroscopy is now considered superior to blind EB, D&C, and ultrasound [1].

Indications of Hysteroscopy [3, 7].

- endometrial thickness is greater than 4 mm on TVS.
- focal endometrial pathology.
- thickened, irregular endometrium, or other concerning features on TVS.
- recurrent or prolonged bleeding.
- if random endometrial sampling has been nondiagnostic.

Office hysteroscopy

Office hysteroscopy is a minimally invasive procedure allowing direct visualization of uterine pathology without the need for general anesthesia and the use of an operating room, generating cost savings in the long run and greater compliance among patients [5]. Office hysteroscopy appears safe and feasible and allows accurate diagnosis of focal intrauterine pathologies, which may otherwise be misdiagnosed with blind procedures [5].

In outpatient hysteroscopy, the vaginoscopy approach should be the standard technique, as it is better tolerated by women compared to conventional hysteroscopy. Biopsy guided by office hysteroscopy has better accuracy than other blind sampling methods, like D&C and Pipelle, that could fail to sample a significant proportion of the endometrial cavity [5].

18.4.3.5 Advances in Diagnostic Techniques

Blood biomarkers are being developed for endometrial cancer. A panel of protein biomarkers, including CA125 and HE4, shows promise. CA125 is elevated in advanced cases but is unreliable for early detection. Genomic biomarkers like CTCs, ctDNA, and miRNA may help in diagnosis and monitoring, though their low early-stage concentrations limit current applicability [3].

The SIR-En index, a new biomarker which combines systemic inflammatory indices with endometrial thickness, can effectively differentiate between endometrial hyperplasia and carcinoma in menopausal women with abnormal uterine bleeding, with high specificity (94%) and positive predictive value (96%). Further studies are required to validate these findings and optimize clinical application [8].

18.5 Management

Atrophy: For treating moderate to severe symptoms of vaginal atrophy, low-dose vaginal estrogen therapy (ET) is considered the most successful treatment option. For mild symptoms, lubricants and moisturizers are considered first-line. Progesterone is not required with vaginal ET. Atrophic endometritis can be treated with systemic estrogen therapy. The addition of progesterone is necessary if the uterus is intact.

Polyp: During an office hysteroscopic examination, it is recommended to evaluate the following parameters of a polyp—number, dimensions, consistency, location, and characteristics of the base of implantation. These features may provide information about the malignancy risk and thus influence the method of removal of the polyp [5].

Submucous myoma: Office hysteroscopic myomectomy is the first-line surgical treatment for submucosal myomas. It is minimally invasive, safe, cost-effective, and associated with high patient satisfaction. It is an effective, and preferred approach for appropriately sized submucosal fibroids. The size limitations for hysteroscopic removal are for FIGO Type 2 fibroids up to 4 cm and Type 0–1 fibroids up to 5 cm [5].

Endometrial hyperplasia and carcinoma: Hyperplasia without atypia should be treated conservatively (normalization of the cycle through weight loss, metformin, oral contraceptives, cyclical progestogens, or Levonorgestrel IUD). Preventive hysterectomy is advised only in exceptional cases (e.g., extreme obesity without any prospect of weight loss). The surgery should be a total hysterectomy, i.e., it must include removal of the cervix [6].

Atypical hyperplasia is not reversed with progesterone. Patients with atypical hyperplasia/endometrioid intraepithelial neoplasia, or EC, should be referred to a gynecological oncology unit for treatment. Treatment is almost always surgical with staging of disease—hysterectomy with salpingo-oophorectomy and bilateral pelvic and para-aortic lymphadenectomy [6].

18.6 Special Considerations

Certain circumstances require particular attention or adjustments in management strategies and include:

(a) Recurrent PMB.
(b) PMB in women on MHT.
(c) Tamoxifen-treated women.
(d) Asymptomatic postmenopausal women with thick endometrium.
(e) Incidental finding of endometrial fluid on ultrasound.

18.6.1 Recurrent PMB

Any bleeding happening 6 weeks or more after a previously investigated episode of PMB is defined as a recurrent PMB [9]. Recurrent PMB can occur in 6–25% of postmenopausal women who have experienced a previous episode of PMB. Factors that are predictive of recurrent PMB include the use of MHT and benign polyps at the first PMB. Women with recurrence of PMB were more commonly diagnosed with benign polyps and less commonly diagnosed with malignancies compared to patients with only a single episode [9]. Recurrent PMB does not always indicate cancer, but it still requires proper evaluation.

All women who experience unexplained, persistent, or recurrent PMB should be evaluated by hysteroscopy and repeat endometrial biopsy, even if the previous investigations were normal or reassuring. A low threshold for reinvestigating these women should be maintained [7].

If PMB persists or recurs, histologic evaluation (endometrial biopsy or hysteroscopy with biopsy) is necessary even if ET is <3 mm because rare cases of endometrial carcinoma (particularly type II) can present with an endometrial thickness of less than 3 mm [4].

Other risk factors (older age, obesity, diabetes, use of Tamoxifen, Lynch syndrome, or history of unopposed estrogen exposure) further justify a lower threshold for biopsy.

18.6.2 PMB in Women on Menopause Hormone Therapy

The risk of malignancy in women who are on appropriate MHT is lower than in those not taking MHT [2]. In a recent retrospective cohort study, the EC detection rate in women under 60 years with PMB who were using MHT was very low (0.47%) as opposed to that in women who were not using MHT (2.18%) [10]. Continuous regimens have a lower risk of malignancy than sequential regimens. All women on MHT should be investigated if their bleeding is persistent [7]. The most common reasons for unscheduled bleeding on MHT include polyps and submucous fibroids [2]. The approach to postmenopausal bleeding (PMB) in women using MHT varies based on the type of regimen.

18.7 Women on Cyclical Estrogen-Progestogen Therapy (Sequential MHT)

The bleeding should occur in a cyclic pattern, similar to withdrawal bleeding. Women on sequential MHT should be evaluated if they experience irregular bleeding despite adjustment of dose, if their bleeding increases in heaviness or duration, or if more than 3 months have passed since initiating treatment [7].

For patients on sequential therapy, TVS should be performed in the first half of the cycle, with an endometrial thickness of 8 mm serving as the threshold for biopsy in cases of unscheduled bleeding [2].

18.8 Women on Continuous Combined MHT (Estrogen + Progestogen Daily)

Irregular bleeding is common in the first 6 months of initiation of therapy. Any bleeding persisting beyond 6 months, or new-onset bleeding after a significant period of amenorrhea requires investigation. The causes of PMB may include endometrial atrophy, endometrial hyperplasia, polyps, or malignancy.

There is an ongoing debate regarding the recommendation of upper limit of normal ET in patients on continuous MHT regimens. An ET of ≤5 mm is generally considered indicative of atrophy in a bleeding patient, requiring no further investigation [2, 11]. In women with PMB on MHT available data suggest that office hysteroscopy-guided endometrial sampling should be performed if the ET is ≥8 mm [11].

1. Where additional risk factors exist, clinical discretion may be used for an earlier evaluation [7].
2. Women on Unopposed Estrogen (e.g., estrogen-only MHT).

Unopposed estrogen stimulates the endometrium and increases the risk of endometrial hyperplasia and carcinoma. Any postmenopausal bleeding in these women requires immediate evaluation (TVS and/or endometrial biopsy).

18.8.1 Tamoxifen-Treated Women

Tamoxifen induces a benign subepithelial stromal hypertrophy and glandular cystic atrophy that is often subendometrial or contained within polyps; therefore, there is very little correlation between TVS measurement of ET and abnormal pathology [11].·Routine endometrial surveillance is not recommended for asymptomatic women on tamoxifen [1, 11].

Tamoxifen increases EC risk by up to three- to six-fold by stimulating endometrial estrogen receptors [11]. Any abnormal uterine bleeding in tamoxifen-treated women should be investigated by diagnostic hysteroscopy with endometrial sampling independently of ET [11]. In these women, TVS is not a useful tool for triage [7].

18.8.2 Asymptomatic Postmenopausal Women with Thick Endometrium

Endometrial thickness >4 mm on TVS in asymptomatic postmenopausal women (those without bleeding) does not always require evaluation [4, 11]. Investigations should be individualized based on patient risk factors (e.g., obesity, diabetes, history of unopposed estrogen use, Lynch syndrome) [4, 11]. TVS is not a screening tool for EC in asymptomatic women, as incidental findings of increased ET do not necessarily indicate malignancy [4]. In postmenopausal women without bleeding incidental finding of endometrial thickness ≥11 mm on TVS, requires further investigation [7].

18.8.3 Incidental Finding of Endometrial Fluid on Ultrasound

The incidental finding of endometrial fluid on ultrasound in asymptomatic postmenopausal women is typically benign unless the endometrial thickness exceeds 4 mm [1]. A study by Topçu et al. involving 141 asymptomatic postmenopausal women found that fluid in the endometrial cavity is benign when the endometrial lining is <4 mm [12].

Key Points

- PMB needs prompt and thorough evaluation to exclude or diagnose endometrial cancer or precancer. The dictum is—it is cancer unless proven otherwise. The aim is to identify the small proportion of women who have endometrial cancer or precancer while minimizing the use of invasive procedures in those with benign causes of PMB.
- A complete history and physical assessment is the first step, imaging is the second step, with biopsy or hysteroscopic evaluation indicated for those with abnormal imaging or additional risk factors for EC.
- TVS is a good modality for an initial evaluation with an NPV of 99% for EC in low-risk women with the first episode of PMB.
- Thin endometrium does not exclude cancer in all patients with recurrent bleeding.
- Recurrent bleeding with inadequate endometrial sample warrants hysteroscopy and endometrial biopsy.
- Strong suspicion, thorough evaluation and early diagnosis reduce morbidity and mortality due to PMB.

Long Answer Questions (LAQs)

1. Describe the causes of postmenopausal bleeding (PMB) and discuss their relative frequency and clinical significance.
2. Discuss the risk factors and associations for PMB, and describe the approach for the evaluation and diagnosis of a woman presenting with PMB.
3. Describe the advances in diagnostic techniques and management strategies for postmenopausal bleeding.
4. How should postmenopausal bleeding be evaluated and managed in a woman currently receiving menopausal hormone therapy (MHT)?

Short Answer Questions (SAQs)

1. What are the most common benign causes of postmenopausal bleeding?
2. What new diagnostic tools have improved safety and accuracy for PMB assessment?
3. How will you evaluate postmenopausal bleeding in a breast cancer survivor on tamoxifen?
4. How will you manage a patient with recurrent PMB?
5. What is the first-line investigation for evaluating postmenopausal bleeding?

Multiple Choice Questions (MCQs)

1. All are true about endometrial hyperplasia except:

   A. In hyperplasia without atypia, the chances of coexisting invasive cancer at diagnosis are 10%
   B. In hyperplasia without atypia, the risk of progression to cancer is 1–3% if estrogen excess persists
   C. Atypical hyperplasia is a precursor to endometrioid endometrial cancer
   D. Up to 60% of patients with atypical hyperplasia have coexisting invasive cancer or are at high risk of developing it

2. Which statement is true regarding first-line investigation for evaluating PMB?

   A. Dilatation and curettage (D&C) is the first step for evaluating PMB
   B. Endometrial thickness of 4 mm or less on TVS generally excludes endometrial cancer in an average-risk woman
   C. Hysterosalpingography is a new diagnostic tool for evaluating PMB

D. Endometrial thickness of 5 mm or more on TVS generally excludes endometrial cancer in an average-risk woman

3. Which of the following is not a risk factor for endometrial cancer in postmenopausal women?

   A. Increasing age
   B. Obesity
   C. Smoking
   D. Use of unopposed estrogen

4. Which of the following is a limitation of blind endometrial sampling?

   A. It is very expensive
   B. It cannot detect endometrial polyps
   C. It can miss focal pathology in more than 50% of the cavity
   D. It requires general anesthesia

5. Which of the following new diagnostic tools combines systemic inflammatory indices with endometrial thickness to differentiate between hyperplasia and carcinoma?

   A. CA125
   B. HE4
   C. SIR-En index
   D. MRI

6. Which of the following is a common iatrogenic cause of PMB?

   A. Metformin
   B. Tamoxifen
   C. Labetalol
   D. Thyroxine

7. A 56 year-old woman presents with vaginal bleeding 6 years after her last menstrual period. She is not on hormone replacement therapy. On examination, there are no visible lesions on the vulva or cervix. Transvaginal ultrasound shows an endometrial thickness of 3 mm. What is the most likely cause of her bleeding?

   A. Endometrial cancer
   B. Endometrial polyp
   C. Vaginal atrophy
   D. Cervical erosion

8. A 65-year-old woman with a history of breast cancer treated with tamoxifen presents with PMB. TVS shows a heterogeneous endometrial echo and a polypoid lesion. What is the most appropriate diagnostic procedure?

   A. Endometrial sampling using Pipelle
   B. Office hysteroscopy with directed biopsy

   C. Repeat TVS in 6 months
   D. Start estrogen therapy

9. A 70-year-old woman presents with recurrent postmenopausal bleeding. She had a negative endometrial biopsy 2 months ago, but symptoms persist. What should be the next step?
   A. Repeat endometrial biopsy
   B. Hysteroscopy
   C. Start antibiotics
   D. No further action needed only reassurance

10. A 68-year-old obese woman with a history of hypertension presents with PMB. TVS shows an endometrial thickness of 6 mm and a focal intracavitary lesion. Which of the following is the most likely diagnosis?
    A. Endometrial polyp
    B. Cervical cancer
    C. Vaginal atrophy
    D. Tubercular endometritis

Answers

1. A
2. B
3. C
4. C
5. C
6. B
7. C
8. B
9. B
10. A

References

1. Carugno J. Clinical management of vaginal bleeding in postmenopausal women. Climacteric. 2020;23(4):343–9. https://doi.org/10.1080/13697137.2020.1739642.
2. D. Black diagnosis and medical management of abnormal premenopausal and postmenopausal bleeding. Climacteric. 2023;26(3):222–8. https://doi.org/10.1080/13697137.2023.2178893.
3. Jones ER, O'Flynn H, Njoku K, Crosbie EJ. Detecting endometrial cancer. Obstetr Gynaecol. 2021;23:103–12. https://doi.org/10.1111/tog.12722.

4. ACOG. Committee opinion summary: the role of transvaginal ultrasonography in evaluating the endometrium of women with postmenopausal bleeding. Obstet Gynecol. 2018;131(5):945–6.
5. Giampaolino P, Della Corte L, Di Filippo C, Mercorio A, Vitale SG, Bifulco G. Office hysteroscopy in the management of women with postmenopausal bleeding. Climacteric. 2020;23(4):369–75. https://doi.org/10.1080/13697137.2020.1754389.
6. Emons G, Beckmann MW, Schmidt D, Mallmann P. Uterus commission of the Gynecological Oncology Working Group (AGO). New WHO classification of endometrial hyperplasias. Geburtshilfe Frauenheilkd. 2015;75(2):135–6. https://doi.org/10.1055/s-0034-1396256. PMID: 25797956; PMCID: PMC4361167.
7. Duffy A, Ní Bhuinneain M, Burke N, Murphy C. National clinical practice guideline: assessment and management of postmenopausal bleeding. National Women and Infants Health Programme and The Institute of Obstetricians and Gynaecologists. December 2022.
8. Ronsini C, Iavarone I, Vastarella MG, Della Corte L, Andreoli G, Bifulco G, Cobellis L, De Franciscis P. SIR-EN—new biomarker for identifying patients at risk of endometrial carcinoma in abnormal uterine bleeding at menopause. Cancer. 2024;16:3567. https://doi.org/10.3390/cancers16213567.
9. van Maldegem LDPR, van der Zande JA, van Werkhoven LA, Ewing-Graham PC, Heemskerk-Gerritsen BAM, van Doorn HC. Recurrent postmenopausal bleeding: pathological findings and predictive factors. A multicentre, prospective, observational study. Acta Obstet Gynecol Scand. 2024;103:1283–91. https://doi.org/10.1111/aogs.14851.
10. Buchanan C, Robinson M, Macdonald M. Endometrial cancer ratein hormone replacement therapy users with postmenopausalbleeding: retrospective cohort study. Post Reprod Health. 2022;28(3):143–8.
11. Saccardi C, Spagnol G, Bonaldo G, Marchetti M, Tozzi R, Noventa M. New light on endometrial thickness as a risk factor of cancer: what do clinicians need to know? Cancer Manag Res. 2022;14:1331–40. https://doi.org/10.2147/CMAR.S294074. PMID: 35401014; PMCID: PMC8985823.
12. Topçu HO, Taşdemir Ü, İslimye M, Bayramoğlu H, Yılmaz N. The clinical significance of endometrial fluid collection in asymptomatic postmenopausal women. Climacteric. 2015;18(5):733–6. https://doi.org/10.3109/13697137.2015.1031214. Epub 2015 Apr 14.

Evaluation of Adnexal Mass in Menopause

19

Nisha Singh and Deepshikha Rajput

Abstract

Adnexal masses in post-menopausal women pose a diagnostic and therapeutic challenge due to their significantly higher risk of malignancy compared to pre-menopausal women. A systematic approach is essential, beginning with detailed history, clinical examination, and imaging—most notably transvaginal ultrasound (TVUS), which remains the first-line modality. Serum CA-125 is the most widely used tumour marker, though its limited specificity necessitates adjunctive use with other biomarkers such as HE4 and multimodal scoring systems, including the Risk of Malignancy Index (RMI), ROMA, and IOTA rules, which aid in risk stratification. When malignancy is suspected, further imaging with MRI or CT is warranted to evaluate disease extent and operability. Management decisions are guided by risk assessment, symptoms, and patient factors, with surgical intervention being the cornerstone of treatment. In post-menopausal women, even benign-appearing lesions often warrant surgical removal due to the increased baseline risk of malignancy. Multidisciplinary evaluation, appropriate risk stratification, and individualized treatment strategies remain crucial for optimizing outcomes in this population.

Keywords

Adnexal mass · Post-menopausal women · Ovarian cancer · Risk of Malignancy Index · Transvaginal ultrasound

---

N. Singh (✉) · D. Rajput
Department of Gynaecological Oncology, King George's Medical University, Lucknow, India
e-mail: nisha@kgmcindia.edu

R. Malik et al. (eds.), *Menopause Essentials*,
https://doi.org/10.1007/978-981-95-7498-8_19

19.1 Introduction

Adnexal masses in post-menopausal women pose a significant challenge in diagnosis and management for primary care providers and gynaecologists due to the high risk for malignancy in this age group. The evaluation of an adnexal mass in a post-menopausal female requires a systematic approach to differentiate between benign and malignant aetiologies. Usually noted incidentally, the finding may represent a benign, borderline, or malignant neoplasm of the reproductive tract, metastasis from a distant site, or a non-neoplastic process. This chapter will provide a comprehensive overview of the evaluation of adnexal masses in post-menopausal women, including epidemiology, clinical presentation, diagnostic workup, and management strategies.

19.2 Incidence and Prevalence

Adnexal masses are relatively common, with an estimated prevalence of 18% in post-menopausal women. Most of these masses are benign, with only a small proportion being malignant. However, the risk of malignancy increases with age, and the risk in menopausal women is 30% compared to 7% in premenopausal women [1].

19.3 Differential Diagnosis

Among the differential diagnosis of an adnexal mass, ovarian cancer is the most common which is the fifth leading cause of cancer-related deaths in women. The lifetime risk of developing ovarian cancer is approximately 1 in 78, with most cases occurring in women over the age of 50.

The various differential diagnoses of adnexal mass in a menopausal woman that should be kept in mind while evaluating a case are as follows:

19.3.1 Gynaecological Causes

1. *Ovarian Diseases*
   Malignant Neoplasms

   - Epithelial ovarian cancer: This is the most common ovarian malignancy that may be serous, mucinous, endometrioid or clear cell type in histology.
   - *Sex cord-stromal tumours*: The adult granulosa cell tumour is common in menopausal women followed by Sertoli-Leydig cell tumour.
   - *Germ cell tumours* like dysgerminoma, yolk sac tumour, and immature teratoma are rarely seen in menopausal women.
   - *Metastatic cancer* like Krukenberg tumour from primary gall bladder, stomach, or breast cancer.

Benign Neoplasms

- *Serous cystadenoma*: Thin-walled, serous fluid-filled cyst.
- *Mucinous cystadenoma*: Larger, multi-loculated cyst with mucinous fluid.
- *Fibroma*: Solid, benign tumour; may be associated with Meigs syndrome (ascites, pleural effusion).
- *Mature cystic teratoma (dermoid cyst)*: rarely seen in menopausal women.

Borderline Tumours—exhibit proliferative activity and atypia but lack stromal invasion.

- *Serous borderline tumours*—most common subtype, often bilateral, may show micropapillary features.
- *Mucinous borderline tumours*—usually unilateral and large with intestinal and endocervical subtypes.
- *Endometroid borderline tumours*—rare, associated with endometriosis.
- *Clear cell borderline tumours*—very rare.
- *Seromucinous borderline tumours*—mixed features of serous and mucinous differentiation.
- *Borderline Brenner Tumours*—transitional cell (urothelial like) epithelium.

2. *Tubal Diseases*
   - *Hydrosalpinx*: Fluid-filled, blocked fallopian tube mostly due to tuberculosis.
   - *Pyosalpinx*: Pus-filled fallopian tube due to infection (e.g. PID).
   - *Tubo-ovarian abscess*: Complication of PID or genital tuberculosis.
3. *Paraovarian/Paratubal Diseases*
   - *Para ovarian cysts*: Arise from remnants of the Wolffian or Müllerian ducts.
   - *Para tubal cysts*: Similar to paraovarian cysts but located near the fallopian tube.
4. *Uterine Fibroids*: Subserous broad ligament or pedunculated fibroids may mimic an adnexal mass.

19.3.2 Non-Gynaecologic Causes

1. *Gastrointestinal diseases*
   - Appendiceal abscess or mucocele.
   - Diverticular abscess.
   - Colonic or rectal cancer.
   - Mesenteric cyst or tumour.
   - GIST (gastrointestinal stromal tumour).
2. *Urinary Tract diseases*
   - Pelvic kidney.
   - Ureteric or bladder diverticulum.

3. *Peritoneal diseases*

   - Peritoneal inclusion cysts.
   - Pelvic adhesions and fibrosis.

4. *Lymphadenopathy*: Enlarged Pelvic Lymph Nodes

19.4 Protective Factors for Ovarian Cancer

Certain factors that may reduce the risk of ovarian cancer are:

- *Oral contraceptives*: Long-term use of birth control pills is associated with a reduced risk. Use of OCPs for 5 years decreases the risk by 50%.
- *Pregnancy, breastfeeding, and tubal ligation* are shown to lower the risk.

19.5 Symptoms

Another important aspect to be recorded in history is the presenting complaint. Post-menopausal women with adnexal mass may present with a variety of symptoms, although many are asymptomatic and the mass is discovered incidentally during imaging studies. Common symptoms include:

- *Pelvic Pain*: Dull, aching pain in the lower abdomen or pelvis.
- *Abdominal Distension*: Feeling of fullness or bloating is usually associated with large tumours.
- *Urinary Symptoms* (frequency, urgency, or difficulty urinating) and *Gastrointestinal Symptoms* (changes in bowel habits, constipation, or diarrhoea) are pressure symptoms due to the enlarging pelvic mass.
- *Vaginal Bleeding*: Post-menopausal bleeding, although less common, may be associated with hormone producing ovarian tumours.

19.6 Clinical Examination

Clinical examination plays a crucial role in identifying the organ of origin and its nature (benign or malignant) in a case presenting as an adnexal mass. A thorough physical examination is essential in the evaluation of an adnexal mass. Key components of the examination include:

- *General examination*: Signs of systemic illness like fever, tachycardia, and hypotension may indicate infection or rupture of an adnexal mass. Enlarged lymph nodes in supra clavicular, axillary, or inguinal regions may suggest metastatic disease or infection.

- *Abdominal examination*: Abdominal distension or asymmetry may suggest a large mass. Tenderness or guarding is a sign of peritoneal irritation, torsion or rupture. Palpation of a mass, its location, shape, size, laterality, consistency, surface, margins and mobility help in identifying organ of origin. Signs of fluid thrill and shifting dullness indicate ascites that might be associated with malignancy, rupture of a cyst, or genital tuberculosis.
- *Pelvic examination*: Rule out any cervical or vaginal masses, which could cause similar symptoms. Palpation of the uterus is important to assess the size, shape, mobility, and excluding a subserous or broad ligament fibroid.
- The pelvic adnexal mass may be appreciated as unilateral or bilateral indicating stage of disease.
- Soft or cystic masses are often benign, while firm, irregular masses may raise suspicion for malignancy. Fixed, immobile masses could be a sign of malignancy, while mobile masses are usually benign.
- *Rectal examination:* This is mandatory for masses in the posterior pelvic space and helps in ruling out rectal mucosal involvement.

19.7 Diagnostic Workup

19.7.1 Imaging Studies

Imaging plays a crucial role in the evaluation of adnexal masses. The primary imaging modalities include:

1. *Sonography–Transvaginal (TVS) or Transabdominal sonography (TAS)*—TVS is the first-line imaging modality for evaluating an adnexal mass. It provides detailed images of the pelvic structures, helps in identifying organ of origin and differentiating between benign and malignant masses based on characteristics such as:

    - *Size*: Larger masses (above 6 cm) are more likely to be malignant.
    - *Morphology*: Complex masses with solid components, septations, or papillary projections are more suspicious for malignancy.
    - *Doppler Flow*: Increased vascularity within the mass suggests neovascularization, which is a sign of malignancy.

    TAS is supplementary to TVS when the mass extends beyond TVS view. Standardization of USG reporting should be done by IOTA or O-RADS US.

International Ovarian Tumour Analysis (IOTA). This reporting system was formulated in 1999 by Dirk Timmerman, Lil Valentin, and Tom Bourne. They published a consensus statement on terms, definitions, and measurements to describe

Table 19.1 IOTA simple rules

	M-rules		B-rules
M1	Irregular solid tumour	**B1**	Unilocular cyst
M2	Presence of ascites	**B2**	Presence of solid components where the largest solid component has the largest diameter <7 mm
M3	At least four papillary structures	**B3**	Presence of acoustic shadows
M4	Irregular multilocular solid tumour with the largest diameter >100 mm	**B4**	Smooth multilocular tumour with the largest diameter <100 mm
M5	Very strong blood flow (colour score 4)	**B5**	No blood flow (colour score 1)

the sonographic features of adnexal masses. Simple IOTA rules [2] are used to differentiate benign and malignant masses as described in Table 19.1.

How the rules work?

- If one or more M features are present without any B-features, the mass is malignant.
- If one or more B features are present without any M-features, the mass is benign.
- If both B and M features are present, or no features are present, the result is inconclusive and a second test is needed.

Ovarian-Adnexal Reporting and Data System Ultrasound (O-RADS US) [3], introduced by the American College of Radiology in 2018, forms the ultrasound component of ORADS. This system aims to ensure that there are uniform, unambiguous sonographic evaluations of ovarian or other adnexal lesions, accurately assigning each lesion to a risk category of malignancy being present, which informs the appropriate management to be instituted. The ORADS evaluation classifies ovarian masses into classes 0–5 as follows:

O-RADS US 0—An incomplete evaluation.
O-RADS US 1—Physiologic category <3 cm diameter.
O-RADS US 2—Benign category (<1% risk of malignancy).
O-RADS US 3—Low risk of malignancy (1% to <10%).
O-RADS US 4—Intermediate risk of malignancy (10% to <50%).
O-RADS US 5—Lesions with a high risk of malignancy (≥50%).

Doppler Colour scoring (CS) indicator should be added to classes 4 and 5—CS1: no flow, CS2: minimal flow, CS3: moderate flow, CS4: strong flow.

USG features of Borderline ovarian tumours: They typically appear as complex cystic adnexal masses with both benign and malignant features. They are often multilocular with thin septations, and internal papillary projections, especially in *serous types*. These projections may show mild vascularity on colour Doppler. *Mucinous subtypes* are usually large, multilocular with 'honeycomb' appearance due to numerous fine septae, but lack solid invasive components.

Unlike invasive carcinomas, borderline tumours have smooth external walls, minimal or no ascites, and rarely show peritoneal spread. While ultrasound alone cannot confirm the diagnosis, these characteristic findings should raise suspicion for a borderline tumour.

2. *Magnetic Resonance Imaging (MRI)*

   MRI is particularly useful for characterizing complex adnexal masses. It provides superior soft tissue contrast and can help identify tissue characteristics and local invasion of the disease. MRI can differentiate between solid and cystic components, as well as identify fat, blood, or other tissue types. MRI can assess for invasion of adjacent structures, such as the bladder or rectum.

   The reporting system best suited is the *Ovarian-Adnexal Reporting and Data System Magnetic Resonance Imaging (O-RADS MRI)* [4] which forms the MRI component of ORADS as follows:

   O-RADS MRI 0—Incomplete evaluation
   O-RADS MRI 1—Risk of malignancy N/A; normal ovaries
   O-RADS MRI 2—Risk of malignancy <0.5%; almost certainly benign
   O-RADS MRI 3—Risk of malignancy ~5%; low risk
   O-RADS MRI 4—Risk of malignancy ~50%; intermediate risk
   O-RADS MRI 5—Risk of malignancy ~90%; high risk
3. *Computed Tomography (CT)*—It is often used for staging in cases where malignancy is suspected. Contrast-enhanced CT (CECT) provides detailed images of the abdomen and pelvis, allowing for the assessment of:
   - *Tumour Extent*: Size and location of the mass, as well as involvement of surrounding structures.
   - *Lymph Node Involvement*: Enlarged lymph nodes may indicate metastatic disease.
   - *Distant Metastases*: CT can detect metastases to the liver, lungs, or other distant sites.

   It particularly helps in deciding the operability, whether the patient should go for surgery or neoadjuvant chemotherapy, and what surgical extent is needed.

19.7.2 Tumour Markers

A *tumour marker* is a biomarker that can be used to indicate the presence of cancer or the behaviour of cancers, measure progression or response to therapy. They can be found in body fluids or tissues. Markers can help with assessing prognosis, surveilling patients after surgical removal of tumours, and even predicting drug-response and monitor therapy. The commonly used tumour markers for adnexal mass diagnosis are:

1. *Cancer Antigen 125 (CA-125)*

   CA-125 is the most widely used tumour marker for diagnosis and prognosis of ovarian cancer. First described in 1981 by Bast and colleagues, it is an epitope of a larger glycoprotein (MUC16), coded by gene on chromosome 19p. It is found in amniotic fluid and chorionic membrane of foetus and can also be expressed in different tissues of Mullerian origin (endocervix, endometrium) and Coelomic origin (pleura, pericardium, peritoneum, intestine, lungs).

   Elevated levels of CA-125 are seen in epithelial ovarian cancer, although it can also be elevated in benign conditions such as endometriosis, pelvic inflammatory disease, and even in some non-gynaecological conditions like liver disease or heart failure.

   - *Normal Range*: <35 U/mL.
   - *Elevated Levels*: Levels >35 U/mL are more suggestive of malignancy, particularly in post-menopausal women.

2. *Human Epididymis Protein 4 (HE4)*

   HE4 is a newer tumour marker that has shown promise in the evaluation of adnexal masses. It is product of WFDC2 gene (chromosome 20). It is less likely to be elevated in benign conditions like endometriosis, making it a useful adjunct in the diagnosis of ovarian cancer. It is more specific and sensitive than CA 125.

   - *Normal Range*: 60–150 pmol/L.
   - *Elevated Levels*: Higher levels are associated with an increased risk of malignancy.

3. *AFP (Alpha-Fetoprotein)*—This tumour marker is elevated in germ cell tumours particularly those with yolk sac components. Normal values range from 0 to 10 ng/mL.
4. *hCG (Human Chorionic Gonadotropin)*—Like AFP, hCG is associated with germ cell tumours, particularly choriocarcinoma and embryonal carcinoma. The normal values range from 0 to 5 mIU/mL.
5. *LDH (Lactate Dehydrogenase)*—LDH is often elevated in dysgerminoma, normal values ranging from 140 to 280 U/L.
6. *CA 19-9 (Carbohydrate Antigen 19-9)*—Elevated in mucinous ovarian tumours, pancreatic and gastrointestinal cancers. The normal values range from 0 to 37 U/mL.
7. *CEA (Carcinoembryonic antigen)*—CEA is protein normally produced during foetal development. It is often elevated in mucinous ovarian cancer, colorectal cancer and pancreatic cancer. The normal values range from 0 to 5 ng/mL.
8. *Serum Inhibin B*—It is hormone produced by granulosa cells of the ovaries. It is typically elevated in granulosa cell tumour (sex cord-stromal tumour). The normal values range from 10 to 200 pg/mL.

19.7.3 Multimodal Tests

Several scoring systems and risk indices have been developed to assess the likelihood of ovarian malignancy based on USG, MRI findings and tumour markers. These systems help standardize the evaluation of ovarian masses and guide clinical decision-making that helps in planning management strategies. Below are the most commonly used scoring systems and risk indices:

1. *Risk of Malignancy Index (RMI)*

   RMI was introduced to evaluate the likelihood of ovarian cancer based on clinical, ultrasound, and laboratory data [5]. The clinical parameter is menopausal status and laboratory value is for CA 125. Ultrasound features include multi-locularity, solid areas, intra-abdominal metastasis, ascites, and bilaterality.

   $$\text{RMI} = \text{CA} - 125\,\text{Level} \times \text{USG score} \times \text{Menopausal score}$$

   There are four versions of the RMI system that have been developed over time: RMI 1, RMI 2, RMI 3, and RMI 4 as shown in Table 19.2. These versions primarily differ in their scoring for ultrasound findings, and menopausal status.

   A score above 200 indicates malignancy with RMI 1, 2, and 3, while a score above 450 is used in RMI 4 that includes size of lesion as an extra parameter.

   RMI 1 had the highest AUC (0.825, 95% CI: 0.790–0.856) among the four RMIs in the borderline ovarian tumour group. *RMI 1 has the highest specificity (87.6%), while RMI 2 has the highest sensitivity (69.75%).*
2. *ROMA—Risk of ovarian malignancy algorithm* [6]: Moore et al. described ROMA in 2009. It is a paid algorithm that includes CA125, HE4 and menopausal status.

Table 19.2 Scoring system for RMI 1, RMI2, RMI3, and RMI4

Variants	RMI 1 score (Jacobs et al. 1990)	RMI 2 score (Tingulstadt et al. 1996)	RMI 3 score (Tingulstadt et al. 1999)	RMI 4 score (Yamamoto et al. 2009)
USG findings				
0	0	1	1	1
1	1	1	1	1
≥2	3	4	3	4
Pre-menopausal	1	1	1	1
Post-menopausal	3	4	3	4
Size of tumour				
<7 cm	–	–	–	1
≥7 cm	–	–	–	2
Cut-off	200	200	200	450

A score of 1.31 in pre-menopausal women and score of 2.77 in post-menopausal females indicates malignancy. *The test has a sensitivity of 92% and specificity of 76%.*

3. *OVA 1* [7]—OVA 1 is the first generation multivariate index assay that was introduced by Ueland et al. in 2011. It is a combination of 5 tumour markers—CA 125, Transferrin, apolipoprotein A1, transthyretin, beta 2 macroglobulin. It is a computer based program that takes each variable to create an ovarian malignancy risk score. Malignancy is indicated with score of 5 for premenopausal women and 4.4 for post-menopausal women. *The test has a sensitivity of 94.2% and specificity of 53.5%.*
4. *IOTA ADNEX Model* [8] *(Assessment of Different NEoplasia in adneXa)* is another predictive model introduced in 2014. It is used to assess the likelihood of malignancy in an adnexal mass based on ultrasound findings and other parameters. It comprises a mathematical algorithm with nine predictors as shown in Table 19.3. It differentiates between subtypes of malignant masses. Score can be calculated with or without CA 125. *Its sensitivity is 100%, and specificity is 82.2%.*
5. *CPH-I—Copenhagen index* [9]: Karlsen et al. described CPH I in 2015. It includes CA 125, HE4 and age of the patient. *Cut off value is −0.070 with sensitivity of 95% and specificity of 78.4%.*
6. *OVERA*—In 2016, FDA approved OVERA was introduced as a second-generation multivariate index assay (MIA2G). It is based on CA 125, Transferrin, apolipoprotein A1, FSH and HE4 assays. Because FSH is a part of panel, determining menopausal status is not required. OVERA risk score ranges from 0.0 to 10.0. *Single cut off value of 5 has a sensitivity of 91.3% and specificity of 69.1%.*
7. *OVA1+(plus)*—It is a reflex test where OVA1 is performed first followed by OVERA if results fall in the intermediate range 4.4–6.0 (post-menopausal) or 5.0–7.0 (pre-menopausal). *It has a sensitivity of 96% and specificity of 98%.*
8. *Triple screen* [10]—Goff et al. described Triple screen test in 2017. It is considered positive if two out of three conditions are fulfilled:

   (i) Symptom index—given by Goff et al. in 2007. He identified symptoms which are independently associated with ovarian cancer by logistic regression model—pelvic or abdominal pain, increased abdominal size, bloating,

Table 19.3 IOTA ADNEX MODEL variables

Clinical variables	Ultrasound variables
1. Age	4. Maximum diameter of lesion
2. CA 125	5. Maximum diameter of largest solid part of tumour
3. Type of centre	6. More than 10 cyst loculi
	7. No. of papillary projections
	8. Acoustic shadows
	9. Ascites

difficult eating and feeling full. It was considered positive if these 6 symptoms were reported >12 a month but were present for <1 year.

(ii) CA125— $\geq$ 35 U/mL.

(iii) HE4— $\geq$ 140 pmol/L.

Triple screen has a sensitivity of 79% and specificity of 91%.

19.7.4 Comparative Summary of Various Scoring Systems

IOTA Simple rules and ORADS US are the best imaging-based scoring systems while RMI is the best multimodal scoring system for gynaecologists at large because they have high diagnostic accuracy, are straightforward and easily applicable, especially in resource-limited setting.

CPH-I and triple screen are simple and easy to use but not validated globally in comparison to other models; hence, they are not commonly utilized.

IOTA ADNEX and ORADS MRI are useful for complex or uncertain cases, particularly when ultrasound findings are inconclusive but advanced imaging is needed.

ROMA, OVA 1, and OVERA are particularly useful for post-menopausal women as they incorporate both biomarkers and menopausal status, improving risk stratification but are expensive and not easily available.

19.7.5 Summary of Diagnostic Workup

The management of an adnexal mass in a post-menopausal woman depends on the clinical presentation, imaging findings and tumour markers that help in identifying organ of origin and assessment of risk of malignancy.

As per RCOG 2016, there is currently not enough evidence to support the routine clinical use of tumour markers except CA 125 to assess the risk of malignancy in post-menopausal ovarian cysts [11].

MRI should be used as the second-line imaging modality for the characterization of indeterminate ovarian cysts when ultrasound is inconclusive.

If, from the clinical picture, ultrasonographic findings and tumour markers, malignant disease is suspected, a CT scan of the abdomen and pelvis should be arranged, with onward referral to a gynaecological oncology multidisciplinary team.

Asymptomatic, simple, unilateral, unilocular ovarian cysts, less than 5 cm in diameter, have a low risk of malignancy. In the presence of normal serum CA125 levels, these cysts can be managed conservatively, with a repeat evaluation in 4–6 months. It is reasonable to discharge these women from follow-up after 1 year if the cyst remains unchanged or reduces in size, with normal CA125, taking into consideration a woman's wishes and surgical fitness [11].

19.8 Treatment of Ovarian Mass

19.8.1 Strategies

- For asymptomatic, physiological, ovarian cysts, conservative management with close surveillance may be appropriate. This typically involves regular follow-up with imaging and if there is any change, repeat tumour markers. Persistent or complex adnexal mass (>5 cm) that does not resolve on follow-up needs surgery.
- In post-menopausal females, bilateral salpingo-oophorectomy should be done even if it is a unilateral benign ovarian mass.
- Symptomatic painful masses with features suggestive of torsion or rupture need urgent medical and surgical attention.
- Endometriomas are treated with hormonal therapy or surgical excision depending on symptoms and size.
- Tubercular masses are treated with antitubercular therapy after diagnostic confirmation with surgery reserved for complications. Sometimes diagnostic laparoscopy may be required for confirmation of diagnosis.
- Benign or malignant ovarian tumours need surgical removal in cases with Suspicion of malignancy and operable disease. Advanced malignancy may need confirmation with trucut biopsy and referral to medical oncologist for neo adjuvant chemotherapy.
- Appendiceal/ diverticular abscess is treated with broad spectrum IV antibiotics followed by percutaneous drainage for localized abscess if needed. Surgical intervention is usually delayed with an interval appendectomy performed 6–8 weeks later once the infection resolves.
- Intestinal tumours like colorectal cancer or GIST are managed by gastro surgeons with surgical resection and if necessary, chemotherapy or targeted therapy.
- Indications for hysterectomy in a post-menopausal woman with ovarian mass which is apparently benign:

    1. Co-existing uterine pathology (e.g. fibroids, endometrial hyperplasia, abnormal bleeding, adenomyosis, CIN lesions.
    2. Ovarian masses with high suspicion of malignancy—staging laparotomy or debulking surgery which includes total abdominal hysterectomy should be done.
    3. Ovarian mass may be sent for frozen section analysis. If frozen report suggestive of malignancy/ borderline tumours, complete staging laparotomy with TAH and BSO should be done.

19.8.2 Treating Expert

Patients with ovarian tumours should be stratified into low, intermediate, or high risk for malignancy.

Women with an intermediate or high risk of malignancy should be referred to a gynaecological oncologist for further management.Women with low risk for malignancy may be managed by general gynaecologist with backup of a gynaecological oncologist.

19.8.3 Type of Surgical Intervention

The type of surgery depends on the age, fertility status, risk of malignancy and the patient's overall health.

- *Minimally Invasive Surgery (Laparoscopy)*—Cases with low risk of malignancy (e.g. premenopausal women with benign-appearing mass on imaging, small to moderate-sized masses) may be managed through cystectomy especially in younger women to preserve ovarian function. Unilateral salpingo-oophorectomy is preferred in large, complex or recurrent cysts. If malignancy is discovered during laparoscopy, conversion to laparotomy is necessary for complete the surgery. Intraoperative frozen section analysis if available, should be utilized to rule out malignancy in suspicious cases.
- *Laparotomy*—This is indicated in cases with high risk of malignancy, large masses (>10 cm) or masses suspicious for torsion or rupture and with inability to perform safe laparoscopy due to extensive adhesions.

In post-menopausal women, the threshold for surgical intervention is lower, particularly for complex or persistent masses. Even apparently benign lesions in this group warrant careful evaluation, and bilateral salpingo-oophorectomy (BSO) is often performed due to the higher baseline risk of malignancy.

In cases where borderline ovarian tumours are suspected or confirmed, the surgical approach is complete staging that includes omentectomy, peritoneal washings, and biopsies. Frozen section analysis, if available intraoperatively, can significantly influence the extent of surgery, especially in uncertain cases. However, it has limitations in mucinous and borderline tumours, and caution must be exercised in interpreting the results.

If malignancy is suspected based on clinical, radiologic, or intraoperative findings, more extensive surgery is indicated. Here, the preferred approach is laparotomy, which allows complete staging and reduces the risk of intra operative rupture and spillage.

The standard surgical procedure includes total abdominal hysterectomy (TAH), bilateral salpingo-oophorectomy (BSO), omentectomy, peritoneal washings, and peritoneal biopsies from all quadrants. Any enlarged or suspicious lymph nodes should be sampled or removed. In early-stage disease, systematic surgical staging is essential for accurate diagnosis and further management. The goal of surgery is optimal cytoreduction, i.e. removal of all visible disease, which has a direct impact on prognosis.

In advanced-stage disease, if complete resection is not feasible upfront, patients may be considered for neoadjuvant chemotherapy followed by interval debulking surgery.

In conclusion, surgical management of ovarian masses must be individualized, balancing oncologic treatment and patient safety. Proper surgical staging and complete resection, when indicated, remain the cornerstone of effective management.

19.9 Conclusion

The evaluation of an adnexal mass in a post-menopausal woman requires a systematic and multidisciplinary approach. Given the increased risk of malignancy in this population, a thorough diagnostic workup, including imaging and tumour marker assessment, is essential. Risk stratification tools help guide management decisions. Surgical intervention remains the cornerstone of treatment, particularly when malignancy is suspected.

Key Points

1. In post-menopausal women, adnexal masses have a higher likelihood of being malignant. Evaluation aims to assess this risk through clinical, radiological, and laboratory findings.
2. Transvaginal ultrasound (TVUS) is the preferred imaging technique to assess adnexal masses. It helps differentiate between benign and malignant masses based on characteristics like size, cystic or solid components, and septations or nodules.
3. The serum level of CA-125 is often measured as it can be elevated in ovarian cancer. While a high level is suggestive of malignancy, it is not specific and may also be elevated in benign conditions, thus necessitating further investigation.
4. Various scoring systems and multimodal tests have been developed over years that incorporate clinical symptoms, ultrasound findings, and tumour marker levels that can help stratify the risk and guide management decisions.
5. If malignancy is suspected or the mass is symptomatic, surgical removal (often by laparotomy or laparoscopy) is indicated and should be preferably handled by a gynaecological oncologist. The type of surgery depends on the extent of the disease and fertility needs.

Long Answer Questions (LAQs)

1. A p2 + 0(11) 70-year-old female presented to the OPD with a unilateral adnexal mass. On examination, a solid cystic multilocular mass of approximately 8 cm with irregular margins is felt in the right adnexa. CA-125 is 158. The rest tumour markers were normal. Discuss the approach to the management of this patient.
2. Discuss investigation modalities useful in the evaluation of an adnexal mass in post-menopausal females.
3. How will you manage a case of a 65-year-old post-menopausal female with bilateral adnexal masses?
   Ca 125: 346
   CEA: 7 ng/mL
   LDH: 150
   AFP: 2.4
   Hcg: 0.78
   Ca 19.9: 55
4. Describe various scoring systems and their significance in the diagnosis of ovarian malignancies.

Short Answer Questions (SAQs)

1. What are IOTA rules and their significance?
2. Enumerate the differential diagnosis of a unilateral adnexal mass.
3. Write a short note on risk factors and protective factors for ovarian malignancies.
4. Write a short note on limitations of minimally invasive surgery in the context of ovarian masses.
5. Enumerate conditions where CA-125 can be raised (gynaecological and non-gynaecological).

Multiple Choice Questions (MCQs)

1. What is the risk of malignancy in post-menopausal women?

   A. 18%
   B. 7%
   C. 30%
   D. 40%

2. Which imaging modality is considered the first-line investigation in the evaluation of an adnexal mass?
   A. CT scan abdomen and pelvis
   B. MRI pelvis
   C. Transvaginal ultrasound (TVS)
   D. Abdominal X-ray

3. which of the following is not the component of triple screening?
   A. LDH
   B. CA-125
   C. Symptom index
   D. HE-4

4. Which tumour marker is elevated in granulosa cell tumours of the ovary?
   A. LDH
   B. Inhibin B
   C. CA-125
   D. CEA

5. Sensitivity of ROMA as an algorithm in ovarian malignancy is:
   A. 40–45%
   B. 50–55%
   C. 65–70%
   D. 85–90%

6. In context to iota rules, identify the wrong one.
   A. If one or more m features are present without any b features, mass is malignant.
   B. If one or more b features are present without any m features, the mass is benign.
   C. If one feature is benign and two features are malignant, mass is malignant.
   D. If no features are present, result is inconclusive.

7. Which of the following is not a characteristic of m rules in iota?
   1. Presence of ascites
   2. Presence of acoustic shadows
   3. Multilocular >10 cm
   4. 3 papillary structures

   A. 1, 4
   B. 1, 2
   C. 3, 4
   D. 2, 4

8. In a premenopausal woman with a 4 cm simple ovarian cyst, asymptomatic and found incidentally, the next step is:

   A. Immediate surgical removal
   B. Start chemotherapy
   C. Repeat ultrasound in 6–8 weeks
   D. Order CT abdomen

9. Which of the following factors reduces the risk of ovarian cancer

   A. Menopausal age
   B. History of Endometriosis
   C. OCP intake for 5 years or more
   D. Nulliparity

10. What is the full form of ORADS?

    A. Ovarian risk assessment and diagnostic scale
    B. Ovarian-adnexal reporting and data system
    C. Ovarian radiology and detection scale
    D. Ovarian adnexal reporting and data stratification

Answers

1. C
2. C
3. A
4. B
5. D
6. C
7. D
8. C
9. C
10. B

References

1. Berek JS, Renz M, Kehoe S, Kumar L, Friedlander M. Cancer of the ovary, fallopian tube, and peritoneum: 2021 update. Int J Gynaecol Obstet. 2021;155(Suppl 1):61–85. https://doi.org/10.1002/ijgo.13878.
2. Dang Thi Minh N, Nguyen Van T, Duong Duc H, Nguyen Tuan M, Duong Thi Tra G, Do Tuan D, et al. IOTA simple rules: an efficient tool for evaluation of ovarian tumors by non-experienced but trained examiners – a prospective study. Heliyon. 2024;10(2):e24262.

3. Andreotti RF, Timmerman D, Strachowski LM, Froyman W, Benacerraf BR, Bennett GL, et al. O-RADS US risk stratification and management system: a consensus guideline from the ACR Ovarian-Adnexal Reporting and Data System Committee. Radiology. 2020;294(1):168–85.
4. Jacobs I, Fairchild A, Ogunyemi, O, Slack J. Calculation of a risk of malignancy index in assessment of adnexal masses. The Lancet, 1990;336(8720), 910–913.
5. Sadowski EA, Thomassin-Naggara I, Rockall A, Maturen KE, Forstner R, Jha P, et al. O-RADS MRI risk stratification system: guide for assessing adnexal lesions from the ACR O-RADS Committee. Radiology. 2022;303(1):35–47.
6. Bryce C. Risk of ovarian malignancy algorithm (ROMA) for assessing likelihood of ovarian cancer. Am Fam Physician. 2023;107(3):303–4.
7. Reilly GP, Gregory DA, Scotti DJ, Lederman S, Neiman WA, Sussman S, et al. A real-world comparison of the clinical and economic utility of OVA1 and CA125 in assessing ovarian tumor malignancy risk. J Comp Eff Res. 2023;12(6):e230025. https://doi.org/10.57264/cer-2023-0025. Epub 2023 May 22.
8. Giourga M, Pouliakis A, Vlastarakos P, Stavrou S, Tsiriva M, Gerede A, et al. Evaluation of IOTA-ADNEX model and simple rules for identifying adnexal masses by operators with varying levels of expertise: a single-center diagnostic accuracy study. Ultrasound Int Open. 2023;9(1):E11–7.
9. Song Z, Wang X, Fu J, Wang P, Chen X, Zhang D. Copenhagen index (CPH-I) is more favorable than CA125, HE4, and risk of ovarian malignancy algorithm (ROMA): nomogram prediction models with clinical-ultrasonographic feature for diagnosing ovarian neoplasms. Front Surg. 2023;9:1068492.
10. Goff BA, Agnew K, Neradilek MB, Gray HJ, Liao JB, Urban RR. Combining a symptom index, CA125 and HE4 (triple screen) to detect ovarian cancer in women with a pelvic mass. Gynecol Oncol. 2017;147(2):291–5.
11. Royal College of Obstetricians and Gynaecologists. (2016). Ovarian cysts in postmenopausal women (green-top guideline No. 34). London: RCOG.

20 Premature Ovarian Insufficiency

Deepti Goswami and Anshul Solanki

Abstract

Premature ovarian insufficiency (POI) is characterized by the cessation of ovarian function before the age of 40. Etiology is multifactorial, including genetic, autoimmune, iatrogenic, metabolic, infectious, and environmental factors. Seventy-five to ninety percent of cases may be idiopathic. The diagnosis is based on elevated serum FSH (>25 IU/L) on two occasions, at least 1 month apart. POI manifests mostly as secondary amenorrhea or as primary amenorrhea. Estrogen deficiency causes vasomotor, genitourinary, and neuropsychiatric symptoms and long-term systemic complications like osteoporosis and increased risk of fractures, cardiovascular diseases, and metabolic dysfunction. Infertility is the other distressing symptom. The management aims to reduce estrogen deficiency symptoms, prevent long-term complications, and address fertility concerns. Hormone replacement therapy (HRT) with estrogen-progesterone until the natural age of menopause (~50 years) is the mainstay of management. Oral contraceptive pills can be used for hormone replacement; however, its benefit over sequential HRT for bone health is questionable. Annual assessment of blood pressure, lipid profile, and metabolic parameters is recommended. Dual-Energy X Ray Absorptiometry (DXA) helps in baseline bone marrow density (BMD) assessment and is repeated not before 2 years. Spontaneous pregnancy is rare and mostly occurs in the early years of diagnosis. Oocyte donation with in vitro fertilization (IVF) is the most effective fertility treatment.

Keywords

Ovarian insufficiency · Ovarian failure · Hormone replacement · Amenorrhea

D. Goswami (✉) · A. Solanki
Obstetrics & Gynaecology, Maulana Azad Medical College, New Delhi, India

R. Malik et al. (eds.), *Menopause Essentials*,
https://doi.org/10.1007/978-981-95-7498-8_20

20.1 Introduction

Premature ovarian insufficiency (POI) is characterized by the cessation of ovarian function before the age of 40, leading to hypoestrogenism and anovulation with a prevalence of 1–3.7% [1]. The nomenclature for this condition has undergone the same change over time. For decades, it was known as "primary ovarian failure" (POF) [2], and then "primary ovarian insufficiency" [3] was suggested. Lately, to avoid confusion with primary amenorrhea the proposed terminology is "premature ovarian insufficiency."

20.2 Diagnosis

POI is characterized by amenorrhea or oligomenorrhea for at least 4 months and an elevated serum FSH >25 IU/L. FSH assessment needs to be done twice, at least 4 weeks apart [1].

20.3 Causes

POI has a multifactorial etiology, including genetic, autoimmune, iatrogenic, metabolic, infectious, and environmental factors. Despite extensive research, the cause cannot be identified in nearly 75–90% that are called idiopathic.

20.3.1 Genetic Causes

Genetic abnormalities, particularly those involving X chromosome abnormalities and autosomal mutations account for a significant subset of POI cases.

- X chromosome disorders like Turner Syndrome (45XO or mosaicism), X chromosome trisomy, or structural defects. A past study by the author has reported a 3.8% prevalence of triple X karyotype in POI [4].
- X-Autosome Translocations and Deletions: POI1 and POI2 are specific regions on the X chromosome linked to POI. POI 1 is located at Xq24–Xq27, and POI 2 is at Xq13–Xq21. Chromosomal breakage in these regions, particularly during meiosis, may cause X-autosome translocations, disrupting ovarian function. Genetic testing can detect these translocations, aiding in POI diagnosis.
- Fragile X Premutation: The FMR1 gene encodes the fragile X mental retardation protein (FMRP), which is mainly expressed in the brain, testes, and ovaries. This gene contains a CGG trinucleotide repeat, normally ranging from 10 to 40 repeats. A premutation (55–200 repeats) results in excessive and abnormal FMR1 mRNA, disrupting protein function and leading to POI. It is the most prevalent single-gene disorder associated with POI, reported in up to 7.5% of sporadic cases and up to 13% of cases with a family history. However, it is less

common in Asian populations, compared to Western populations. A prevalence of less than 1% has been reported in the Chinese population [5]. In India, studies from Hyderabad and Mumbai identified no FMR1 premutation in POI, whereas a small study from Lucknow found one case of this premutation among 25 cases [6–8]. An ongoing study being conducted by the author has yielded findings similar to those of a Chinese study. Information about FMR1 premutation is of help in providing genetic counseling and fertility guidance for these women.

- Autosomal Gene Mutations: FOXL2 (Forkhead Box L2) is essential for ovarian development and follicular maintenance, with mutations leading to blepharophimosis-ptosis-epicanthus-inversus syndrome (BPES) and POI. NOBOX, FIGLA, BMP15, and GDF9 are involved in oocyte maturation and folliculogenesis and mutations in these genes have also been implicated in POI.

20.3.2 Autoimmune Causes

Autoimmune POI arises due to autoantibody-mediated destruction of ovarian tissue or associated endocrinopathies. It often coexists with adrenal insufficiency (Addison's disease) in APS (autoimmune polyglandular syndrome) type 1 and type 2 and is also associated with thyroid disorders (Hashimoto's thyroiditis, Graves' disease), type 1 diabetes mellitus, and SLE. The author's earlier published data show that the prevalence of hypothyroidism in Indian women with POI is 24% [9].

20.3.3 Iatrogenic Causes

Gonadotoxic therapies can induce POI by directly damaging ovarian follicles.

- Chemotherapy: Alkylating agents (e.g., cyclophosphamide) and platinum-based compounds (e.g., cisplatin) have high ovarian toxicity. The risk is dose-dependent and influenced by age and ovarian reserve.
- Radiotherapy: Pelvic and whole-body irradiation (e.g., for hematologic malignancies) can lead to irreversible ovarian damage, particularly with higher radiation doses (>20 Gy).
- Surgical Interventions: Bilateral oophorectomy leads to immediate ovarian failure. Ovarian cystectomy and endometriosis surgery may compromise ovarian reserve by inadvertently damaging functional ovarian tissue.

20.3.4 Metabolic and Enzymatic Disorders

Rare metabolic disorders can disrupt ovarian function by impairing hormone biosynthesis or follicular development like galactosemia (GALT deficiency), Perrault syndrome (an autosomal recessive disorder characterized by sensorineural hearing loss and POI), 5α-reductase, and aromatase deficiency (disrupts estrogen synthesis, impairing normal follicular maturation).

20.3.5 Infectious Causes

Certain infections can trigger oophoritis and ovarian failure, either through direct viral invasion or immune-mediated destruction. Such infections include mumps and oophoritis. It is the most well-documented infectious cause of POI, occurring in up to 7% of postpubertal females with mumps. CMV, TB, and HIV are less commonly implicated but can contribute to ovarian dysfunction through chronic inflammation.

20.3.6 Environmental and Toxic Exposures

- Tobacco Smoke: Polycyclic aromatic hydrocarbons (PAHs) are directly toxic to oocytes and may induce apoptosis.
- Industrial Chemicals: Bisphenol A (BPA), phthalates, pesticides, and heavy metals disturb endocrine pathways.
- High-Risk Occupational Exposures: Radiation, solvents, and agricultural chemicals may increase the risk of POI.

20.3.7 Idiopathic POI

In approximately 75–90% of cases, no identifiable cause is found despite extensive evaluation [1]. Ongoing research suggests that epigenetic regulation, mitochondrial dysfunction, and immune dysregulation may play roles in unexplained POI. In the largest-scale WES study of POI, the rate of contribution to POI by genetic variations reached 23.5% [15].

20.4 Clinical Features

POI manifests with multisystemic symptoms, including menstrual disturbances, estrogen deficiency-related complications, and infertility. Due to persistent hypoestrogenemia, affected women have several long-term health risks.

20.4.1 Menstrual Irregularities

Disruptions in the menstrual cycle are the hallmark of POI, reflecting impaired ovarian function with a majority (about 86%) presenting as secondary amenorrhea and 14% as primary amenorrhea [10]. Preceding menstrual cycles are often irregular with increased intervals between periods.

20.4.2 Symptoms of Estrogen Deficiency

Estrogen deficiency leads to a range of systemic and vasomotor symptoms, affecting quality of life:

- Vasomotor Symptoms: Hot flashes, night sweats, and temperature dysregulation due to hypothalamic instability similar to menopausal symptoms but often more severe in younger women.
- Genitourinary Syndrome of Menopause (GSM): Vaginal dryness, dyspareunia, and recurrent urinary tract infections due to urogenital atrophy. Decreased lubrication and loss of vaginal elasticity, contribute to sexual dysfunction.
- Neuropsychiatric Symptoms: Mood disturbances, including anxiety, depression, and irritability, often exacerbated by hormonal fluctuations. Cognitive complaints such as difficulty with concentration and memory (often termed "brain fog").

20.4.3 Infertility and Subfertility

POI is a significant cause of infertility. Women need to be counseled that spontaneous pregnancy is rare and not possible to predict. Bidet et al. (2008) observed five pregnancies in a cohort of 302 POI women all of which occurred less than a year after the diagnosis of POI [11]. Over the author's 18 years of experience in nearly 400 patients with well-established amenorrhea due to POI, only two cases of spontaneous pregnancy have been observed, one of which occurred in a woman with chemotherapy-induced POI. In one of the studies published by the author in the journal "Human Reproduction," 11% of women with POI exhibited episodic declines in serum FSH levels but none had a return of menses or conception [12].

It is also seen that in young women, combined oral contraceptives (COCs) are frequently prescribed without proper evaluation of amenorrhea, leading to the misdiagnosis of POI as polycystic ovary syndrome (PCOS). This misdiagnosis results in inappropriate treatment, delaying required interventions for fertility and bone health.

20.4.4 Long-Term Health Consequences

Chronic estrogen deficiency predisposes women with POI to long-term systemic complications:

1. Osteoporosis and Increased Fracture Risk: Estrogen deficiency increases bone resorption by reducing osteoblast function, enhancing osteoclast activity, and activating T-cells, leading to higher cytokine and oxidative stress levels. This contributes to osteoporosis (BMD T-score <−2.5) affecting 5–17% of non-iatrogenic POI cases and osteopenia (T-score −1.0 to −2.5). The pattern of bone

loss in POI is characterized by greater susceptibility of trabecular bone compared to cortical bone, increasing the risk of vertebral fractures [13].

While low BMD is linked to fractures in postmenopausal women, studies on POI-specific fractures remain uninvestigated. In a recent study published by the author, BMD, trabecular bone score (TBS), and prevalence of vertebral fractures (VFs) were assessed using dual-energy X-ray absorptiometry in 70 POI women. These women exhibited significantly lower BMD, degraded microarchitecture, and higher VF prevalence (15.7%). Age, amenorrhea duration, and vitamin D levels were key determinants of bone health. BMD at the lumbar spine, hip, and forearm was reduced by 11.5, 11.4, and 9.1%, degraded microarchitecture was observed in 66.7% of patients and 15.7% of the POI had vertebral fractures [14].

1. Cardiovascular Disease (CVD): POI, early menopause (before age 45), and surgical menopause a significant female-specific risk factors for CVD. Studies and meta-analyses consistently show an increased risk of coronary artery disease, stroke, and CVD-related mortality in affected women, likely due to reduced exposure to cardioprotective endogenous estrogen.
2. Metabolic Dysfunction: In POI, there is an increased risk of insulin resistance, type 2 diabetes, central adiposity, and altered energy metabolism leading to weight gain and increased waist-hip ratio. A meta-analysis of 21 studies in 2022 with 1573 POI women found that they exhibited significantly higher waist circumference, total cholesterol, low-density lipoprotein, high-density lipoprotein, triglycerides, and fasting glucose levels. These findings emphasize the need for early screening and lifelong metabolic health management in women with POI.
3. Emotional distress and reduced quality of life due to infertility, hormonal imbalances, and chronic health risks. There is also a higher risk of depressive and anxiety disorders.

20.5 Clinical Approach and Diagnosis

The diagnosis of POI is based on clinical and biochemical criteria that confirm ovarian dysfunction before the age of 40.

20.5.1 Clinical

- Menstrual Disturbances: Secondary amenorrhea or oligomenorrhea persisting for at least 4–6 months in a woman less than 40 years. In cases of primary amenorrhea, failure to achieve menarche by the age of 14 years warrants further investigation.
- Symptoms of Estrogen Deficiency: Vasomotor symptoms, genitourinary atrophy, mood disturbances, and cognitive complaints.
- Infertility or Subfertility: Young women with amenorrhea are prescribed COC pills.

20.5.2 Biochemical and Endocrine Assessment

- *Elevated FSH (>25 IU/L on two occasions, at least 1 month apart) is the hallmark of POI.* FSH levels in the menopausal range (>40 IU/L) indicate advanced ovarian dysfunction.
- Low estradiol levels (<50 pg/mL or < 180 pmol/L) confirm hypoestrogenism. A persistently low E2 in the presence of high FSH supports the diagnosis.
- Elevated LH levels often accompany high FSH, but FSH remains the primary diagnostic marker.
- AMH though not a diagnostic test is nevertheless a marker of decreased ovarian function. Low or undetectable AMH levels (<0.5 ng/mL) are expected in POI.
- Thyroid function tests (TSH, free T4, T3) to exclude autoimmune thyroid disease.
- Morning cortisol to assess for autoimmune adrenal insufficiency (Addison's disease), particularly in autoimmune POI.

20.5.3 Genetic and Autoimmune Investigations

- Karyotype Analysis (Chromosomal Studies): It is recommended for women diagnosed with POI at an early age. However, there is no strict age cutoff for testing, as recent findings suggest that chromosomal abnormalities are often underdiagnosed in older POI women. It detects Turner syndrome (45XO or mosaicism), X-autosome translocations, and triple X syndrome.
- FMR1 Premutation Testing: Screening for fragile X premutation (CGG repeats 55–200) may detect premutation in about 1–2% of POI cases. Daughters of such patients should be counseled about their risk of developing POI, allowing them to plan for conception before ovarian failure occurs.
- Autoimmune Antibody Screening: Adrenal antibodies and antithyroid peroxidase (TPO) antibodies to assess for adrenal and thyroid autoimmunity. There is no role in testing for antiovarian antibodies.

20.6 Role of Imaging

Imaging studies are not required to make the diagnosis of POI.

20.7 Management

The key step after a POI diagnosis is to sensitively inform the patient, provide accurate information, and offer appropriate referrals. The management of POI aims to reduce estrogen deficiency symptoms, prevent long-term complications, and address fertility concerns. Given the significant impact of POI on bone health, cardiovascular function, mental well-being, and reproductive potential, a multidisciplinary approach is required.

20.8 Hormone Replacement Therapy

20.8.1 Principles of HRT

1. HRT aims to closely mimic natural physiological hormone replacement.
2. If the uterus is present, both estrogen and progestogen are needed to prevent endometrial hyperplasia.
3. Using nonoral routes (e.g., transdermal) bypasses liver metabolism, reducing thrombotic risks.
4. Younger women often require higher estrogen doses than those typically used at menopause to maintain BMD and match physiological needs.

20.8.2 Components of HRT

Estrogen

There are four primary types of estrogen used in HRT:

- Estradiol (the primary ovarian estrogen).
- Ethinylestradiol (a synthetic form).
- Conjugated equine estrogen (CEE).
- Newer estetrol-based products.

Given the long-term nature of HRT in POI management, an optimal risk-benefit ratio is important. While experts recommend HT that closely mimics natural ovarian hormone production (estradiol), guidelines differ by region, and there is no single agreed-upon guideline for HRT.

Progesterone

The major types of progesterone are:

- micronized progesterone,
- medroxyprogesterone acetate.

Progesterone plays a crucial role in protecting the endometrium from the proliferative effects of estrogen for POI women. Micronized progesterone is considered first-line in many studies done on postmenopausal women. Many clinicians use medroxyprogesterone acetate. There is limited evidence on the type and role of various progesterone preparations in POI patients.

For those desiring bleed-free HRT and contraception, the 52 mg levonorgestrel intrauterine device combined with appropriate estrogen replacement is an option, as it is approved for both endometrial protection and contraception in many countries.

Less commonly used progesterones for HRT include oral dydrogesterone and norethisterone acetate as suggested from data on HRT in women with usual age menopause.

20.8.3 Route

Estrogen: The administration of systemic estrogen can be achieved through oral intake, transdermal patches, sprays, gels, and implants, though availability varies across regions. Local estrogen therapy for vulvovaginal atrophy and genitourinary syndrome of menopause includes estrogen-releasing vaginal rings, creams, and pessaries. Transdermal estrogen offers the advantages of bypassing first-pass metabolism and minimizing venous thromboembolism risk. Since there is little evidence on the best route for estrogen, patient preference and compliance are important factors.

Progesterone: It can be administered orally, transdermally via patches, or intrauterine. Micronized progesterone is available in oral, vaginal, and transdermal forms, with only the oral route approved for endometrial protection. Vaginal administration may offer reduced side effects while maintaining protection, though the evidence remains inconclusive. Transdermal progesterone cream has been found inadequate for preventing estrogen-induced endometrial proliferation and should not be used in POI patients.

20.8.4 Dose

For estrogen therapy in women with POI, a minimum dose of 2 mg oral estradiol or 100 μg transdermal estradiol per day is necessary to prevent bone loss, as lower doses suitable for older postmenopausal women are insufficient. Estrogen dosage should ideally be titrated against physiological estradiol levels (200–400 pmol/L) rather than solely vasomotor symptom relief, as some women with POI may have minimal symptoms despite estrogen deficiency. Women with minimal or no symptoms may start with lower doses, increasing as needed based on tolerance, serum estradiol, and BMD.

For progestogen therapy, the required dose depends on the estrogen dose and regimen. Progesterone can be given in a continuous combined or sequential manner. For continuous combined regime, 2.5 mg medroxyprogesterone acetate (MPA) or 100 mg micronized progesterone is given combined with estrogen. For a sequential regime, medroxyprogesterone acetate 10 mg is added to the last 10–12 days of estrogen each month. These recommendations are based on studies in women with usual age menopause, ensuring pharmacokinetic efficacy and endometrial safety.

20.8.5 Duration of HRT

Unlike postmenopausal women, HRT is continued at least until the natural age of menopause (~50 years) to prevent premature estrogen deficiency complications. Long-term benefits outweigh the risks in women with POI.

20.8.6 COCs as HT

OCPs are another common and easily available form of hormone therapy in POI. However, its benefit over sequential HRT is questionable, particularly over bone health. Furthermore, it contains ethinyl estradiol which being a synthetic estrogen may have unfavorable effects on lipid profile and hemostasis, adversely affecting the thromboembolic risk.

20.8.7 Risks of HRT

1. Women with POI generally have a lower risk of breast cancer compared to women with later menopause due to reduced estrogen exposure. HT with physiological doses of estradiol does not appear to increase this risk. While continuous combined estrogen-progestogen regimens may carry a higher risk in postmenopausal women, data for POI are limited. Women with BRCA1/2 mutations may use HT after risk-reducing surgery, but HT is generally contraindicated for breast cancer survivors.
2. Estrogen-only HT increases the risk of endometrial hyperplasia and endometrial cancer in postmenopausal women, and while this has not been studied specifically in POI women, the same risk is assumed. Therefore, higher doses of estrogen in POI treatment require proportional increases in progestogen for endometrial protection.
3. Estrogen deprivation in POI or early surgical menopause is linked to increased stroke risk, which appears to be reduced by HRT. In women with usual age menopause, HRT slightly increases thrombotic stroke risk, but this is not observed with standard or low-dose transdermal estradiol.
4. Any clinical concern regarding the risk of thromboembolism needs to be addressed. An observational study reported a higher venous thromboembolism (VTE) risk with oral CEE than with oral E2 (estradiol). A nested case–control study found a lower VTE risk with E2 versus CEE. However, a 2021 retrospective cohort study found no significant VTE risk difference between CEE and oral/transdermal E2 [16]. The author has prescribed mostly CEE to nearly 400 POI patients over the past 20 years and none showed any signs or symptoms of VTE.

20.8.8 Contraindications

- Active hormone-sensitive malignancies (e.g., breast cancer).
- Severe liver disease or thromboembolic disorders.

20.9 Role of Androgen Therapy

Testosterone therapy in women with POI is primarily indicated for hypoactive sexual desire disorder (HSDD) when symptoms persist despite HT. While androgen levels decline with age, there is debate regarding their decline in POI. Testosterone can be administered transdermally (gel/patch/cream), orally, or via implant. Oral administration may negatively impact lipid profiles, whereas transdermal administration may cause skin irritation, and excess hair growth, leading to discontinuation in some users.

Androgen replacement should not use male dosages, as these result in supraphysiological levels in women with unknown safety and efficacy. Studies on androgen therapy for HSDD suggest that a 300 μg testosterone patches daily is optimal.

Monitoring testosterone levels every 3–6 months is recommended to avoid excessive dosing. If no symptom improvement occurs within 6 months, discontinuation is advised.

20.10 Bone Health and Osteoporosis Prevention

HRT is a key intervention for BMD preservation in women with POI. Discontinuation or delayed initiation of HRT is associated with lower BMD and increased fracture risk. Pharmacological treatments, including bisphosphonates, SERMs, and denosumab are effective in reducing fracture risk in postmenopausal women but have not been studied in POI women. They are therefore reserved for severe osteoporosis when HRT is contraindicated. Additional benefits have been seen from lifestyle modifications and adequate vitamin D and calcium intake (calcium: 1000–1500 mg/day, Vitamin D: 800–2000 IU/day). Weight-bearing exercises like resistance training and impact exercises help maintain BMD.

20.11 Cardiovascular Health

Estrogen therapy has demonstrated beneficial effects on vascular endothelium, lipid metabolism, endothelial function, and cardiovascular physiology in women with POI. However, long-term data on HT in POI is limited. Additionally, estrogen influences cardiac function, insulin resistance, and lipid oxidation. Lipid and glucose screening is recommended at diagnosis and regularly thereafter. Lifestyle modifications include regular exercise, smoking cessation, and healthy diet.

20.12 Role of Nonhormonal Therapies

Pharmacological treatments included antidepressants (SSRIs and SNRIs), gabapentinoids, clonidine, oxybutynin, and neurokinin receptor antagonists, among others.

Nonpharmacological interventions included cognitive behavioral therapy (CBT), hypnosis, and stellate ganglion blockade.

No RCTs, cohort, or case–control studies specifically evaluated nonhormonal treatments for women with POI. Further research is needed to establish the efficacy and safety of these interventions in the POI population.

20.13 Lifestyle Management Options

Given the impact of POI on both short-term symptoms and long-term health, there is increasing interest in lifestyle interventions to decrease adverse effects and improve quality of life (QoL). While evidence for lifestyle interventions in POI is limited, broader research on menopausal women suggests potential benefits.

Regarding dietary interventions, adherence to a high-quality diet rich in vegetables, fruits, and whole grains is associated with lower symptom severity, whereas processed and high-fat foods correlate with worsened symptoms.

Cardiovascular health benefits of exercise interventions were well-documented across multiple studies, with improvements in cardiorespiratory fitness, lipid metabolism, body composition, and blood pressure regulation. Resistance and combined aerobic-resistance training were particularly effective in reducing metabolic risk factors and enhancing muscle strength.

20.14 Fertility Management

Up to 5–10% of women with POI experience intermittent ovarian function and spontaneous pregnancy; however, spontaneous pregnancy is rare and mostly occurs in the early years of diagnosis. Oocyte donation with IVF is the most effective fertility treatment. Gonadotropin stimulation is ineffective due to ovarian follicle depletion [17]. Emerging therapies include stem cell therapy and in vitro activation (experimental).

20.15 Psychological and Psychosocial Support

Cognitive behavioral therapy and counseling for emotional distress, peer support groups, and patient education centers should be made available. Daisy Network is the sole UK charity dedicated to POI, offering medical and psychological support, promoting awareness, and facilitating research on its causes and treatments.

20.16 Prevention of POI in Iatrogenic Cases

All women receiving cancer treatment (surgical/chemotherapy/radiotherapy) should be counseled about the potential risks of ovarian failure, adverse pregnancy outcomes, and the importance of HRT to preserve the physiological functions of estrogen. A few fertility preservation techniques to decrease this risk of imminent ovarian failure in such women include surgical ovarian transposition (oophoropexy) which involves repositioning the ovaries outside the radiation field, to a higher abdominal location, administration of GnRH agonists theoretically reduces gonadotoxicity by suppressing ovarian activity. Other techniques include embryo cryopreservation and ovarian tissue cryopreservation followed by transplantation.

20.17 Monitoring and Follow-Up

- Annual assessment of blood pressure, lipid profile, and metabolic parameters including glucose levels.
- Fertility counseling and referral as needed.
- DXA helps in baseline BMD assessment but is not mandatory. The optimal interval for repeat measurements remains unclear. Existing guidelines recommend repeating DXA at intervals of approximately 2 years, depending on risk factors and ongoing treatment. Alternative imaging modalities include trabecular bone score (TBS), quantitative ultrasound (QUS), and quantitative computed tomography (QCT). TBS, a DXA-derived assessment of lumbar spine trabecular microarchitecture, serves as an independent predictor of fracture risk. Women with POI demonstrate a higher prevalence of degraded TBS compared to controls and increased fracture prevalence. This recent study done by the author is the first in the world to have systematically assessed trabecular bone score and vertebral fractures in women with POI [14].

20.18 Puberty Induction in POI

Puberty induction is required in individuals who present with primary amenorrhea and lack of sexual characteristics due to POI.

20.18.1 Timing and Rationale for Estrogen Initiation

Initiation at 11–12 years of age to promote uterine and breast development, facilitate growth, optimize BMD, and support neurocognitive development [18].

20.18.2 Estrogen Preparations, Delivery Methods, and Dosages

Preferred estrogen formulations include natural estrogens, particularly 17β-estradiol, administered orally which includes estrabet 1–2 mg to mimic physiological puberty [18]. Combined oral contraceptive pills are discouraged due to synthetic estrogen and progesterone interference with optimal development. The recommended initial estrogen dose is one-tenth to one-eighth of the adult replacement dose, with gradual increases over 2–4 years. Both oral and transdermal estrogens induce typical breast development. Progesterone introduction is advised after 18–24 months of estrogen therapy or upon breakthrough bleeding [18]. At the end of puberty induction, treatment should transition to long-term hormone replacement therapy tailored to individual needs. Late-diagnosed patients may require an accelerated induction protocol to optimize secondary sexual development. Given high rates of HRT discontinuation in adulthood, continuity of care is essential to prevent osteoporosis and maintain feminization.

POI, once considered rare, is now increasingly recognized due to advancements in diagnostic capabilities. While it is extensively studied in Western countries, data in India remains limited. Timely diagnosis is crucial, as a delayed or misdiagnosis can lead to serious complications, including impaired cardiovascular and bone health, as well as infertility. The genetic component of POI highlights the need for vigilance among female relatives of affected women. Most importantly, HRT offers an effective treatment that, when initiated timely and for the correct duration, can decrease the long-term health risks associated with POI.

Key Points

- POI occurs when the ovaries lose function before the age of 40.
- It can be caused by genetic factors (e.g., Turner syndrome, Fragile X premutation), autoimmune diseases, chemotherapy, or idiopathic reasons.
- Symptoms include oligomenorrhea or amenorrhea, hot flashes, night sweats, vaginal dryness, infertility, mood swings, and decreased libido.
- Diagnosis is based on symptoms, medical history, and FSH (>25 IU/L on two occasions, at least 4 weeks apart). Estradiol and AMH levels have a supporting role.
- Long-term complications include increased risk of osteoporosis, cardiovascular diseases, dyslipidemias, emotional distress, and mental health challenges.
- HRT is the primary treatment for POI. Supportive management includes maintenance of bone health, egg donation and ARTs, a healthy lifestyle, and emotional support.

Long Questions

(a) Describe the pathogenetic factors implicated in the development of POI. What preventive measures can be considered?
(b) What are the long-term health consequences of POI in young women? How should healthcare providers address these issues?
(c) Discuss the various modalities and preparations for hormone replacement in the management of POI.
(d) A 28-year-old woman presents with amenorrhea and symptoms of estrogen deficiency. Outline a stepwise diagnostic workup to confirm POI and exclude other causes.

Short Questions

(a) What is the definition of premature ovarian insufficiency?
(b) What are the strategies for the prevention and management of bone loss in patients with POI?
(c) Can women with POI become pregnant naturally? Briefly explain:
(d) How does POI impact lipid profile?
How can one differentiate between amenorrhea due to POI and that due to hypogonadotropic hypogonadism?

Multiple Choice Questions

1. Which hormonal pattern is most indicative of POI?

   A. Low FSH, high LH, high estrogen
   B. High FSH, low estradiol
   C. Low LH, normal estradiol
   D. High prolactin, low FSH

2. Which of the following is NOT a typical clinical feature of POI?

   A. Amenorrheabr
   B. Hot flashes
   C. Galactorrhea
   D. Infertility

3. What is the primary goal of HRT in women with POI?

   A. To initiate ovulation
   B. To prevent polycystic ovarian syndrome
   C. To replace estrogen and reduce long-term health risks
   D. To increase testosterone levels

4. POI is associated with which of the following autoimmune conditions?

    A. Addison's disease
    B. Type 2 diabetes mellitus
    C. Myasthenia gravisbr
    D. Celiac disease

5. Why is estrogen therapy initiated at low doses and gradually increased in adolescent girls with POI?

    A. To prevent breast tenderness
    B. To avoid premature epiphyseal closure and mimic normal pubertal growth
    C. To reduce the risk of acne
    D. To induce ovulation progressively

6. Which of the following symptoms is least likely to be caused by POI?

    A. Vaginal dryness
    B. Night sweats
    C. Acne and hirsutism
    D. Mood disturbances

7. Women with POI are at increased risk for which of the following long-term complications?

    A. Hyperthyroidismbr
    B. Endometrial hyperplasiabr
    C. Osteoporosis and cardiovascular disease
    D. Breast cancer

8. Which of the following non-hormonal therapies is important in managing POI?

    A. GnRH analoguesbr
    B. Calcium and vitamin D supplementationbr
    C. Androgen blockersbr
    D. Aromatase inhibitors

9. What is the most effective fertility treatment for women with established POI?

    A. Clomiphene citrate stimulation
    B. In vitro fertilization using donor oocytes.
    C. Intrauterine inseminationbr
    D. Ovulation induction with metformin

10. What is the primary goal of estrogen therapy in puberty induction for girls with POI?

    A. To restore ovulation.
    B. To stimulate breast development and uterine growth.
    C. To induce menarche immediately
    D. To suppress gonadotropin levels permanently

Answers MCQ

1. B
2. C
3. C
4. A
5. B
6. C
7. C
8. B
9. B
10. B/p

References

1. European Society for Human Reproduction and Embryology (ESHRE) Guideline Group on POI, Webber L, Davies M, Anderson R, Bartlett J, Braat D, Cartwright B, et al. ESHRE guideline: management of women with premature ovarian insufficiency. Hum Reprod. 2016;31(5):926–37.
2. Goswami D, Conway GS. Premature ovarian failure. Hum Reprod Update. 2005;11(4):391–410.
3. Welt CK. Primary ovarian insufficiency: a more accurate term for premature ovarian failure. Clin Endocrinol. 2008;68(4):499–509.
4. Goswami R, Goswami D, Kabra M, Gupta N, Dubey S, Dadhwal V. Prevalence of the triple X syndrome in phenotypically normal women with premature ovarian failure and its association with autoimmune thyroid disorders. Fertil Steril. 2003;80(4):1052–4.
5. Lu CL, Li R, Chen XN, Xu YY, Yan LY, Yan J, et al. The 'normal' range of FMR1 triple CGG repeats may be associated with primary ovarian insufficiency in China. Reprod Biomed Online. 2017;34(2):175–80.
6. Chatterjee S, Maitra A, Kadam S, Patel Z, Gokral J, Meherji P. CGG repeat sizing in the FMR1 gene in Indian women with premature ovarian failure. Reprod Biomed Online. 2009;19(2):281–6.
7. Tosh D, Rao KL, Rani HS, Deenadayal DA, Murty US, Grover P. Association between fragile X premutation and premature ovarian failure: a case-control study and meta-analysis. Arch Gynecol Obstet. 2014;289(6):1255–62.
8. Muthuswamy S, Dean DD, Agarwal S. Molecular screening of intellectually disabled patients and those with premature ovarian failure for CGG repeat expansion at FMR1 locus: implication of combined triplet repeat primed polymerase chain reaction and methylation-specific polymerase chain reaction analysis. Neurol India. 2016;64(6):1175–9.
9. Goswami R, Marwaha RK, Goswami D, Gupta N, Ray D, Tomar N, et al. Prevalence of thyroid autoimmunity in sporadic idiopathic hypoparathyroidism in comparison to type 1 diabetes and premature ovarian failure. J Clin Endocrinol Metab. 2006;91(11):4256–9.
10. Jiao X, Zhang H, Ke H, Zhang J, Cheng L, Liu Y, Qin Y, Chen ZJ. Premature ovarian insufficiency: phenotypic characterization 6571 within different etiologies. J Clin Endocrinol Metab. 2017;102:2281–90.
11. Bidet M, Bachelot A, Touraine P. Premature ovarian failure: predictability of intermittent ovarian function and response to ovulation induction agents. Curr Opin Obstet Gynecol. 2008;20(4):416–20.

12. Goswami D, Arif A, Saxena A, Batra S. Idiopathic primary ovarian insufficiency: a study of serial hormonal profiles to assess ovarian follicular activity. Hum Reprod. 2011;26(8):2218–25.
13. Meczekalski B, Niwczyk O, Bala G, Szeliga A. Managing early onset osteoporosis: the impact of premature ovarian insufficiency on bone health. J Clin Med. 2023;12(12):4042.
14. Dhakate M, Goswami D, Goswami R, Saha S, Kandasamy D, Arora M. Bone mineral density, vertebral fractures and trabecular bone score in primary ovarian insufficiency. J Endocrinol Investig. 2023;46(9):1865–74.
15. Ke H, et al. Landscape of pathogenic mutations in premature ovarian insufficiency. Nat Med. 2023;29:483–92.
16. LaVasseur C, Neukam S, Kartika T, Samuelson Bannow B, Shatzel J, DeLoughery TG. Hormonal therapies and venous thrombosis: considerations for prevention and management. Res Pract Thromb Haemost. 2022;6(6):e12763.
17. Kalantaridou SN, Davis SR, Nelson LM. Premature ovarian failure. Endocrinol Metab Clin N Am. 1998;27(4):989–1006.
18. Nordenström A, Ahmed SF, van den Akker E, Blair J, Bonomi M, Brachet C, et al. Pubertal induction and transition to adult sex hormone replacement in patients with congenital pituitary or gonadal reproductive hormone deficiency: an Endo-ERN clinical practice guideline. Eur J Endocrinol. 2022;186(6):G9–G49.

Delayed Menopause

21

Jyothi Unni

Abstract

There is a variation of age at natural menopause in Indian women based on several sociocultural and epidemiological factors. Women who have not attained menopause by the age of 55 years are considered to have delayed menopause. Some factors associated with delayed menopause include multiparity, longer breastfeeding, alcohol and caffeine consumption, obesity, and use of combined oral contraceptives. Women with polycystic ovarian syndrome also have an increased chance of attaining menopause late. The risks of delayed menopause include an increase of estrogen-dependent cancers such as breast, endometrial, and ovarian cancer. Women who attain menopause late should be encouraged to get screened annually for cancers. However, there are some advantages of longer years of estrogen exposure. These include a reduction in osteoporosis and cardiovascular disease. There is also an increase in life expectancy and decrease in all-cause mortality.

Keywords

Delayed menopause · Late menopause

Introduction The age at natural menopause varies significantly between different populations and ethnic groups. In India, there are differences between states, as well as among rural and urban women, and women of different socioeconomic backgrounds. According to the WHO Fact Sheet 2024, natural menopause occurs between ages 45 and 55 years. The Clinical Practice Guidelines of the Indian

J. Unni (✉)
Department of Obstetrics and Gynecology, Jehangir Hospital, Pune, Maharashtra, India

R. Malik et al. (eds.), *Menopause Essentials*,
https://doi.org/10.1007/978-981-95-7498-8_21

Menopause Society state that delayed menopause is not defined, but it can be taken as two standard deviations (SD) above the natural age of menopause in that population, so in India, we may consider it to be beyond 54 years [1].

Prevalence The longitudinal aging study in India (LASI-1) considered women who had attained natural menopause after the age of 55 years as having had delayed menopause. They studied data from 25,356 women from all 35 states and union territories of India and found a prevalence of 4.4% of delayed menopause. It was the highest in Sikkim at 9.8%. The mean and SD in this study for late menopause were 59.38 and 3.74 years, respectively [2].

Global prevalence estimates vary from 5% to 17% depending on the age cut-off used. The variation could also be due to different causes and several sociocultural influences on the natural age of menopause. The importance lies in the fact that there may be an increase in some risks, particularly of estrogen-dependent cancers in such a situation.

Associated Factors There are some factors that are known to be associated with late menopause.

- Women whose mothers have delayed menopause are more likely to have late menopause themselves. It is unclear whether this is due to genetic influences or environmental factors which are common to mother–daughter pairs.
- Increasing parity has been implicated in delaying menopause. Large population studies have shown an association between late menopause and combined oral contraceptive use, being parous, number of pregnancies and live births, and longer breastfeeding duration. The mechanism postulated is that since there is a fixed pool of follicles and a certain number of ovulatory cycles in a woman's lifetime, all these factors which cause anovulation delay the menopause.
- Data from the Study of Women's Health Across the Nation (SWAN) has shown that there are ethnic differences too. Japanese have later menopause than Caucasians and Hispanics. This could be due to dietary factors since phytoestrogen-rich diets are known to delay the onset of natural menopause.
- Several authors have shown that overweight and obese women are at increased risk of having delayed menopause. This is presumed to be due to an increase in the aromatization of estrogen in the adipose tissue.
- It is thought that regular exercise increases hormone production and thus may delay menopause, though literature reveals that excessive exercise is a factor in causing early and premature menopause.
- Consumption of alcohol in moderation increases estrogen levels, and this could lead to late menopause. Caffeine intake of a cup per day delays menopause by 2–3 years.

Schoenmaker et al. in a review of lifestyle factors and socioeconomic parameters across six continents found that higher education and high occupation level were associated with later menopause as was living in more developed countries [3].

A meta-analysis published in 2020 found that previous ever use of oral contraceptives (HR = 0.87, CI = 0.82–0.93), age at menarche ≥13 years (HR = 0.90, CI = 0.84–0.96), and having at least one live birth (HR = 0.79, CI = 0.74–0.85) were associated with a later age of natural menopause. The authors suggest that these factors could be markers of later ovarian aging. It could be that oral contraceptives suppress FSH and thus lead to a delay in natural menopause [4].

Vatankhah H et al. studied age of menopause in women in Iran and found that older women (OR 8.65, 95% CI = 5.31–14.08) and women with a history of diabetes (OR 2.42, 95% CI = 1.63–3.60), hypertension (OR 2.06, 95% CI = 1.42–2.97), thyroid disease (OR 1.85, 95% CI = 1.07–3.20), and depression (OR 2.00, 95% CI = 1.35–2.97) were more likely to have delayed menopause. The authors suggested that since the age of menopause can affect subsequent health in women, understanding the determinants of menopausal age is important and should be pursued [5].

A large study has been done to investigate the possibility of modifying factors that are implicated in affecting the age of natural menopause. A total of 87,349 postmenopausal women were studied. It was found that 16.7% of these women had late menopause, which was defined as menopause occurring at or after age 53 years. Increased physical activity, cessation of smoking, and consuming a diet high in phytoestrogens, meat, and dairy products delay the onset of menopause [6].

Women with PCOS attained menopause 4 years later than non-PCOS women in a Swedish study. However, using AMH to predict age at menopause, a study from Iran suggested that the reproductive lifespan of PCOS women could be 2 years longer, i.e., they were likely to reach menopause 2 years later than women without PCOS.

A study looking at gene variants found that there are some common variants between PCOS and the age of menopause, and thus, women with PCOS may have genetic factors in common with women who have delayed menopause [7].

Hormonal Changes The decline in inhibin levels seems to start later in women with late menopause compared with those with average age of natural menopause. High LH levels also occur later in these women, even when FSH levels are elevated to menopausal levels. And it is only when LH is also high that they attain menopause. Once they are menopausal, these women have a similar hormonal profile to those who attained menopause earlier.

Risks of Delayed Menopause Due to the continued exposure to estrogen for a longer period, women with late menopause are at higher risk of getting endometrial, ovarian, and breast cancers.

Unopposed estrogen exposure is known to cause endometrial hyperplasia and subsequently increase the risk of endometrial cancer. Delayed menopause is potentially associated with increased exposure to estrogen. A recent publication, looking at the association of reproductive factors and endometrial cancer risk, found that late menopause (≥55 years) showed an HR of 2.84 (95% CI = 1.78–4.55; *P* for trend <0.001) compared with the youngest age category for menopause (<45 years) [8].

Repeated exposure to an inflammatory environment on the surface of the ovary and tube following ovulation is postulated to increase the ovarian cancer risk. It has been reported that ovarian cancer risk increased by 14% for every 5-year increase in lifetime ovulatory years [9]. So, delayed menopause, by increased estrogen due to more ovulatory years, increases the risk of ovarian cancer.

Early age at menarche and late age at menopause have been implicated as risk factors for the development of breast cancer due to increased exposure to estrogen. Each year of delay of menopause increases the breast cancer risk by 3% [10]. A scoping review in 2021 found that there is a positive correlation between late menopause and certain subtypes of breast cancer, mainly ER+, PR+, and HER2+ subtypes.

Interestingly, a systematic review found that there was an increased risk of lung cancer in women with delayed menopause, and contrary to the risk of lung cancer usually found in smokers, the higher risk of lung cancer associated with late menopause was seen among nonsmokers.

Advantages of Delayed Menopause There are advantages too. Estrogen protects these women from dyslipidemia, coronary artery disease, and osteoporosis. It also increases life expectancy and decreases all-cause mortality [2].

Estrogen lowers total cholesterol and LDL cholesterol, causes vasodilatation of the coronary arteries, increases fibrinolysis, and thus has a favorable impact on coronary artery disease. The risk of ischemic cardiovascular disease, ischemic and hemorrhagic stroke, and death from coronary artery disease is significantly lower in women who have delayed menopause due to the cardioprotective effects of estrogen.

It is well known that estrogen increases bone mineral density, leading to a slower rate of bone loss and osteopenia as well as osteoporosis. This also decreases sarcopenia and fracture risk. Women who attain menopause late have better hand grip strength and functional efficiency of the upper and lower limbs.

It is also thought that estrogen may have an impact on cognition and delay the onset of cognitive decline.

21.1 Management

A detailed history and a thorough clinical examination should be done. Her BMI and waist circumference should be recorded, as well as her blood pressure. A detailed systemic and pelvic examination must be performed.

Investigations

If a woman with late menopause presents to a clinician, we should use the opportunity to investigate her for noncommunicable diseases, including cancer screening.

Hemogram, HbA1C, Lipid Profile, Renal and Liver Function Tests
Cervical Smear
Ultrasound of Abdomen and Pelvis, including TVS
Mammography
Bone Densitometry by DEXA

It is prudent to screen women with delayed menopause for endometrial and breast cancer. A transvaginal ultrasound should be performed for all women with late menopause, and if the endometrial thickness is >4 mm, they should undergo an endometrial biopsy. If focal lesions are visualized on ultrasound, it would be better to perform a hysteroscopy, so that the lesion can be visualized and biopsied or resected.

Mammography should be performed annually for these women so that malignancies can be picked up early and treated.

Unfortunately, since there is no definite screening strategy for ovarian cancer yet, we are unable to screen effectively for this in low-risk women. An abdominal ultrasound may show an ovarian tumor, but often ovarian cancer is only diagnosed in late stages. Multimodal screening of the general population has led to earlier detection and downstaging, but no mortality benefit has been demonstrated. Risk-reducing salpingo-oophorectomy in individuals with greater than 4–5% lifetime risk of developing ovarian cancer has been shown to reduce ovarian cancer incidence and mortality.

Women with delayed menopause should be counseled that they should report to their doctor at the earliest if they have any of the following symptoms:

- Heavy or prolonged vaginal bleeding
- Lump in the breast or retraction of the nipple
- Discharge from the nipple, especially if blood-stained
- Distention of the abdomen or bloating
- Change in bowel or bladder habits

Key Points

1. Women who have not attained menopause by the age of 55 years are considered to have late or delayed menopause.
2. The advantages of continued estrogen exposure for a few additional years include a reduction in cardiovascular risk and osteoporosis.
3. However, there are also concerns regarding the increased risk of estrogen-dependent cancers such as endometrial, ovarian, and breast cancer.

Women with delayed menopause should be screened annually or earlier if symptoms develop, to identify cancers at an early stage to reduce morbidity and mortality.

Long Questions

1. Discuss the advantages of delayed menopause.
2. What are the risks of attaining menopause late?
3. What investigations would you advise to a 56-year-old woman who is still menstruating?

Short Questions

1. Define delayed menopause.
2. What is the prevalence of delayed menopause?
3. What are the factors which may cause late menopause?

Multiple Choice Questions (MCQs)

1. Which of the following is NOT a potential factor in delaying menopause?
   A. Breastfeeding for an extended period
   B. Regular exercise
   C. Smoking
   D. Consuming a phyto-estrogen rich diet
2. Delayed menopause causes:
   A. Increase in cardiovascular risk
   B. Decrease in cardiovascular risk
   C. Decrease in breast cancer risk
   D. Increase in osteoporosis risk
3. RRSO stands for:
   A. Relative risk of salpingo-oophorectomy
   B. Risk rate of salpingo-oophorectomy
   C. Risk reducing signs of ovaries
   D. Risk reducing salpingo-oophorectomy
4. Women who reach menopause late have a higher risk of:
   A. Endometrial cancer
   B. Breast cancer
   C. Ovarian cancer
   D. All of the above

5. Factors associated with delayed menopause include:

   A. Obesity
   B. Early menarche
   C. Nulliparity
   D. Sedentary lifestyle

Answers

1. C
2. B
3. D
4. D
5. A

References

1. Meeta M, Digumarti L, Agarwal N, Vaze N, Shah R, Malik S. Clinical practice guidelines on menopause: an executive summary and recommendations: Indian menopause society 2019–2020. J Midlife Health. 2020;11(2):55–95.
2. Halder P, Kansal S, Mamgai A, Rathor S. Untimely menopause, state wise prevalence and determinants: insights from longitudinal aging study in India (LASI-1). J Obstet Gynecol India. 2025; https://doi.org/10.1007/s13224-024-02094-1.
3. Schoenaker DA, Jackson CA, Rowlands JV, Mishra GD. Socioeconomic position, lifestyle factors and age at natural menopause: a systematic review and meta-analyses of studies across six continents. Int J Epidemiol. 2014;43(5):1542–62.
4. Roman Lay AA, do Nascimento CF, Horta BL, Dias Porto CFA. Reproductive factors and age at natural menopause: a systematic review and meta-analysis. Maturitas. 2020;131:57.
5. Vatankhah H, Khalili P, Vatanparast M, Ayoobi F, Esmaeili-Nadimi A, Jamali Z. Prevalence of early and late menopause and its determinants in Rafsanjan cohort study. Sci Rep. 2023;13(1):1847.
6. Wang M, Kartsonaki C, Guo Y, Lv J, Gan W, Chen ZM, Li LM, Hu CG, Yang L, Yu M. Factors related to age at natural menopause in China: results from the China Kadoorie Biobank. Menopause. 2021;28(10):1130–42.
7. Saxena R, Bjonnes AC, Georgopoulos NA, Koika V, Panidis D, Welt CK. Gene variants associated with age at menopause are also associated with polycystic ovary syndrome, gonadotrophins and ovarian volume. Hum Reprod. 2015;30(7):1697–703.
8. Katagiri R, Iwasaki M, Abe SK, Islam MR, Rahman MS, Saito E, et al. Reproductive factors and endometrial cancer risk among women. JAMA Netw Open. 2023;6(9):e2332296.
9. Trabert B, Tworoger SS, O'Brien KM, Townsend MK, Fortner RT, Iversen ES, et al. Ovarian Cancer Cohort Consortium (OC3). The risk of ovarian cancer increases with an increase in the lifetime number of ovulatory cycles: an analysis from the Ovarian Cancer Cohort Consortium (OC3). Cancer Res. 2020;80(5):1210–8.
10. Korzets Y, Yariv O, Mutai R, Moore A, Shochat T, Yerushalmi R, et al. The impact of endogenous estrogen exposures on the characteristics and outcomes of estrogen receptor positive, early breast cancer. Discov Oncol. 2021;12(1):26.

Cancer Screening Guidelines for Menopausal Women

22

Pranav Mohan Singhal and Monal Garg

Abstract

The benefits of screening for breast and cervical cancers are well-established, while those for endometrial and ovarian cancers depend on individual risk factors especially family history. Regular cancer screening after menopause is crucial due to heightened risks, particularly for cervical and endometrial cancers. Postmenopausal women should stay alert to symptoms such as unusual bleeding, which may signal uterine cancer, and persistent bloating, which could indicate ovarian cancer. In India, it's advised that women aged 30 and older undergo cervical cancer screenings, which can be conducted through methods like visual inspection with acetic acid (VIA), Pap smears, or HPV DNA tests. Each of these methods has specific intervals for testing, starting from age 30 and continuing until age 65. For women living with HIV, screening is recommended to begin earlier, that is by the age of 25. When it comes to breast cancer screening, guidelines suggest that women aged 25 to 40 should have clinical breast examinations (CBE) every 1 to 3 years, while those over 40 should aim for annual CBEs and mammograms. It's essential for women to regularly review and update their cancer screening plans during menopause to ensure they remain proactive about their health.

Keywords

Cancer screening · Menopause · Cancer · Women · Detection

P. M. Singhal (✉)
Thoracic Surgical Oncology, National Cancer Center, Goyang, South Korea

M. Garg
Gynaecological Oncology, National Cancer Center, Goyang, South Korea

R. Malik et al. (eds.), *Menopause Essentials*,
https://doi.org/10.1007/978-981-95-7498-8_22

22.1 Introduction

Studies have indicated a significant connection between age and cancer. Menopause is a normal aspect of aging and generally does not heighten the risk of gynecological cancers unless it happens after the age of 55 [1]. Given the worldwide increase in cancer occurrences, there is an immediate necessity for enhanced cancer screening techniques, especially in our country, where there is an absence of organized, population-based screening initiatives. This article explores the most recent guidelines for screening the two most prevalent cancers impacting women: cervical cancer and breast cancer.

Efforts in cancer screening ought to emphasize enhancing cancer prevention while reducing the risks associated with excessive testing and overtreatment. An optimal screening test should possess high sensitivity and specificity, be user-friendly, and cost-effective. At present, screening for cervical and breast cancer is being conducted in India. Nevertheless, guidelines for screening colorectal cancer have been established in the Western world and have yet to be embraced in India. There are several recommendations for screening that are available which are as follows:

22.2 Cervical Cancer Screening

22.2.1 Current Status of Cervical Cancer

In 2022, there were an estimated 662,044 cases of cervical cancer worldwide, resulting in an age-standardized incidence rate (ASIR) of 14.12 cases per 100,000 individuals. This led to approximately 348,709 deaths, corresponding to an age-standardized mortality rate (ASMR) of 7.08 per 100,000. Cervical cancer is the fourth leading cause of cancer-related illness and death among women globally. Notably, 42% of the cases and 39% of the deaths occurred in China, which accounted for 23% of the cases and 16% of the deaths, and India, which accounted for 19% of the cases and 23% of the deaths.

Focusing on India, the GLOBOCAN 2022 data shows that there were 127,356 new cervical cancer cases, making it the second most prevalent cancer among women in the nation. On a global scale, there were 662,301 new cases, placing India second in terms of incidence. The GLOBOCAN 2022 estimates pointed out that there were 348,709 deaths due to cervical cancer around the world [2].

The global objective of the WHO's Cervical Cancer Elimination Initiative is to lower incidence rates to below 4 per 100,000 women-years within this century, thereby eradicating the disease as a significant public health concern [3]. Currently, just 10 countries—all situated in the Eastern Mediterranean—report incidence rates beneath this threshold as of 2022.3 Given the high incidence rates and concerning trends in numerous transitioning countries, modeling studies propose that achieving the goal of eradicating cervical cancer by the end of the century may be unattainable unless there is a substantial enhancement in preventive strategies and treatment initiatives, especially in HPV screening and vaccination. The Cervical Cancer Elimination Initiative has established ambitious national goals of 90–70–90 for nations striving to eradicate cervical cancer by 2030. These objectives indicate that 90% of girls should complete the full series of the HPV vaccine by the age of 15, 70% of women must undergo screening with a high-performance test at ages 35 and 45, and 90% of women diagnosed with precancerous lesions or invasive cancer should receive proper treatment. Fortunately, there is encouraging evidence that utilizing a self-sampling method could boost screening rates among women who are either under-screened or have never been screened, along with the potential efficacy of a single-dose vaccine to simplify the implementation of these programs [3]. Additionally, three important guidelines concerning cervical cancer screening are outlined in Table 22.1 (Tables 22.2 and 22.3).

Table 22.1 Guidelines for cervical cancer screening

	ACS (2020) [4]	FOGSI (2018) [5] Good resource	FOGSI (2018) [5] Limited resource	WHO (2021) [6]
Modality	Primary HPV testing If not available then cotesting (HPV + PAP) or cytology alone	A—Primary HPV testing B—Cytology C—Colposcopy and Bx D—VIA	A—VIA B—Colposcopy +/_ Bx	HPV DNA testing If not available can use VIA or cytology
Age to start/Target	25 years/25–65 years	25 years/25–65 years Cytology/Pri HPV at 25 Cotest at 30 years	30 years/30–65 years	30 years/30–49 years
Frequency	HPV testing, Cotest every 5 years Cytology alone every 3 years	HPV testing, Cotest every 5 years Cytology alone every 3 years	Every 5 years (At least 1–3 times in life)	HPV DNA testing Every 5–10 years VIA /cytology every 3 years
Age to stop	65 years A—No H/O intraepithelial neoplasia grade 2 or more severe diagnosis with in past 25 years and B—Adequate negative prior screening in the 10-year period before age 65 years	65 years Consistent negative result in last 15 years Women with no prior screening should undergo test once at 65 years if negative should exit screening.		After 50 years After 50 years if 2 consecutive negative screening result consistent with recommended regular screening interval (60–70 years) Screening even just twice in a lifetime is beneficial (While transitioning to program)

**ACS* American Cancer Society, *FOGSI* Federation of Obstetrics and Gynaecologic Societies of India, *WHO* World Health Organization

Table 22.2 Cervical cancer screening modalities

Molecular	Cytologic	Visual inspection
Nucleic acid amplification tests (NAAT) HR-HPV mRNA	Conventional Pap smear	Visual inspection with acetic acid or with Lugol's iodine (VIA/VILI) Naked eye Magnified by colposcope or camera
DNA methylation	Liquid-based cytology (LBC)	Automated visual evaluation of digital images
Protein biomarkers HPV antibodies Oncoproteins	Dual staining to identify p16 and Ki-67	

Table 22.3 Primary HPV screening tests [7]

Indication	Test name	Manufacturer	Results
Primary HPV testing	Cobas HPV	Roche	Pooled 14 HR-HPV: +/– Genotype specific: 16, 18, and type group 31, 33, 35, 39, 45, 51, 52, 56, 58, 59, 66, and 68
Primary HPV testing	BD HPV Onclarity	BD	Pooled 14 HR-HPV: +/– (Genotype specific: 16, 18, 31, 45, 51, 52, and type groups (33/58), (35/39/68), (56/59/66))
Triage after ASCUS cytology or cotesting with cytology	Cervista HPV HR	Hologic Gen-Probe	Positive, negative, indeterminate
Triage after ASCUS cytology or cotesting with cytology, where the Cervista HPV HR test was used as the triage test	Cervista HPV 16/18	Hologic Gen-Probe	Positive for genotype, negative, indeterminate
Triage after ASCUS cytology	Aptima HPV	Hologic Gen-Probe	Positive, negative, invalid
Triage after ASCUS cytology or cotesting with cytology, where the Aptima HPV HR test was used as the triage test	Aptima HPV 16/18/45	Hologic Gen-Probe	Positive for genotype, negative, invalid
Reflex triage after ASCUS cytology	Digene Hybrid Capture 2 HPV DNA	Qiagen	Positive/negative

22.3 Breast Cancer Screening

Why is screening important?

- Screening lowers the chances of dying from breast cancer and allows for the early initiation of treatment.
- Research indicates that screening asymptomatic women for breast cancer can decrease the mortality rate by 20–30% [8].
- Evaluating a person's risk for breast cancer is essential.

22.3.1 Risk Assessment

To develop an appropriate screening strategy, the first step is to evaluate risk levels (average, moderate, high). It is essential to determine whether a woman has an average or increased risk of breast cancer to guide counseling regarding breast cancer monitoring, advanced screening options such as Magnetic Resonance Imaging (MRI) screening, risk reduction methods, and genetic testing. The risk categories are established based on the lifetime probability of being diagnosed with breast cancer (rather than the risk of dying from breast cancer). These categories are classified as average (less than 15%), moderate (approximately 15% to 20%), or high (more than 20%) lifetime risk [9]. The main risk factors include:

- Personal history of breast, ovarian, tubal, or peritoneal cancer
- Family history of breast, ovarian, tubal, or peritoneal cancer
- Ancestry (for example, Ashkenazi Jewish) associated with breast cancer 1 or 2 mutations
- Known carrier of a pathogenic mutation related to a hereditary breast and ovarian cancer syndrome in oneself or in a family member
- Mammographic breast density
- Previous breast biopsy that showed a high-risk lesion (such as atypical hyperplasia)
- Early onset of menstruation and late onset of menopause (after age 55)
- Chest radiotherapy received between the ages of 10 and 30. Risk assessment tools like Gail and BRCA PRO are easily available.

A lack of awareness, reliance on only "opportunistic screening," and the rising prevalence of breast cancer among women in India emphasize the necessity for greater breast awareness, alongside self-examinations and clinical breast exams at intervals of 1–3 years for women aged 20–39. Studies show that screening mammography reduces the risk of death from breast cancer and encourages the use of early treatment. As per the systematic review conducted by the American Cancer Society (ACS) and the USPSTF (United States Preventive Services Task Force), screening mammography is associated with a decreased risk of breast cancer mortality in randomized controlled trials (relative risk [RR], 0.80–0.82) and in cohort studies (RR, 0.75; 95% CI, 0.69–0.81). Different methods of breast cancer screening include the following:

1. *Breast Self-Examination:*

   There is currently no evidence that breast self-examination (BSE) reduces the mortality rate by detecting breast cancers at an early stage, and many organizations do not recommend it. For women who choose to perform BSE, it should not be done in isolation; clinical breast examinations and mammography should complement it.
2. *Clinical Breast Examination:*

   Several randomized trials have included both mammography and clinical breast examination (CBE), but the independent contributions of these methods remain unclear. Mammography detects approximately 90% of screen-detected cancers, while CBE detects about 50%. Additionally, mammography is more standardized than CBE.

3. *Mammography:*

   Mammography is the best-studied imaging technique that has consistently been shown to reduce breast cancer mortality, as evidenced by multiple randomized trials. It is available in several forms: screen-film mammography, digital mammography, and digital breast tomosynthesis (3D mammography). Mammography and clinical breast examinations (CBE) complement each other, and it is recommended that women have CBEs around the time of their regularly scheduled annual mammograms.

   Mammograms can be categorized into screening and diagnostic types and are typically performed in two views:

   1. Craniocaudal (CC): In this position, the breast is elevated and placed on the plate, with pressure applied from the top (Fig. 22.1a).
   2. Mediolateral oblique (MLO): In this view, the breast is squeezed and captured from the side at a slanted angle (Fig. 22.1b).

Utilizing both perspectives enhances the detection rates of cancer and lowers recall rates. If only a single view can be taken, the MLO view is favored because it encompasses a greater volume of breast tissue than the CC view.

The effective radiation dose from a standard screening mammogram is roughly 0.7 mSv, which is comparable to the amount of natural background radiation received over a 3-month period. Most mammography machines provide an average dose of 0.1 to 0.2 rads (1 to 2 mGy) per exposure.

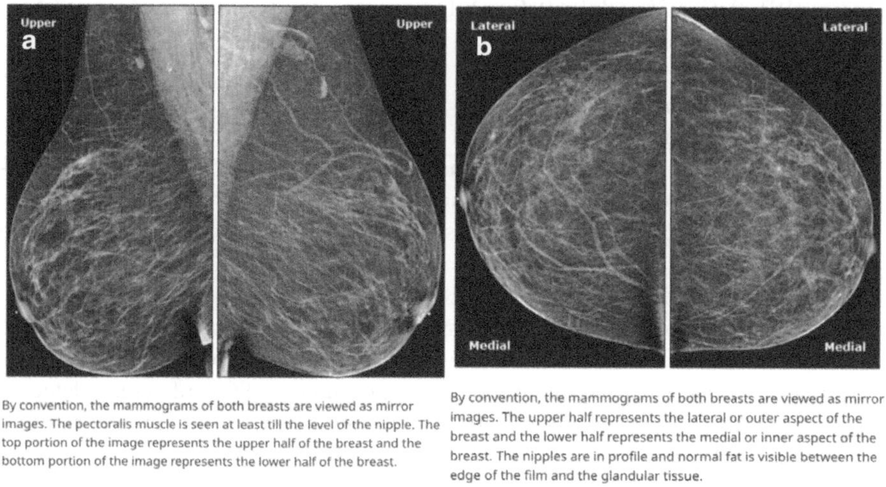

Fig. 22.1 (**a**) Craniocaudal (CC): In this position, the breast is elevated and placed on the plate, with pressure applied from the top. (**b**) Mediolateral Oblique (MLO): In this view, the breast is squeezed and captured from the side at a slanted angle

4. *Other Modalities:*

Ultrasound:

- Useful for dense breast tissue and is utilized to investigate abnormal areas.
- Indications for its use include:
  - Young patients
  - Pregnant individuals
  - Infection or inflammation
- It can differentiate between solid and cystic masses.

MRI (Magnetic Resonance Imaging):

- Produces detailed cross-sectional images.
- Serves as an adjunct to mammography but is less specific than a mammogram.
- Indications for MRI:
  - Unclear findings on a mammogram or ultrasound.
  - Postlumpectomy scarring.
  - Extensive ductal carcinoma in situ (DCIS) or infiltrating lobular cancer.
  - Presence of silicone implants.
  - Monitoring after neoadjuvant chemotherapy (NACT).
  - Screening for individuals with BRCA mutations and a lifetime risk of 20–25% (Tables 22.4 and 22.5).

Table 22.4 BI-RADS (Breast Imaging-Reporting and Data System) categorization [10]

Category	Interpretation	Explanation
BI-RADS 0	Incomplete	Needs additional imaging evaluation and/or prior mammograms for comparison. This category is used when there is not enough information from the views available to derive a conclusion. This is more commonly used in screening studies, which are interpreted as abnormal when the radiologist is not providing immediate reads
BI-RADS 1	Negative	This is a completely negative examination. The woman should continue with screening mammography and clinical breast examination based on current screening guidelines
BI-RADS 2	Benign	Benign masses such as fibroadenomas or cysts or benign vascular or parenchymal calcifications may be reported. There is no concern for malignancy and no further action needs to be taken. The rationale for reporting these findings is to document benignity and to prevent unnecessary evaluation. Routine follow-up is recommended
BI-RADS 3	Probably benign	This category is used when there is a finding that does not have characteristic benign features, but the likelihood of malignancy is less than 2%. Examples of lesions in this category would include a focal asymmetry, a group of round calcifications, or a circumscribed mass that is detected on a baseline screening examination
BI-RADS 4	Suspicious	This category implies that there is a lesion with suspicious features for malignancy. The chance that the imaging finding is a cancer ranges between 2% and 94%. The degree of suspicion or worry for malignancy varies both with the lesion and with the interpreter
BI-RADS 5	Highly suggestive of malignancy	Lesions that have classic worrisome imaging features such as speculations (pleomorphic calcifications and skin retraction are placed in this category. The suspicion of malignancy is 95 to 100%
BI-RADS 6	Known, biopsy-proven malignancy	This includes patients with established biopsy-proven cancers that have yet to be surgically excised who present for further imaging to either evaluate the contralateral breast or assess response to neoadjuvant chemotherapy, or who present for a second opinion with interpretation of outside imaging studies

BI-RADS Breast Imaging—Reporting and Data System
Screening mammograms should only be given BI-RADS assessments of 0, 1, or 2
BI-RADS categories 3–6 are reserved for a diagnostic evaluation

Table 22.5 Guidelines for breast cancer screening [11]

Organization	Mammography			Interval for mammography	Clinical breast exam	Self-breast exam
	40–49	50–74	75+			
US Preventive Services Task Force	Individualized	Yes	Insufficient evidence	Biennial	Insufficient evidence	Not recommended
American College of Obstetrics and Gynaecology	Offered	Yes	Shared decision-making process	Every 1–2 years	Offer 1–3-year screening for women aged 25–39 years; -annually for above 40 years	Not recommended
American Cancer Society	Offered, 40–44 Recommended, 45–49	Yes	Continue screening until life expectancy <10 years	Annual, 40–54; Annual/Biennial, 55+	Not recommended	Not recommended
National Comprehensive Cancer Network	Yes	Yes	Continue screening until life expectancy <10 years	Annual	Every 1–3 years for those aged 25–39, then annually for those above 40 years	Not recommended
American College of Radiology	Yes	Yes	Continue screening until life expectancy <5–7 years	Annual	Not addressed	Not recommended
American College of Physicians	Individualized	Yes	No	Biennial	Not recommended	Not recommended
American Academy of Family Physicians	Individualized	Yes	Insufficient evidence	Biennial	Insufficient evidence	Not recommended

22.4 Colorectal Cancer Screening

In developed nations, the rates of newly diagnosed colorectal cancer (CRC) and related fatalities have declined due to improved understanding, screening, and treatment. There is a troubling increase in colorectal cancer (CRC) among younger people, especially in India, where information about younger patients is scarce. Given India's largely younger demographic, the rise in CRC will primarily affect younger people. A simple fecal immunohistochemical test, with high sensitivity and negative predictive value, can effectively identify those needing further invasive colonoscopies, making it suitable for mass screening [12].

22.4.1 Screening Methods

Almost all colorectal cancers arise from the adenoma–carcinoma pathway, making colonoscopy an effective screening method for early detection, as it can identify and excise polyps before they progress to cancer. Polyps can be hyperplastic, adenomatous, hamartomatous or inflammatory, with adenomatous polyps larger than 10 mm posing the highest risk of malignancy. Despite its proven benefits for survival, colonoscopy usage remains low in Western populations. Flexible sigmoidoscopy is also effective in reducing colon cancer incidence and mortality. A research study conducted in South India found that 12.19% of the 246 patients assessed had polyps. Among individuals aged 40 to 50, 8.7% had adenomas. Additionally, it was noted that one out of every six individuals over the age of 40 had a polyp [13].

The guaiac-based fecal occult blood test (FOBT) is a cost-effective screening tool for colorectal cancer (CRC) that reduces mortality risk by 16%, but it has low sensitivity and can yield false positives. The fecal immunochemical test (FIT) improves sensitivity by detecting human globin, requires only one test, and does not need dietary changes. However, FIT is less available and more expensive, making it underutilized for screening in our country.

Computed tomography (CT) colonography serves as a noninvasive substitute for conventional colonoscopy, demonstrating sensitivity and specificity exceeding 90% for identifying polyps that are greater than 10 mm in size. However, radiation exposure data is lacking, and polyps still require removal through colonoscopy. In India, various screening methods such as the multitarget stool DNA test and SEPT9 DNA test are currently inaccessible, indicating an opportunity to create an affordable blood test for colon cancer screening.

22.4.2 Current Status of CRC Screening in India

Currently, there are no established guidelines for colorectal cancer screening in India. Organizations such as the Indian Council of Medical Research, the Indian Society of Medical and Pediatric Oncology, and the Indian Cancer Society should consider developing these guidelines, as they would undoubtedly benefit the Indian community.

Key Points

- An ideal screening test should be sensitive, specific, easy to use, and financially efficient.
- Seventy percent of women need to be screened for cancer cervix with a high-performance test at ages 35 and 45, and 90% of women with precancerous lesions or invasive cancer should receive appropriate treatment.
- Research indicates that screening asymptomatic women for breast cancer can decrease the mortality rate by 20–30%.
- Currently, there are no established guidelines for colorectal cancer screening in India.

Long Answer Questions (LAQs)

1. What are the WHO strategies for the elimination of cervical cancer?

2. Please elaborate on the FOGSI cervical cancer screening guidelines for both resource-rich and resource-limited regions.

3. Illustrate with a diagram the mechanism by which HPV infection leads to cervical cancer in women.

4. What are the various modalities for screening breast cancer?

Short Answer Questions (SAQs)

1. What are the different methods for testing HPV?
2. What risk factors are associated with the development of breast cancer?
3. Explain the BIRADS system used for breast cancer screening?
4. What are the new WHO recommendations for cervical cancer screening?
5. What are the various guidelines for breast cancer screening?

Multiple Choice Questions (MCQs)

1. When should women be advised to stop routine cervical cancer screening?
   A. After age 60 years with prior negative tests
   B. After age 50 years with prior negative tests
   C. After age 75 years, irrespective of prior negative tests
   D. After age 65 years with prior negative tests

2. According to the latest WHO cervical cancer screening guidelines, what is the target age group?
   A. 25–75 years
   B. 30–49 years
   C. 30–55 years
   D. 21–60 years

3. How does the HPV E6 protein contribute to the development of cervical cancer?
   A. It inhibits the p53 tumor suppressor protein.
   B. It promotes cell differentiation.
   C. It repairs DNA damage.
   D. It suppresses immune responses.

4. What is the mechanism of HPV causing cervical cancer?
   A. Chromosomal replication
   B. Epigenetic modification
   C. Production of cytotoxins
   D. Oxidative stress

5. What is the primary reason HPV vaccination that helps prevent cervical cancer?
   A. It kills existing HPV infections.
   B. It induces immunity against high-risk HPV types before exposure.
   C. It treats existing cervical lesions.
   D. It prevents all sexually transmitted infections.

6. What is the primary goal of breast cancer screening?
   A. To diagnose symptomatic breast lumps
   B. To detect breast cancer at an early, more treatable stage
   C. To prevent breast cancer from developing
   D. To replace clinical breast examinations

7. For women aged 75 years and older, screening recommendations are generally:
    A. Continue annually without exception
    B. Are to stop immediately
    C. Are individualized based on health status and life expectancy
    D. Shift to more frequent screening

8. What is the standard limitation of mammography screening?
    A. It can produce false positives, leading to unnecessary biopsies.
    B. It can miss cancers, especially in dense breast tissue.
    C. It involves exposure to low-dose radiation.
    D. All of the above.

9. Breast self-examination is recommended as a primary screening tool for breast cancer.
    A. True—It is recommended as a screening tool for those aged 25 years or older.
    B. False—It is not advised as a screening tool, but it may help women become familiar with their breasts.
    C. True—It is the best modality for breast cancer screening.
    D. False—it is not helpful because of its very low sensitivity and specificity.

10. A 45-year-old woman underwent a mammogram, which revealed a 2 × 1.5 cm BIRADS 4 lesion in her left breast. What is the next plan of action?
    A. Perform a biopsy of the lesion
    B. Follow up on the lesion after 6 months
    C. Conduct an MRI of the breast for confirmation
    D. Perform a breast ultrasound to confirm the findings

Answers

1. D
2. B
3. A
4. B
5. B
6. B
7. C
8. D
9. B
10. A

References

1. Abulajiang Y, Liu T, Wang M, et al. The influence of menopause age on gynecologic cancer risk: a comprehensive analysis using NHANES data. Front Oncol. 2025;15:1541585.
2. Bray F, Laversanne M, Sung H, et al. Global cancer statistics 2022: GLOBOCAN estimates of incidence and mortality worldwide for 36 cancers in 185 countries. CA Cancer J Clin. 2024;74(3):229–63.
3. Zhou L, Li Y, Wang H, et al. Global cervical cancer elimination: quantifying the status, progress, and gaps. BMC Med. 2025;23(1):67.
4. Fontham ETH, Wolf AMD, Church TR, et al. Cervical cancer screening for individuals at average risk: 2020 guideline update from the American Cancer Society. CA Cancer J Clin. 2020;70(5):321–46.
5. Bhatla N, Singhal S, Saraiya U, et al. Screening and management of preinvasive lesions of the cervix: good clinical practice recommendations from the Federation of Obstetrics and Gynaecologic Societies of India (FOGSI). J Obstet Gynaecol Res. 2020;46(2):201–14.
6. Harlfinger J, Sommer I, Gartlehner G. WHO guideline for screening and treatment of cervical pre-cancerous lesions for cervical cancer prevention (Second Edition). Gesundheitswesen. 2023;85(7):630–4.
7. Harper DM, Bettcher CM, Young AP. It is time to switch to primary HPV screening for cervical cancer. Am Fam Physician. 2024;109(1):8–9. PMID: 38227863.
8. Zielonke N, Gini A, Jansen EEL, et al. Evidence for reducing cancer-specific mortality due to screening for breast cancer in Europe: a systematic review. Eur J Cancer. 2020;127:191–206.
9. Balleyguier C, Ayadi S, Van Nguyen K, Vanel D, Dromain C, Sigal R. BIRADS classification in mammography. Eur J Radiol. 2007;61(2):192–4. https://doi.org/10.1016/j.ejrad.2006.08.033. Epub 2006 Dec 11. PMID: 17164080.
10. Ren W, Chen M, Qiao Y, Zhao F. Global guidelines for breast cancer screening: a systematic review. Breast. 2022;64:85–99. https://doi.org/10.1016/j.breast.2022.04.003. Epub 2022 Apr 19. PMID: 35636342.
11. Practice bulletin number 179: breast cancer risk assessment and screening in average-risk women. Obstet Gynecol. 2017;130(1):e1–e16.
12. Shivshankar S, Patil PS, Deodhar K, et al. Epidemiology of colorectal cancer: a review with special emphasis on India. Indian J Gastroenterol. 2025;44(2):142–53.
13. Khan A, Hasana U, Nadeem IA, et al. Advances in colorectal cancer screening and detection: a narrative review on biomarkers, imaging, and preventive strategies. J Egypt Natl Canc Inst. 2025;37(1):20.

Vaccination at Menopause 23

Nalini Sharma

Abstract

Menopause is a vital stage that increases vulnerability to diseases that can be averted by vaccination. It is characterized by immune system aging, hormonal decline, and an increased risk of comorbidities like diabetes, cardiovascular disease, and chronic respiratory illness. Women in their midlife are more likely to get diseases that can spread to vulnerable groups because of travel, occupational exposure, and caregiving responsibilities. Vaccination during menopause can greatly reduce the risk of influenza, pneumococcal disease, hepatitis A and B, tetanus, pertussis, varicella, herpes zoster, meningococcal infections, and COVID-19.

Various guidelines like World Health Organization, CDC, FOGSI, and the Indian Menopause Society stress upon the significance of yearly influenza vaccination, pneumococcal vaccination for women 65 years of age or older or with comorbidities, recombinant zoster vaccination after age 50, and hepatitis B vaccination for high-risk groups like healthcare workers and women with chronic conditions.

Immunization not only reduces illness, hospital admissions, and healthcare costs but also promotes healthy aging, allowing women to sustain independence and mobility. However, barriers such as limited awareness, inconsistent guidelines, and insufficient counseling continue to hinder vaccination uptake. Strengthening immunization practices during menopause is key to empowering women, protecting families, and supporting global healthy aging goals.

N. Sharma (✉)
Department of Obstetrics and Gynaecology, Geetanjali Medical College and Hospital, Udaipur, Rajasthan, India

R. Malik et al. (eds.), *Menopause Essentials*,
https://doi.org/10.1007/978-981-95-7498-8_23

Keywords

Menopause · Adult immunization · Immunosenescence · Guidelines · Vaccination Hepatitis B vaccines · Herpes zoster vaccine · Influenza vaccines · Pneumococcal vaccines

Due to hormonal decline, inflammation, and immunosenescence, women's immune systems deteriorate with age, increasing their vulnerability to infections [1]. The higher incidence of noncommunicable diseases (NCDs) in this age group, including diabetes, hypertension, chronic respiratory conditions, and cardiovascular disease, exacerbates this vulnerability.

With rising socioeconomic status, many midlife women are financially independent, socially active, and frequently travel abroad for family visits or leisure. Vaccine-preventable illnesses (VPDs) such as influenza, hepatitis A and B, tetanus, typhoid, herpes zoster, *Streptococcus pneumoniae*, and COVID-19 are therefore more likely to affect them. Additionally, immunocompromised family members and infants might contract these illnesses from unvaccinated mothers.

Healthy aging is described by the World Health Organization (WHO) as "the process of developing and maintaining the functional ability that enables well-being in older age." During a woman's menopause, prevention-focused healthcare, such as routine screenings and vaccinations, can greatly enhance her quality of life. Vaccines protect against serious illnesses like hepatitis, tetanus, influenza, and pneumonia, helping reduce hospitalizations, healthcare costs, and mortality. Immunization also enables safe global mobility for midlife and menopausal women by lowering the risk of travel-related infections. Therefore, vaccination during menopause empowers women, safeguards families, reduces economic losses, and aligns with the WHO's vision of healthy aging.

Vaccine-preventable diseases in women at menopause are:

1. Pneumococcal disease
2. Tetanus
3. Influenza
4. Hepatitis A
5. Hepatitis B
6. Varicella
7. Meningococcus
8. MMR
9. Pertussis
10. Covid-19

11. Cholera
12. Japanese encephalitis

Guidelines for Vaccination in India

Vaccination guidelines are not universal in this age group. There are variations in recommendations of various professional bodies of different geographic locations. Few of them are [2–6]:

1. Geriatric Society of India
2. Federation of Obstetric and Gynaecological Societies of India (FOGSI)
3. The Centre for Disease Control and Prevention: The Advisory Committee on Immunization Practices (ACIP) Guidelines (Table 23.1)
4. Indian Medical Association (IMA)
5. Indian Menopause Society (IMS)

Table 23.1 The Centre for Disease Control and Prevention: The Advisory Committee on Immunization Practices (ACIP) Guidelines [2]

Vaccine	19–26 years	27–49 years	50–64 years	≥65 years
COVID–19	1 or more doses of 2025–2026 vaccine (See Notes)			2 or more doses of 2025–2026 vaccine (See Notes)
Influenza inactivated (IIV3, ccIIV3) **Influenza recombinant** (RIV3)	1 dose annually			1 dose annually (HD–IIV3, RIV3, or aIIV3 preferred)
Influenza inactivated (aIIV3; HD–IIV3) **Influenza recombinant** (RIV3)	Solid organ transplant (See Notes)			
Influenza live, attenuated (LAIV3)	1 dose annually			
Respiratory syncytial virus (RSV)	Seasonal administration during pregnancy (See Notes)		60–74 years (See Notes)	≥75 years
Tetanus, diphtheria, pertussis (Tdap or Td)	1 dose Tdap each pregnancy; 1 dose Td/Tdap for wound management (See Notes)			
	1 dose Tdap, then Td or Tdap booster every 10 years			
Measles, mumps, rubella (MMR)	1 or 2 doses depending on indication (if born in 1957 or later)			For health care personnel (See Notes)
Varicella (VAR)	2 doses (if born in 1980 or later)	2 doses		
Zoster recombinant (RZV)	2 doses for immunocompromising conditions (See Notes)		2 doses	
Human papillomavirus (HPV)	2 or 3 doses depending on age at initial vaccination or condition	27–45 years		
Pneumococcal (PCV15, PCV20, PCV21, PPSV23)			See Notes	See Notes
Hepatitis A (HepA)	2, 3, or 4 doses depending on vaccine			
Hepatitis B (HepB)	2, 3, or 4 doses depending on vaccine or condition			
Meningococcal A, C, W, Y (MenACWY)	1 or 2 doses depending on indication (See Notes for booster recommendations)			
Meningococcal B (MenB)	19–23 years; 2 or 3 doses depending on vaccine and indication (See Notes for booster recommendations)			
***Haemophilus influenzae* type b** (Hib)	1 or 3 doses depending on indication			
Mpox	2 doses			
Inactivated poliovirus (IPV)	Complete 3-dose series if incompletely vaccinated. Self-report of previous doses acceptable (See Notes)			

Yellow: Recommended vaccination for adults who meet age requirement, lack documentation of vaccination, or lack evidence of immunity
Purple: Recommended vaccination for adults with an additional risk factor or another indication
Blue: Vaccination is based on shared clinical decision-making
Grey: No Guidance/ Not Applicable

23.1 Pneumococcal Vaccine [7,8]

- For healthy adults, under age of 65 years, pneumococcal vaccine is not recommended.
- It is recommended in adults more than age 65 years old.
- ACIP recommendations differ from Indian guidelines for schedule of PCV13 vaccine (Tables 23.2).

Table 23.2 Vaccines recommended for adults available in India [4, 9]

Vaccine	Abbreviation(s)	Brand names
COVID-19 vaccine	1vCOV–mRNA	CoviShield Covaxin
Haemophilus influenzae type b vaccine	Hib	ActHIB, Hiberix, PedvaxHIB
Hepatitis A vaccine	HepA	Havisure
Hepatitis B vaccine	HepB	GeneVac-B, Revac-B
Hepatitis A and hepatitis B vaccine	HepA–HepB	Twinrix
Human papillomavirus vaccine	HPV	Cervavac, Gardasil 9
Influenza vaccine (inactivated, egg-based)	IIV3	Fluarix Tetra Influvac Tetra
	aIIV3	Fluad
	HD–IIV3	Fluzone High-Dose
Influenza vaccine (inactivated, cell culture)	ccIIV3	Flucelvax
Influenza vaccine (recombinant)	RIV3	Flublok
Influenza vaccine (live, attenuated)	LAIV3	Nasovac-S, Nasovac-S4
Measles, mumps, and rubella vaccine	MMR	M–M–R II, Priorix Tresivac, Tresivac PFS
Meningococcal serogroups A, C, W, Y vaccine	MenACWY–CRM	Menveo
	MenACWY–TT	MenQuadfi
Meningococcal serogroup B vaccine	MenB–4C, MenB–FHbp	Bexsero, Trumenba
Meningococcal serogroup A, C, Y, W-135, X vaccine	MenACWY–TT/ MenB–FHbp	MenFive
Pneumococcal conjugate vaccine	PCV13	Prevnar 13
Pneumococcal polysaccharide vaccine	PPSV23	Pneumosil, Pneumosil PFS
Poliovirus vaccine (inactivated)	IPV	Ipol
Tetanus and diphtheria vaccine	Td	Tenivac
Tetanus, diphtheria, and acellular pertussis vaccine	Tdap	Boostrix
Varicella vaccine	VAR	Varivax
Zoster vaccine, recombinant	RZV	Shingrix

23.1.1 Dosing Frequencies and Intervals

- 0.5 CC intramuscular single dose. For several frequent vaccine serotypes, PCV13 is advised initially because it increases the antipneumococcal response to later administration with PPSV23.
- Single dose of 0.5 CC intramuscular PCV13 is recommended first, as it amplifies the antipneumococcal response to subsequent administration of PPSV23 for many common vaccine serotypes.

Considerations for Special Situations

- A single dose of PCV13 followed by PPSV23 ≥ 8 weeks later is advised for immunocompetent patients with chronic conditions such as chronic heart disease, chronic liver disease, poorly controlled diabetes mellitus, chronic lung disease, current smokers, and alcohol abusers. It is also advised for adults with a history of invasive pneumococcal disease, cochlear implants, cerebrospinal fluid (CSF) leak, sickle cell disease or other hemoglobinopathy, or functional asplenia or hyposplenism.
- A single dose of PCV13 followed by PPSV23 ≥ 8 weeks later is advised for adults with a history of invasive pneumococcal disease, cochlear implants, cerebrospinal fluid (CSF) leak, or impaired splenic function (anatomic asplenia or hyposplenism, sickle cell disease or other hemoglobinopathy, or functional asplenia or hyposplenism).
- A single dose of PCV13 followed by PPSV23 at least 8 weeks later is advised for all immunocompromised individuals, including those with HIV infection, iatrogenic immunosuppression, chronic kidney disease, hematologic malignancy, other solid tumor malignancies with or without metastasis, hematopoietic stem cell transplantation, and solid-organ transplantation. Due to insufficient data, there is no advice for PCV or PPSV23 during pregnancy.

PCV13 should be provided 4 weeks prior to Hajj pilgrimage, whereas PPSV23 should be delivered following return from the Hajj Pilgrimage.

Coadministration Schedule
For adults, PCV13 may be given together with:

- Trivalent/quadrivalent inactivated influenza vaccine
- Tetanus–diphtheria vaccine
- Diphtheria–(DTaP) tetanus–acellular pertussis
- Hepatitis B inactivated polio-Haemophilus influenzae type b.

PCV13 and PPSV23 can be given at the same time as all other recommended vaccines with a different syringe at an anatomically separate site, simultaneously at the same clinic visit, and at any subsequent time (no minimum interval is recommended between doses) without waiting period after the vaccination, unless MCV4-D (quadrivalent meningococcal conjugate vaccine) is used.

Contraindications

- Vaccine virus anaphylaxis, hypersensitivity to any vaccine component and in acute respiratory illness
- Caution should be exercised in vaccination of immunocompromised persons (congenital or acquired asplenia, HIV [human immunodeficiency virus] infection, malignancy, undergoing hematopoietic stem cell transplant, and nephrotic syndrome). In these patients, a decreased antibody response to the vaccine might result in an increased risk for invasive pneumococcal disease.
- Severe allergic reaction to vaccine or component, hypersensitivity to any component of the vaccine, during acute respiratory illness

  Precautions—Moderate or severe acute illness with or without fever.

23.2 Tetanus

Abbreviations—Td, Tdap

Dosing frequencies and intervals—3 doses 2 weeks apart third dose 6–12 months apart.

Considerations for Special Situations

Give the remaining doses (1, 2, or 3 doses) to finish the three-dose primary series for pertussis, diphtheria, or tetanus. One dosage of Tdap is followed by one dose of Td or Tdap at least 4 weeks later, a third dose of Td or Tdap 6 to 12 months later (Tdap is preferable as the initial dose and can be substituted for any Td dose), and then Td or Tdap every 10 years after that.

Special circumstances: One dose of Tdap should be taken during each pregnancy, ideally in the first few weeks of gestation (weeks 27–36).

Wound care: Individuals who have received three or more doses of the vaccine containing tetanus toxoid: Give Tdap or Td if the last dose of the tetanus-toxoid-containing vaccine was more than 10 years ago for clean, minor wounds.

Tetanus, diphtheria, or pertussis: administer remaining doses (1, 2, or 3 doses) to complete 3-dose primary series. One-dose Tdap followed by 1-dose Td or Tdap at least 4 weeks later, and a third dose of Td or Tdap 6–12 months later (Tdap is preferred as first dose and can be substituted for any Td dose), then Td or Tdap every 10 years thereafter.

Special Situations

- *Pregnancy:* One-dose Tdap during each pregnancy, preferably in early part of gestational weeks 27–36

- *Wound management:* Persons with 3 or more doses of tetanus–toxoid-containing vaccine:
  For clean and minor wounds, administer Tdap or Td if more than 10 years since last dose of tetanus–toxoid-containing vaccine;
  for all other wounds, administer Tdap or Td if more than 5 years since last dose of tetanus–toxoid-containing vaccine.

Contraindications—Severe allergic reaction; encephalopathy post-DTP; history of hypersensitivity

Precautions—Guillain-Barre syndrome, Arthus-type reactions, neurological instability, moderate/severe illness

Side effects—Pain, redness swelling at the site of injection, fever, headache, muscle aches

23.3 Influenza

Abbreviations—HiB (Haemophilus Influenzae Type B)

Dosing frequencies and intervals—Annual vaccination before flu season (typically October–November in India). Quadrivalent preferred over trivalent. 0.5 mL dose

Considerations for Special Situations

Asplenia, whether anatomical or functional (including sickle cell disease): One dosage if not previously vaccinated against HIV; elective splenectomy: One dose, ideally at least 14 days prior to splenectomy.

Hematopoietic stem cell transplant (HSCT): 3-dose series spaced 4 weeks apart beginning 6–12 months following a successful transplant, irrespective of prior Hib vaccination history.

Contraindications—Severe allergic reaction to a vaccine component or after a prior dose, such as anaphylaxis

Precautions—Acute sickness, either moderate or severe, with or without temperature

23.4 Hepatitis A [10]

Abbreviations—Hep A

Dosing schedules—0.5 mL of live hepatitis A vaccination administered subcutaneously or inactivated hepatitis A administered intramuscularly. Live hepatitis A vaccine is administered as a single dose, while inactivated immunizations are administered twice at 0 and 6–12 months.

Considerations for Special Situations
A person who is not fully immunized and who is at risk of contracting the hepatitis A virus or developing a serious illness from it should finish the two-dose series HepA or the three-dose series HepA–HepB.

Risk factors

- Hepatitis B, hepatitis C, cirrhosis, fatty liver disease, alcoholic liver disease, autoimmune hepatitis, and alanine aminotransferase (ALT) or aspartate aminotransferase (AST) levels more than twice the upper limit of normal
- HIV infection, homosexuals
- Injection or noninjection drug use
- Persons experiencing homelessness
- Work with hepatitis A virus in research laboratory or with nonhuman primates with hepatitis A virus infection
- Travel in countries with high or intermediate endemic hepatitis A: HepA–HepB (Twinrix) may be administered on an accelerated schedule of 3 doses at 0, 7, and 21–30 days, followed by a booster dose at 12 months.
- Close, personal contact with international adoptee (e.g., household or regular babysitting) in first 60 days after arrival from country with high or intermediate endemic hepatitis A: dose 1 as soon as adoption is planned; preferably at least 2 weeks before adoptee's arrival.

Contraindications—Severe allergic reaction to a component, such as yeast or neomycin

Precautions
Acute sickness, either moderate or severe, with or without fever
Severe allergic reaction to component including neomycin or yeast

23.5 Hepatitis B

Abbreviations—Hep B(ActHIB, Hiberix, and BioHib)

Dosing Frequencies and Intervals
The dosage for adults is 20 μg at 0, 1, and 6 months. Adults who are immunocompetent do not require a booster. When anti-HBs levels fall to less than 10 mIU mL and the patient is older than 65, a booster dosage may be given.

Special Situations
Considerations for special situations—
Four-dose series or 3 dose is recommended for:

- Asplenia, whether anatomical or functional (including sickle cell disease): One dose if the Hib vaccination was not previously administered .Splenectomy by choice: One dose, ideally at least 14 days prior to splenectomy

- Hematopoietic stem cell transplant (HSCT): independent of Hib vaccination history, a 3-dose series spaced 4 weeks apart beginning 6–12 months after a successful transplant
- Hepatitis B surface antigen (HBsAg)-positive individual sexual partners, sexually active individuals who are not in mutually monogamous partnerships, those seeking diagnosis or treatment for an STD, and men who have sex with men
- Individuals on maintenance dialysis (including in-center or home hemodialysis and peritoneal dialysis), people undergoing predialysis, patients with diabetes, residents and employees of facilities for developmentally disabled people, health care and public safety personnel with a reasonably anticipated risk of exposure to blood or blood-contaminated bodily fluids

Contraindications—Severe allergic reaction to a vaccine component or to a prior injection, such as anaphylaxis

Precautions—Acute sickness, either moderate or severe, with or without fever

23.6 Varicella

Varicella (Chickenpox) Vaccine

- The Varicella vaccine is a live attenuated vaccine.
- A single dose provides strong protection, preventing about 95% of moderate disease and 100% of severe disease.
- Two doses are more effective than one, offering enhanced and sustained immunity.

Recommended dosing schedule:
- A 2-dose series, administered 4–8 weeks apart, for individuals who have not previously received a varicella-containing vaccine (VAR or MMRV [measles–mumps–rubella–varicella vaccine]).

Varicella Vaccine—Special Considerations
Special Situations—Vaccination may be considered (2 doses, given 3 months apart).

- Patients with nephrotic syndrome, chronic kidney disease, or those on dialysis
- Healthcare personnel without evidence of immunity to varicella
- HIV-infected individuals with CD4 $\geq$ 15% and CD4 count $\geq$200 cells/mm^3, with no evidence of immunity

Varicella Zoster Immunoglobulin (VZIG)
- *Indications: High-risk individuals such as:*
- Immunocompromised patients
- Patients with neoplastic diseases or undergoing immunosuppressive therapy
- Pregnant women
- *Administration:* Within 96 hours of exposure
- *Dose:* 125 units per 10 kg body weight (maximum 625 units)

- *Monitoring:* Observe for 28 days postexposure, as VZIG prolongs the incubation period of varicella.

Contraindications
- Severe allergic reaction to a previous dose
- Severe immunocompromised state
- Allergy to gelatin or neomycin
- Patients undergoing radiotherapy or chemotherapy
- HIV-positive individuals with CD4 count <200 cells/μL

Precautions
- Moderate or severe acute illness
- Active herpes zoster episode

23.7 Herpes Zoster Vaccine [11]

A nonlive adjuvanted recombinant zoster vaccine (RZV, Shingrix) is recommended in India (Table 23.3) for the prevention of herpes zoster (HZ). All at-risk individuals aged 50 years and above, particularly those with preexisting health conditions such as chronic obstructive pulmonary disease (COPD), diabetes mellitus, cardiovascular disease, chronic renal disease, and systemic lupus erythematosus (SLE), should be considered for vaccination.

Dosing and Schedule
- RZV (Shingrix): Two intramuscular doses, administered 2–6 months apart
- Efficacy: Clinical trials have demonstrated >90% protection in both 50-year-old and 70-year-old populations, with sustained efficacy for approximately 3 years postvaccination.

Common Side Effects
- Local: Injection site pain
- Systemic: Myalgia, headache, shivering, fever, abdominal discomfort, and nausea

23.8 Meningococcus

There are currently 13 serogroups of meningococcus known: A, B, C, E, H, I, K, L, M, X, Y, Z, and W 135. Meningococcal illness is endemic globally. Serogroups B and C are responsible for the majority of infections in developed nations, while serogroups A and, to a lesser extent, C are prevalent in the developing world.

- *Abbreviations—*
  - Meningococcal Conjugate Vaccine (MCV4):(protects against serogroups A, C, Y, and W-135). *Menactra, Menveo.*
  - Meningococcal Polysaccharide Vaccine (MPSV4):(protects against serogroups A, C, Y, and W-135)
  - Meningococcal A Conjugate Vaccine (MenAfriVac):(protects against group A meningococcal disease)

  - Meningococcal B vaccine: (Bexsero, Trumenba): polysaccharide vaccine
  - *MenFive: (pentavalent* vaccine that protects against serogroups A, C, Y, W, and X)

    Meningococcal polysaccharide vaccine (MPSV4) is the preferred vaccine in India for adults older than 55 years.

    When someone 55 years old or younger and has previously received the Meningococcal Conjugate Vaccine (MCV4)

Dosing Frequencies and Special Situations—MenACWY Vaccine

- Anatomical or functional asplenia (including sickle cell disease), HIV infection, persistent complement component deficiency, or use of complement inhibitors (e.g., eculizumab, ravulizumab):
  - Primary series: 2 doses of Menveo, administered at least 8 weeks apart
  - Booster: 1 dose 5 years after the primary series, and every 5 years thereafter if risk persists
- Travelers to high-risk regions (countries with hyperendemic or epidemic meningococcal disease, such as the meningitis belt of sub-Saharan Africa during the dry season [December–June]) or microbiologists routinely exposed to Neisseria meningitidis:
  - Primary series: 1 dose of Menveo
  - Booster: 1 dose 5 years after the primary series, and every 5 years thereafter if risk persists
- First-year college students living in residential housing (if not previously vaccinated at age 16 years or older) and military recruits:
  - Primary series: 1 dose of Menveo

MenB Vaccine—Special Situations

Primary Series

- Vaccines: Bexsero or Trumenba (the same brand must be used for all doses, including boosters)

Schedule:

- 3-dose series at 0, 1–2, and 6 months
- *Exceptions:*
  - If dose 2 is administered ≥6 months after dose 1, then dose 3 is not required.
  - If dose 3 is given <4 months after dose 2, a fourth dose should be administered ≥4 months after dose 3.

Booster Doses

- 1 booster dose 1 year after completion of the primary series
- Repeat boosters every 2–3 years if risk persists

Contraindications

- Pregnancy
- Anaphylaxis or severe allergic reaction with previous dose or to any vaccine component

23.9 MMR

23.9.1 Dosing Frequencies and Special Situations

Special Situations

- Pregnancy with no evidence of rubella immunity:
  - MMR is contraindicated during pregnancy.
  - Administer 1 dose after delivery, ideally before discharge from the health care facility.
- Nonpregnant women of child-bearing age without rubella immunity:
  - 1 dose of MMR.
- HIV infection (CD4 ≥ 15% and CD4 count ≥200 cells/mm^3 for at least 6 months, with no evidence of immunity to measles, mumps, or rubella):
  - 2-dose series, spaced at least 4 weeks apart.
- Students in postsecondary institutions, international travelers, and close contacts of immunocompromised individuals without immunity:
  - If no prior MMR doses → complete a 2-dose series (≥4 weeks apart).
  - If 1 prior dose received → administer 1 additional dose.
- Mumps outbreak settings and healthcare personnel:
  - Ensure completion of the 2-dose schedule.

Contraindications

- Severe allergic reaction to vaccine components (including neomycin)
- Pregnancy
- Severe immunodeficiency, including HIV infection with CD4 < 15% or CD4 count <200 cells/mm^3

Precautions

- Moderate or severe acute illness
- Recent receipt of blood products
- Thrombocytopenia
- Need for concurrent *tuberculosis testing*

23.10 Typhoid

Types of Vaccines

1. Inactivated whole-cell vaccine
2. Live oral lyophilized Ty21a vaccine
   - Available as liquid suspension (sachets) or enteric-coated capsules
3. Injectable Vi polysaccharide vaccine
4. Vi-rEPA conjugate vaccine
   - The Vi polysaccharide vaccine is a subunit vaccine composed of purified Vi capsular polysaccharide.

Dosing Frequencies and Intervals

- *Ty21a (capsules/sachets):*
  - 3 doses administered on alternate days
  - Booster: Repeat series every 3 years
  - Administration:
    Capsules taken orally with safe water
    Sachets dissolved in 100 mL safe water with buffer to protect the B-subunit from gastric acidity
- *Vi polysaccharide vaccine:*
  - Single dose of 0.5 mL (subcutaneous or intramuscular)
  - Revaccination: Every 3 years
- *Typbar conjugate vaccine:*
  - Recommended between 9 and 12 months of age

Special Situations

- During an *outbreak*, the *entire community at risk* should be vaccinated.

Contraindications

- *Ty21a vaccine* should not be used in:
  - Pregnant women
  - Transplant recipients

23.11 Rabies

23.11.1 Rabies Vaccination—Pre-Exposure and Postexposure Protocols

Pre-Exposure Schedule

High-risk individuals include:

- Veterinarians, dog catchers, forest staff, zookeepers
- Laboratory personnel handling rabies virus
- Medical and paramedical staff treating rabies patients
- Postmen, policemen, courier workers
- Schoolchildren in endemic regions

Dose:

- 3 doses on days 0, 7, and 28
- HDCV (Human diploid cell culture vaccine) or PCECV (Purified chick embryo cell vaccine)—1 mL IM
- Purified Vero cell rabies vaccine—0.5 mL IM
- Reconstituted tissue culture vaccine (TCV)—0.1 mL ID
- Vaccine formulations

Monitoring:
- Antibody titers checked every 6 months for those working with live virus in labs
- Antibody titers checked annually for professionals at permanent risk (e.g., veterinarians, animal handlers, wildlife officers)
- Booster dose required if titers fall below 0.5 IU/mL
- Immunity from a 2-dose injection course lasts 2–3 years

Postexposure Prophylaxis

For unvaccinated individuals:

- 5 doses of rabies vaccine on days 0, 3, 7, 14, and 28
- Human rabies immune globulin (HRIG): 20 IU/kg (maximum 1500 IU), administered with the first vaccine dose

For previously vaccinated individuals:

- 2 doses: day 0 and day 3
- Rabies immunoglobulin, if required, should be infiltrated into and around the wound; any remaining amount given IM at a site distant from the vaccine injection

Management of Re-Exposure
- 2 booster doses on days 0 and 3, regardless of exposure category or time since last vaccination
- Incomplete vaccination → treat as a fresh case
- If rabies immunoglobulin is unavailable, administer a double dose of the first vaccine in:
  - Category III exposures
  - Malnourished patients or those on corticosteroids, anticancer drugs, or antimalarials
  - HIV/AIDS patients with CD4+ count <200/mm^3

Additional considerations:

- Antibody titers should be monitored; boosters given if <0.5 IU/mL.
- Immunosuppressed patients should avoid activities requiring rabies pre-exposure prophylaxis.
- In immunosuppressed individuals, antibody titers should be checked after vaccination.
- Collect sera around *day 14 of the vaccine series* and again at completion of prophylaxis.

23.12 Cholera

Two types of vaccines are available:

- Injectable whole-cell vaccine
- Oral cholera vaccine

Among these, oral cholera vaccines are preferred, as the injectable vaccine provides lower efficacy and shorter duration of protection.

Dosing frequencies and intervals—Two separate doses, 2–6 weeks apart. Dukoral. Oral dose. Efficacy 85–90% protection for 6 months

Special situations—People in a high-risk area receive a booster dose 3 years after initial vaccination. Generally safe with mild side effects like malaise and headache

23.13 Japanese Encephalitis

Live attenuated vaccine—Not routinely recommended for adult vaccination, given only when the conditions of the outbreak

Dosing frequencies and intervals—Subcutaneously, single dose 0.5 mL. Booster dose at 1 year

Side-effects—

- Local reactions: Pain, redness, and swelling at the injection site
- Systemic reactions: Fever, headache, nausea, muscle aches, vomiting, and abdominal pain

Menopause, in women's life is a period of rising financial independence and declining familial responsibilities, resulting in more time for her own passions and life work. However, it also has increased vulnerability to diseases and added risk of metabolic/cardiovascular comorbidities. Vaccination can help achieve a crucial balance between these two contrasting forces, ultimately benefitting the woman. Pre-vaccination evaluation is a crucial safety measure for midlife and older women, many of whom exhibit multimorbidity, polypharmacy, or changing immunological function. A ready checklist serves as a standardized screening tool for determining precautions, temporary deferrals, and contraindications before vaccinations are administered (Table 23.3). Special considerations for history of allergic reactions, autoimmune diseases, immunosuppressive treatment, and possible pregnancy should be taken care of during the perimenopausal transition. Maintaining a vaccination diary can help woman as well as health care provider systematically record doses, time of vaccine given, booster intervals, repeat regimens, and lifetime vaccinations. It will serve as a useful document in preoperative or pre-travel exams, yearly health assessments, and outpatient consultations (Table 23.4).

Table 23.3 Screening checklist for contraindications to vaccines for adults [5]

Question	Yes	No	Don't Know
1. Are you sick today?			
2. Do you have allergies to medications, food, a vaccine ingredient, or latex?			
3. Have you ever had a serious reaction after receiving a vaccine?			
4. Do you have a long-term health problem with heart, lung, kidney, or metabolic disease (e.g., diabetes), asthma, a blood clotting disorder, no spleen, complement component deficiency, a cochlear implant, or a spinal fluid leak? Are you on long-term aspirin therapy?			
5. Do you have cancer, leukemia, HIV/AIDS, or any other immune system problem?			
6. Do you have a parent, brother, or sister with an immune system problem?			
7. In the past 3 months, have you taken medicines that affect your immune system, such as prednisone, other steroids, or anticancer drugs; drugs for the treatment of rheumatoid arthritis, Crohn's disease, or psoriasis; or have you had radiation treatments or anticoagulants (blood thinning medications)?			
8. Have you had a seizure or a brain or other nervous system problem?			
9. During the past year, have you received a transfusion of blood or blood products, or been given immune (gamma) globulin or an antiviral drug?			
10. Are you pregnant or is there a chance you could become pregnant during the next month?			
11. Have you received any vaccinations in the past 1 month (4 weeks)?			
12. Are you traveling internationally in foreseeable future?			

Table 23.4 Adult vaccination diary [5]

Name: ______________________			Contact Number: ______________		
Date of Birth: ___________________			Age: _______ years, _______ months		
Vaccine	Dose 1	Dose 2	Dose 3 / Repeat Dose	Dose Frequency	Notes
COVID-19	Today	1 year		Annually, only during pandemic/ epidemic	Not Applicable
Influenza	Today	1 year		Annually	Not Applicable
Repeat Doses					
Vaccine	Dose 1	Dose 2	Dose 3	Repeat Dose	Dose Frequency
Meningococcal Conjugated	Today	14 days (for high risk conditions)	NA[a]	5 year	5-yearly, if at risk

Table 23.4 (continued)

Name: ____________________			Contact Number: ____________		
Date of Birth: ________________			Age: ______ years, ______ months		
Meningococcal PBCP	Today	6 mo.	NA	2 year	2–3 years later, if at risk
Pneumococcal (PCV13 + PPSV23)	Today (PCV13)	1 year (PPSV23)	NA	5 years (PPSV23, if needed)	NA
TdaPǀTd	Today	Not Applicable	NA	10 year	10-yearly
Once in Lifetime					
Vaccine	Dose 1	Dose 2	Dose 3	Repeat Dose	Dose Frequency
Hib	Today	NA	NA	NA	Once in lifetime
Hepatitis A	Today	6–12 mo.	NA	NA	Once in lifetime
Hepatitis B	Today	1 mo.	6 mo.	NA	Once in lifetime
Chickenpox	Today	1 mo.	NA	NA	Once in lifetime
HPV	Today	1 mo.	6 mo.	NA	Once in lifetime
MMR	Today	1 mo.	NA	NA	Once in lifetime
RSV	Today	NA	NA	NA	Once in lifetime
Shingles (Herpes Zoster)	Today	2 mo.	NA	NA	Once in lifetime

[a]*NA* Not Applicable

Key Points

- Midlife and the menopausal transition, in particular, are crucial times for preventive health measures.
- Vaccination plays a pivotal role in protecting women in menopause who are at risk for several vaccine-preventable diseases. It is important for individuals to stay up to date on recommended vaccinations to protect themselves and others in the community.
- Vaccines such as influenza, MMR, Zoster (RZV), Tdap, and pneumococcal (PCV13 and PPSV23) are routinely recommended for midlife and menopausal women, especially those ≥50 years of age. For women traveling internationally, additional vaccines may be needed based on disease endemicity and the destination country's immunization requirements. Hepatitis B vaccination is strongly

advised for healthcare workers and women with specific risk factors such as diabetes or chronic kidney disease.

- Given the physiological vulnerabilities associated with ageing and comorbidities, there is a pressing need to sensitize healthcare professionals and educate target populations regarding the benefits of adult immunization.

Long Answer Questions (LAQs)

1. Enumerate key vaccines recommended for women at menopause according to three professional bodies (include at least one international organization such as CDC, WHO, or ACOG). For each vaccine, provide details on:
   - Recommended dose and schedule
   - Contraindications
   - Special indications or considerations in menopausal women

Short Answer Questions (SAQs)

1. Identify and discuss key barriers that hinder immunization uptake among menopausal women.
2. List three professional bodies (national or international) that provide guidelines on adult immunization and briefly describe one recommendation from each.
3. Describe the recommended pneumococcal vaccination schedule for an immunocompromised adult woman.
4. Explain how vaccination during menopause supports the WHO's concept of "healthy aging."
5. Write short notes on the following vaccines, highlighting epidemiology, indications in mid-life women, and relevant recommendations:
   (a) Pneumococcal vaccine
   (b) Herpes zoster vaccine
   (c) Influenza vaccine
   (d) Tetanus, diphtheria, and pertussis (TT/Tdap)

Multiple Choice Questions (MCQs)

1. Which of the following is the preferred influenza vaccination strategy for adults ≥65 years?
   A. One dose of trivalent vaccine every 2 years
   B. Annual dose of quadrivalent vaccine
   C. Annual high dose of bivalent vaccine
   D. Only vaccinate during outbreaks

2. According to Indian guidelines, what is the recommended pneumococcal vaccine sequence for an immunocompetent adult with chronic heart disease?
   A. Only PPSV23 every 5 years
   B. PCV13 followed by PPSV23 after ≥8 weeks
   C. PCV13 annually
   D. PPSV23 followed by PCV13 after 1 month
3. What is the recommended Tdap schedule for wound management in a menopausal woman who last received Tdap 6 years ago?
   A. No vaccine needed
   B. Tdap only if it's a clean wound
   C. Tdap if wound is major or contaminated
   D. Td every 3 years
4. Which of the following adults is most likely to benefit from hepatitis A vaccination?
   A. Healthy adult with no travel history
   B. Postmenopausal woman with chronic liver disease
   C. Vaccinated healthcare worker
   D. Elderly woman with no known risk factors
5. Which of the following women is NOT a candidate for Hepatitis A vaccination?
   A. A woman with chronic liver disease and elevated liver enzymes
   B. A woman with HIV infection and no prior HepA vaccination
   C. A woman planning travel to a Hepatitis A endemic country
   D. A healthy postmenopausal woman with no known risk factors and no travel history
6. What is the correct dosing schedule for the recombinant zoster vaccine (RZV) in adults >50 years?
   A. Three doses, 0, 1, 6 months
   B. Two doses, 4–8 weeks apart
   C. Three doses, 0, 2, 6 months
   D. Single dose, annually
7. Which adult woman should NOT receive the varicella vaccine?
   A. HIV+ woman with CD4 ≥200
   B. Dialysis patient with no varicella history
   C. Postmenopausal woman undergoing chemotherapy
   D. Health worker without evidence of immunity
8. Which statement about coadministration of PCV13 and influenza vaccine is CORRECT?
   A. Must be separated by 4 weeks
   B. Can be given at the same visit at different sites
   C. Only influenza vaccine should be given first
   D. Contraindicated in adults >65 years

9. According to FOGSI's adult immunization schedule, which vaccine should be given annually to women over 50?
   A. Hepatitis B
   B. Varicella
   C. Influenza
   D. MMR
10. According to the CDC 2025 adult immunization schedule, which of the following statements is TRUE regarding zoster vaccination?
   A. Zoster vaccine is recommended annually after age 60.
   B. Zoster vaccine is not recommended for immunocompromised individuals.
   C. Two doses of recombinant zoster vaccine (RZV) are recommended for all adults ≥50 years.
   D. A single dose of live zoster vaccine is preferred over recombinant vaccine.

Answers

1. B
2. B
3. C
4. B
5. D
6. B
7. C
8. B
9. C
10. C

References

1. Hou Y, Chen M, Bian Y, Liu Y, Yang J, Wang W, et al. Insights into vaccines for elderly individuals: from the impacts of immunosenescence to delivery strategies. NPJ Vaccines. 2024;9:77. https://doi.org/10.1038/s41541-024-00874-4.
2. Recommended Adult Immunization Schedule for Ages 19 Years or Older, United States, 2025. [Internet]. Available from: https://www.cdc.gov/vaccines/hcp/imz-schedules/adult-age.html.
3. Federation of Obstetric and Gynaecological Societies of India (FOGSI). FOGSI Focus Plus: Adult Vaccination [Internet]. Available from: https://www.fogsi.org/fogsi-focus-plus-adult-vaccination.pdf.
4. Meeta M, Digumarti L, Agarwal N, Vaze N, Shah R, Malik S. Clinical practice guidelines on menopause: an executive summary and recommendations: Indian Menopause Society 2019-2020. J Midlife Health. 2020;11(2):55–95. https://doi.org/10.4103/jmh.JMH_137_20. PMID: 33281418; PMCID: PMC7688016.
5. Adult vaccination booklet: a guide for healthcare professionals in India [internet]. New Delhi: Indian Medical Association; 2024 [cited 2025 Aug 1]. Available from: https://www.emvac.in/wp-content/uploads/2024/06/Adult-Vaccination-Booklet.pdf.

6. Agarwal A, Arora N, Bhattacharya S, Chatterjee P, Kumar A, Rao SV. Vaccination in older adults: an Indian perspective. J Assoc Physicians India. 2015;63(5):42–8.
7. Guidelines for vaccination in normal adults in India. Indian J Nephrol. 2016;26(Suppl 1):S7–S14. PMCID: PMC4928530.
8. Dhar R, Ghoshal AG, Guleria R, Sharma S, Kulkarni T, Swarnakar R, et al. Clinical practice guidelines 2019: Indian consensus-based recommendations on pneumococcal vaccination for adults. Lung India. 2020;37(Suppl):S19–29. https://doi.org/10.4103/lungindia.lungindia_272_20. PMID: 32830790; PMCID: PMC7703813.
9. Murthy N, Wodi AP, McNally VV, et al. Advisory Committee on Immunization Practices. Recommended adult immunization schedule, United States, 2024. Ann Intern Med. 2024; https://doi.org/10.7326/M23-3269. World Health Organization. Healthy ageing and functional ability: Questions and answers [Internet]. Geneva: WHO; [cited 2025 Jun 27]. Available from: https://www.who.int/news-room/questions-and-answers/item/healthy-ageing-and-functional-ability.
10. Shenoy B, Andani A, Kolhapure S, Agrawal A, Mazumdar J. Endemicity change of hepatitis A infection necessitates vaccination in food handlers: an Indian perspective. Hum Vaccin Immunother. 2022;18(1):1868820. https://doi.org/10.1080/21645515.2020.1868820. PMID: 33595412; PMCID: PMC8920195.
11. Ramasubramanian V, Vora A, Lagoubi Y, Lecrenier N, Chugh Y. Proceedings of the expert consensus group meeting on herpes zoster disease burden and prevention in India: an opinion paper. Hum Vaccin Immunother. 2023;19(2):2220608. https://doi.org/10.1080/21645515.2023.2220608. PMID: 37293792; PMCID: PMC10332180.

Contraception in Midlife

24

Anuradha Singh

Abstract

Midlife contraception is often ignored in clinical practice, yet it is crucial for women facing the challenges of perimenopause and early postmenopause. This chapter looks at the changing contraceptive needs of women aged 40 and older, highlighting the dual goals of preventing unintended pregnancies and improving long-term health. Fertility may decrease, but ovulation can continue unpredictably, making contraception important until menopause is confirmed. The chapter reviews hormonal and nonhormonal options, such as combined hormonal contraceptives, progestin-only methods, intrauterine devices, and permanent solutions, with a focus on cardiovascular risk, cancer prevention, and bone health. It also highlights the noncontraceptive benefits of certain methods, including menstrual regulation, management of hot flashes, and prevention of endometrial hyperplasia. Clinical decision-making depends on individual risk assessment, existing health conditions, and patient preferences. The chapter discusses counseling strategies, transitioning off contraception, and the role of contraception in general midlife care, including STI prevention and sexual health. By combining evidence-based guidance with practical guidance, this chapter helps clinicians provide informed and suitable contraceptive care for midlife women.

Keywords

Contraception in midlife · Menopausal transition · Combined hormonal oral contraceptives · LARCs · Intrauterine devices · Implants

A. Singh (✉)
Department of Obstetrics and Gynaecology, Lady Hardinge Medical College, New Delhi, India

R. Malik et al. (eds.), *Menopause Essentials*,
https://doi.org/10.1007/978-981-95-7498-8_24

24.1 Introduction

The perimenopause is the transition from reproductive years to menopause. It is marked by hormonal fluctuations and menstrual irregularities that begin in the late 30s to 50s and span several stages as defined by the STRAW+10 system. This phase, lasting 4 to 8 years, presents physiological and clinical complexities that influence contraceptive needs. Although ovulation becomes inconsistent, around 25% of extended cycles may still result in ovulation, which means the risk of unintended pregnancy continues until menopause is confirmed. Additionally, pregnancy during this stage carries higher health risks for women, making contraceptive planning crucial. The approach to contraception should be personalized, considering unpredictable cycle patterns, evolving health status, and the possibility of using hormones to relieve perimenopausal symptoms. Understanding these changes is crucial for delivering safe, effective, and personalized contraceptive care [1, 2].

24.2 Hormonal Changes and Symptoms in Perimenopause

Perimenopause is marked by significant hormonal changes that impact both physical and emotional well-being. During this time, the production of estrogen and progesterone by the ovaries becomes unpredictable. Estrogen, a key hormone regulating the menstrual cycle, fluctuates drastically, leading to symptoms like irregular periods, lighter or heavier bleeding, mood swings, and hot flashes. Progesterone levels also decline, which affects the maintenance of endometrial thickness and further contributes to menstrual irregularities. These unpleasant symptoms can affect a woman's quality of life. As perimenopause progresses, menstrual cycles may become infrequent or stop for months, only to return unpredictably. This irregularity makes it challenging for women to predict their menstrual patterns or reproductive status, adding to the physical and emotional challenges of this phase.

The ovarian environment also undergoes significant changes that affect hormone levels, ovulation, and fertility. The number of primordial follicles declines due to reduced levels of inhibin B and anti-Müllerian hormone (AMH), leading to a gradual shrinkage in ovarian size and weight. As estradiol (E2) and inhibin B levels fall, the hormonal feedback loop is disrupted, causing an increase in follicle-stimulating hormone (FSH). Low E2 levels also fail to trigger the luteinizing hormone (LH) surge necessary for ovulation, resulting in more frequent anovulatory cycles and irregular menstrual patterns. Although fertility decreases, the unpredictability of ovulation contributes to a higher risk of unintended pregnancies. These changes in hormones highlight the complicated phase of perimenopause and its effects on women's reproductive health [3–5].

The fluctuating levels of hormones also bring a spectrum of physical, emotional, and cognitive symptoms that can complicate contraceptive choices in midlife. Women may experience hot flashes, sleep disturbances, mood swings, and physiological changes like vaginal dryness and weight gain, which not only affect quality of life but may also influence adherence to certain contraceptive methods.

Furthermore, the increased risk of osteoporosis and cardiovascular disease during this transition demands careful consideration when prescribing hormonal contraception. As fertility, though declining, remains possible, individualized contraceptive strategies are essential, balancing symptom management, underlying health risks, and evolving reproductive goals during this complex life stage [6, 7].

24.3 Why Contraception in Perimenopause? Clinical Rationale and Broader Benefits

1. Continued Fertility Risk
   - The ovulation remains unpredictable during perimenopause, making natural fertility difficult to assess.
   - Despite declining fertility, unintended pregnancies still occur—27% of those in women over 40 end in termination [8].
2. Age-Related Health Considerations
   - Women over 40 face increased risks of cardiovascular disease, obesity, breast and gynecological cancers, which influence contraceptive choice.
   - Advanced maternal age is linked to poor oocyte quality, chromosomal abnormalities, spontaneous abortion, ectopic pregnancy, gestational diabetes, and preeclampsia.
   - Late-age pregnancies carry higher rates of elective abortion, caesarean delivery, low birth weight, and preterm birth [9].
3. Psychosocial and Maternal Health Impacts
   - Older maternal age can lead to psychological, social, and domestic challenges that compound physical risks.
   - Effective contraception reduces maternal morbidity and mortality, with risks of pregnancy often exceeding those of most contraceptive methods.
4. Therapeutic Benefits of Hormonal Contraception
   - Hormonal methods help manage perimenopausal symptoms such as abnormal uterine bleeding (AUB), cycle irregularity, and heavy menstrual loss.
   - These benefits enhance quality of life and provide dual protection—both contraceptive and therapeutic.
5. Limitations of Natural Methods
   - Fertility awareness-based methods are unreliable due to erratic ovulation and cycle variability [10].

24.4 Principles of Counseling for Contraceptive Use in Perimenopause

Contraceptive counseling during perimenopause must be delivered with privacy, confidentiality, and with a respectful, nonjudgmental approach, that helps informed decision-making. Providers should use simple language and effective verbal and nonverbal communication to ensure clarity. Women should be informed about all contraceptive options—including oral contraceptives, IUDs, and barrier methods with specific information about benefits and risks.

The counseling in menopause transition must consider age-related comorbidities assessment by medical eligibility criteria, symptom relief, and noncontraceptive benefits [6].

24.5 Contraceptive Options

Selecting appropriate contraception during perimenopause requires a personalized approach. While age alone is not a contraindication, age-related conditions like obesity, hypertension, and diabetes must guide method choice. Cardiovascular disease, hormone-sensitive cancers, and any abnormal bleeding should prompt gynecological evaluation (Table 24.1).

Contraceptive options include combined hormonal contraceptives for cycle control and symptom relief (with caution in smokers over 35), progesterone-based contraceptives like progesterone-only pills, Implants, LNG IUS, DMPA, long-acting intrauterine devices for bleeding reduction (LNG IUS), copper IUD, and hormone-free barrier methods like condoms and diaphragms, which also protect against STIs. Permanent methods like sterilization and vasectomy are also viable options in this age group.

The WHO Medical Eligibility Criteria (MEC) for contraceptive use provides evidence-based guidelines for selecting appropriate contraceptive methods based on a woman's health, age, and reproductive stage, particularly during perimenopause. These guidelines assess factors such as thrombotic risk, hypertension, smoking status, and cardiovascular conditions, categorizing hormonal contraceptives from Category 1 (no restrictions) to Category 4 (unacceptable risk).

Various contraceptive options available in perimenopause are given in the table, each with distinct benefits and risks. These recommendations are aligned with the UK Medical Eligibility Criteria (UKMEC), NNUH (NHS) Perimenopausal Contraception Guidelines (2023) (Table 24.2).

Table 24.1 Medical eligibility for various types of contraception by age

Method	Age (years)	US MEC Category
Estrogen-containing	>/= 40	2
Progestin-only pill	>/= 40	1
Progestin implant	40-45/>45	1/2
DMPA	40 to 45	1
	>45	2
Cu-IUD	40	1
LNG-IUS	40	1

Table 24.2 Contraceptive options during perimenopause, based on recent clinical guidelines and recommendations

Contraceptive method	Key features	Remarks for perimenopause
Combined hormonal contraceptives (CHCs)	Regulate cycles, reduce vasomotor symptoms, offer bone protection	Suitable until age 50 if no contraindications; assess cardiovascular risk
Progestogen-only pills (POPs)	Safe for older women, no estrogen	Can be continued until menopause; may cause irregular bleeding
Levonorgestrel intrauterine system (LNG-IUS)	Long-term option, reduces heavy bleeding, endometrial protection	Highly effective; can be used for contraception and HRT endometrial protection
Copper intrauterine device (Cu-IUD)	Nonhormonal, long-acting	Suitable if hormonal methods contraindicated; may increase bleeding
Depot medroxyprogesterone acetate (DMPA)	Injectable, suppresses ovulation	Use with caution due to bone mineral density concerns in long-term use
Barrier methods	Condoms, diaphragms	Useful for women with contraindications to hormonal methods; less effective
Sterilization (female or male)	Permanent solution	Considered for women who are certain they do not want future pregnancies
Natural methods	Fertility awareness, withdrawal	Not recommended due to cycle irregularity and reduced reliability in perimenopause

24.6 Hormonal Contraception

Combined hormonal contraception (CHC)—available as oral pills, patches, or vaginal rings—is a good option for perimenopausal women up to age 50 who neither smoke nor have cardiovascular risk factors, offering multiple noncontraceptive benefits. UKMEC guidelines advise against CHC for women over 35 who smoke and recommend discontinuing all CHC methods by age 50 in favor of safer alternatives (Table 24.3).

CHCs also improve symptoms like menstrual migraines, hormone-related headaches, and pelvic pain, especially during hormone-free intervals. Additionally, they protect bone health by preventing bone loss and improving bone density, even at low doses [11–13]. They provide long-term protection against ovarian and endometrial cancers (persisting up to 15 years after cessation) and lower the risk of benign breast disease and colorectal cancer.

However, CHC use raises the relative risk of venous thromboembolism from approximately 2 to between 5 and 12 events per 10,000 women-years, making levonorgestrel- or norethisterone-based combined oral contraceptives (COCs) preferred first-line choices in women over 40. Data on CHC-related myocardial infarction and ischemic stroke are mixed and influenced by smoking, hypertension, and migraine with aura; therefore, formulations containing ≤30 μg ethinyl estradiol are

Table 24.3 Age-based guidance for CHC

Age group	MEC category	Recommendation	Clinical considerations
Menarche through 40	Category 1	Can use CHC without restriction	Healthy individuals benefit from CHC for cycle regulation, acne control, and contraception; monitor lifestyle factors.
40 years and older	Category 2	Generally can use CHC; benefits outweigh risks	Assess cardiovascular risk (smoking, hypertension, diabetes, migraine with aura); discontinue by age 50

Table 24.4 CHC guidance table (NHS)

Category	Details
Eligibility and Duration	Use up to age 50 in nonsmokers without cardiovascular risk factors. Discontinue at 50 and switch to a safer method.
Noncontraceptive Benefits	Maintains bone density; reduces menstrual pain, bleeding, and menopausal symptoms.
Cancer protection	Lowers ovarian and endometrial cancer risk (protective effect lasts 15 years postuse); reduces benign breast disease and colorectal cancer incidence.
VTE risk	Increases from ~2 to 5–12 events per 10,000 women-years. First-line agents for women >40: COCs with levonorgestrel or norethisterone due to lower VTE risk.
Cardiovascular and stroke risk	Conflicting data on myocardial infarction and ischemic stroke. Risk modifiers include smoking, hypertension, and migraine with aura. COCs with ≤30 μg ethinylestradiol preferred in women >40 without cardiovascular risks.
Breast cancer risk	Slightly elevated during COC use; returns to baseline by 10 years after stopping.
Formulation recommendations	First line: levonorgestrel- or norethisterone-based COCs and ≤30 μg ethinylestradiol formulations for lower thrombotic and cardiovascular risks. Patches and rings follow similar risk profiles.
Age and smoking considerations	UKMEC restricts CHC for women >35 who smoke—risks outweigh benefits.
Discontinuation	Advise all CHC users to stop by age 50 and transition to nonhormonal or progestogen-only methods.

recommended [11]. The various studies indicate a slight increase in breast cancer risk during COC use, which returns to baseline within 10 years of stopping.

Risk factors-based CHC usage guide is given in (NHS) (Table 24.4).

24.6.1 MOA and Failure Rates

Combined hormonal contraceptives (CHCs) contain an estrogenic component, such as ethinyl-estradiol (EE), E2, or the newer estetrol (E4), along with various progestins derived from natural progesterone, 19-nor-testosterone, or spironolactone.

These contraceptives work by inhibiting ovulation, stabilizing endometrial proliferation, and altering cervical mucus, making it hostile to sperm migration.

CHCs are highly effective when used correctly, with a perfect-use failure rate of 0.3%. However, their effectiveness decreases with inconsistent use, leading to a typical-use failure rate of 7–9% in reproductive-age women. Regular intake is essential for maintaining contraceptive efficacy.

It is important to know that perimenopausal women experience a lesser difference between perfect and typical use effectiveness due to the natural decline in fertility with age. Their risk of unintended pregnancy is lower than that of younger women, even when usage is imperfect. Despite their effectiveness, CHCs require adherence to routine intake, and individual health risks should be considered when selecting a contraceptive method.

24.6.2 Types of Combined Hormonal Contraceptives

24.6.2.1 Combined Oral Contraceptives (COC)

COCs are available in:

- Cyclic regimens, composed of 21 active pills and 7 inactive pills/no assumption
- A shortened hormone free interval (HFI regimen), composed of 24–26 active pills and 2–4 inactive pills
- An extended regimen, which includes 84 active pills and 7 inactive pills
- A continuous regimen, which is made up of a 365-day active pill regimen

The MEC for COCs based on various high-risk factors is provided in Table 24.5.
Contraindications MEC 4

- Age > 35 years with >15 cigarettes per day
- Uncontrolled hypertension
- Diabetes with vascular disease
- Stroke
- Current or history of ischemic heart disease
- Migraine with aura
- The risk of ischemic stroke decreases with decreasing EE dose.
- Smoking and hypertension independently elevate the risk of MI and stroke; therefore, CHC options should thus be used with caution or not at all in women who smoke or who have hypertension.
- CHCs can be used by women with migraine without aura but are contraindicated for contraceptive use in women with migraine with aura since both COCs and aura are independent risk factors for ischemic stroke.

Table 24.5 Medical Eligibility Criteria for COCs based on various high risk factors

Medical condition	US MEC category
Smoking age > 35 years	
<15 cigarettes/day	2
≥15 cigarettes/day	4
Obesity	
BMI 30–34.9	2
BMI ≥35	2
Hypertension	
Controlled hypertension	3
Elevated BP: systolic 140–159 or diastolic 90–94 mm Hg	3
Systolic ≥160 or diastolic ≥95 mm Hg	4
Vascular disease	4
Diabetes	
Without vascular disease	2
With vascular disease or duration >20 years	3 or 4 (depends on severity)
Stroke	4
Current or history of ischemic heart disease	4
Multiple cardiovascular risk factors (age, smoking, obesity, diabetes, etc.)	3 or 4 (depends on severity)

24.6.3 Effects of COCs on Gynecologic and Hormone-Related Cancers

24.6.3.1 Ovarian Cancer

COCs significantly reduce the risk of ovarian cancer, with protective effects increasing with longer duration of use and lasting decades after discontinuation. A systematic review showed at least a 50% risk reduction with COC use (<40 μg EE). A collaborative reanalysis of 45 studies found a 20% decrease in ovarian cancer risk per 5 years of COC use, particularly impactful near the perimenopausal peak incidence. This reduction in risk persisted for more than 30 years after oral contraceptive use, but became somewhat attenuated over time-the proportional risk reductions per 5 years of use were 29% (95% CI 23–34%) for use that had ceased less than 10 years previously, 19% (14–24%) for use that had ceased 10–19 years previously, and 15% (9–21%) for use that had ceased 20–29 years previously [14].

Endometrial Cancer The relative risk reduction ranges from 50% to 70%, most notably for endometrioid and serous subtypes, and persists for at least 15 years after ≥12 months of use [15].

Functional Ovarian Cysts & Benign Tumors Observational data suggest COC use is associated with a lower incidence of functional cysts and benign ovarian tumors, which are common in reproductive-age women [16].

Chemoprophylaxis in BRCA Carriers COCs may serve a chemopreventive role in younger women with BRCA1/BRCA2 mutations, with no conclusive evidence of added breast cancer risk for this group [17].

Breast Cancer Data remain mixed. Earlier high-dose formulations showed a slightly elevated breast cancer risk (RR 1.24–1.30), which declined after cessation of hormonal contraception and was not significant after 10 years. Low-dose pills show minimal risk, though a meta-analysis revealed a small but statistically significant increase with extended use (RR 1.07 per 5 years; RR 1.14 per 10 years) [18]. Regarding age-dependent risk profile, the breast cancer risk increases with age, with baseline risk rising from 1 in 500 at age 35 to 1 in 100 by age 40 [18]. Thrombotic risks, including venous thromboembolism, also rise with age and are highest during the first months of COC use.

Other Oncologic Considerations For women with HPV infection, continuous use of COCs for over 5 years may increase the risk of cervical cancer. Hence, individualized risk–benefit assessment is crucial. Despite controversial data in the literature, several population studies suggest a possible increase in the incidence of Cervical cancer and its precursor lesions for those who have used COCs for > 5 years.

24.6.4 COCs and Cardiovascular Risk

The combined oral contraceptive (COC) use is associated with a slight increase in the relative risk of thromboembolic events, approximately two to three times higher than in nonusers, with the highest risk occurring within the first 3 months of initiation (OR 12, 95% CI 7.1–22.4). The incidence of venous thromboembolism (VTE) rises notably after age 40, underscoring the influence of age. Although the absolute risk of thrombotic stroke (TS) and myocardial infarction (MI) remains low in reproductive-aged women, it escalates with advancing age, higher doses of ethinyl estradiol (EE), and additional cardiovascular risk factors such as smoking, hypertension, diabetes, obesity, and hyperlipidemia. During counseling, it is crucial to weigh these risks against the increased maternal morbidity and mortality associated with pregnancy in older women, especially since many contraindications to hormonal contraceptive use also elevate the risk of significant pregnancy-related adverse events [19].

24.6.5 Nonoral Combined Hormonal Contraceptives

24.6.5.1 Hormonal Contraceptive Patch

The transdermal contraceptive patch is a combined hormonal method applied once a week for 3 weeks, followed by a week without the patch to trigger withdrawal bleeding. It contains ethinylestradiol (35 mcg) and norelgestromin (150 mcg), and delivers hormones through the skin to suppress ovulation, offering a convenient, nondaily alternative to pills. Though its use in perimenopausal women is limited, there are no age-specific contraindications in current guidelines. However, due to higher systemic estrogen exposure than combined oral contraceptives (COCs), studies suggest a slightly increased risk of venous thromboembolism (VTE), especially in older women. Unlike this, transdermal estrogen used for menopausal symptoms delivers lower doses of 17β-estradiol and does not carry the same VTE risk, highlighting different clinical roles and safety profiles [19, 20].

24.6.5.2 Vaginal Ring

The contraceptive vaginal ring, a combined hormonal contraceptive (CHC), offers an alternative to daily pills through cyclic (3 weeks in, 1 week off) or continuous use. It provides 3 weeks of continuous hormone release—delivering 15 mcg of ethinyl estradiol (EE) and 120 mcg of etonogestrel per day—followed by a 1-week ring-free interval to allow for withdrawal bleeding. This monthly regimen offers a user-controlled and discreet contraceptive option.

The vaginal ring helps prevent symptoms of estrogen deficiency in perimenopausal women, while still working well as a contraceptive. Compared to COCs, it causes fewer side effects like nausea, acne, mood changes, and depression. However, some women report more cases of vaginal infections and itching. Bleeding patterns with the ring vary from person to person, and there isn't enough data to compare its cardiovascular risks with those of COC.

One important advantage is that the ring improves vaginal moisture and healthy bacteria—98% of users noticed better lubrication after three cycles, which can help with dryness and cycle control. Still, some women stop using it because of issues like vaginal discharge, the ring falling out, or feeling like there's something foreign in the vagina [19].

24.6.5.3 Progestogen-Only Contraception

The available Progesterone-only contraceptive (POC) methods include oral pills (POP), injectable DMPA, subdermal implants (SDI), and the levonorgestrel-releasing intrauterine system (IUS). These options can alleviate dysmenorrhoea, and the IUS may be used to treat heavy menstrual bleeding after excluding pathology. Altered bleeding patterns are common with POC use, and women over 45 experiencing excessive bleeding should undergo endometrial evaluation.

24.6.5.4 Types of POC

- Progestin-Only Pills (POP)

Progestin-only pills (POPs) are estrogen-free contraceptives suitable for perimenopausal women with contraindications to combined hormonal contraceptives, such as those with obesity, migraines with aura, or cardiovascular risk factors. They act by altering cervical mucus, endometrial development, and tubal motility, and may inhibit ovulation. Desogestrel (75 μg) is the most effective in suppressing ovulation among traditional POPs. With age-related fertility decline, POPs become increasingly effective and are not associated with elevated risks of venous thromboembolism (VTE), stroke, or myocardial infarction (MI). Importantly, they do not negatively affect bone mineral density and are generally well tolerated.

A newer formulation containing 4 mg drospirenone (DRSP) offers improved cycle control and flexibility in dosing. DRSP's anti-mineralocorticoid effects may reduce fluid retention and blood pressure, while its antiandrogenic properties may benefit cardiovascular health. Compared to desogestrel-based POPs, DRSP-only pills show higher rates of scheduled bleeding and amenorrhea, and significantly lower rates of unscheduled spotting, enhancing bleeding predictability. Although breast cancer risk remains debated, any potential increase appears minimal and diminishes after discontinuation. DRSP-only POPs thus represent a promising option for perimenopausal women seeking estrogen-free contraception with improved tolerability and adherence.

- DMPA

Depot medroxyprogesterone acetate (DMPA) is a long-acting injectable contraceptive containing 104–400 mg of medroxyprogesterone acetate, effective for 3 months. It is given as 3 monthly intramuscular or subcutaneous injections. Its use during perimenopause is limited globally, especially after the age of 45 years, due to concerns about bone mineral density (BMD) loss—a critical issue during the climacteric period. Although BMD typically recovers after discontinuation, the potential for accelerated bone loss warrants caution in older users. Despite this, DMPA remains a viable option for women who cannot use estrogen-containing methods and prefer a low-maintenance contraceptive.

DMPA's relatively high progestin dose offers unique advantages, including reduced drug interactions with hepatic enzyme inducers and higher amenorrhea rates—up to 50% after 1 year, increasing with continued use. However, delayed return to fertility, averaging 10 months postinjection, may be a drawback for those planning pregnancy. Its pharmacokinetic profile and bleeding suppression make it suitable for perimenopausal women prioritizing convenience and menstrual regulation [21].

- Etonogestrel Subdermal Implants (ESI)

Etonogestrel subdermal implants (ESIs), such as Nexplanon, are highly effective long-acting contraceptives with a Pearl Index of 0.05/100 woman-years. Inserted subdermally by trained providers, they release etonogestrel at levels sufficient to suppress ovulation within days. ESIs are particularly useful for women with contraindications to estrogen and may benefit conditions like endometriosis by halting ovarian activity.

Their efficacy is unaffected by body weight, making them suitable for women with a BMI >30 kg/m^2. Unlike IUDs, they require replacement every 3 years and do not offer endometrial protection, making them less suitable for women at risk of endometrial hyperplasia.

While ESIs are not associated with bone loss or adverse metabolic effects, bleeding irregularities remain a common reason for discontinuation. Around 15% of users request removal due to unpredictable bleeding, with prolonged or frequent bleeding affecting up to 20% of users. Despite this, ESIs maintain high satisfaction in obese women due to stable hormone distribution. However, they are contraindicated in women with a history of breast cancer and are not retained beyond 3 years in perimenopausal users [5].

- The Levonorgestrel Intrauterine System (LNG IUS)

The levonorgestrel intrauterine system (LNG-IUS 52 mg) is a highly effective contraceptive option for perimenopausal women, lasting up to 7 years with a failure rate of just 0.1% per year. It works by thickening cervical mucus and suppressing the endometrium, making it useful for both contraception and treating abnormal uterine bleeding (AUB), heavy periods, and dysmenorrhea. LNG-IUS 52 mg is considered a first-line treatment for heavy menstrual bleeding in women over 40, with amenorrhea rates reaching 50% within 1 year. It also helps manage endometrial hyperplasia and early-stage cancer when fertility preservation is desired. While generally safe, it should be avoided in women with active breast cancer and used cautiously in those with a history of the disease. Mood changes may occur during the climacteric period, so individualized care is important.

The Faculty of Sexual and Reproductive Healthcare (FSRH) recommends that extended LNG-IUS may be used until age 55 if inserted at age 45 or older, provided it is not serving as the progestogen component of hormone replacement therapy (HRT). Additionally, women who have undergone endometrial ablation should be cautioned about the potential risks associated with intrauterine contraceptive use due to possible complications.

24.6.6 Clinical Guidance on Progestogen-Only Contraception (POC) in Perimenopausal Women

- POC and Cardiovascular Disorders

Progestogen-only contraceptives (POCs) like the POP and subdermal implant (SDI) are not linked to higher risks of stroke, heart attack, or venous thromboembolism (VTE). However, DMPA may affect lipid levels more than other POCs, so caution is advised, especially in women with cardiovascular risk factors. Women without such risks can use DMPA until age 50. After 50, alternative methods should be considered, though continued use may be appropriate in select cases after assessing risks and benefits.

- POC and Breast Cancer

Breast cancer: The evidence of an association between breast cancer and POC is inconclusive, with only small sample sizes. Some studies suggest a risk broadly similar to that of combined hormonal contraception (CHC), while others have suggested no increased risk or a very small increased risk. Overall, most evidence is reassuring about breast cancer and POC.

- POC and Bone Health

Progestogen-only contraceptives (POCs) generally do not affect bone health, except for the injectable form, depot medroxyprogesterone acetate (DMPA). Long-term use of DMPA can lower bone mineral density (BMD), but this usually improves after stopping the injection. Other POCs, like progestogen-only pills (POP) and subdermal implants (SDI), have not shown any negative impact on BMD. The bone loss caused by DMPA is not worsened by menopause. However, women with high risk for osteoporosis due to lifestyle or medical conditions should consider alternative contraceptive methods. Regular review is advised for women over 40 using DMPA to weigh its risks and benefits.

24.6.7 Intrauterine Devices IUD

- CU IUD

Copper intrauterine devices (Cu-IUDs) are hormone-free contraceptives that function by inducing a local inflammatory response in the endometrium, increasing vascular permeability and macrophage activity, while copper ions exert spermicidal effects. They are also effective as emergency contraception if inserted within 5 days of unprotected intercourse. They have a cumulative expulsion rate of about 10% over 3 years and are contraindicated in cases of pelvic infection, malignancy, or uterine abnormalities. CU IUDs are not suitable for women with heavy menstrual bleeding or dysmenorrhea, as they may exacerbate these symptoms, with submucosal fibroids or distorted uterine cavities.

Rare procedural risks include uterine perforation (2/1000), infection (<1/300), and device displacement (5%).

The Faculty of Sexual and Reproductive Healthcare (FSRH) recommends extended use of copper IUD until menopause if inserted at age 40 or above [5].

24.7 LARC and Perimenopause

Long-acting reversible contraceptives (LARCs), including levonorgestrel-releasing intrauterine systems (LNG-IUS), etonogestrel subdermal implants, and copper intrauterine devices (Cu-IUDs), offer highly effective, estrogen-free contraception suitable for perimenopausal women. These methods work via progestin-only mechanisms or mechanical inflammatory effects, avoiding the cardiovascular and thromboembolic risks associated with estrogen-containing contraceptives. LARCs are particularly advantageous in this age group due to their long duration of action, minimal systemic effects, and lack of estrogen-related contraindications. Recent evidence supports their safety and efficacy, with LNG-IUS also offering therapeutic benefits such as reduced menstrual bleeding and endometrial protection [8].

24.7.1 Irreversible Contraception—Sterilization

Sterilization remains a highly effective, permanent contraceptive option for women who have completed childbearing, with added benefits such as potential reduction in ovarian cancer risk through procedures like tubal ligation or salpingectomy. However, it does not affect menstruation, and discontinuation of prior contraceptive methods may alter bleeding patterns. Due to its irreversible nature and associated surgical risks—especially in older women with comorbidities—it requires thorough counseling. While hysteroscopic methods like Essure were once considered less invasive, safety concerns have limited their use in recent years.

Vasectomy has a lower failure rate after proven azoospermia (1 in 2000), and lower complication rates, although chronic postvasectomy pain occurs in up to 14% of men. Female sterilization has a failure rate of 1:200. Other than preventing pregnancy, sterilization confers none of the other benefits of hormonal contraceptives, and is associated with surgical risks.

The rise of long-acting reversible contraceptives (LARCs), which offer comparable efficacy with lower procedural risks and reversible options, has led to more selective recommendations for sterilization. Consideration of ovarian reserve, fertility goals, and individual health profiles is essential, with informed consent playing a critical role in the decision-making process [5, 21].

24.8 Emergency Contraception

Women over 40 who still require contraception should be offered emergency contraception after unprotected sexual intercourse, but it is not as effective and consistent as the use of other contraceptives.

Emergency contraception options include a single 1.5 mg levonorgestrel (LNG) tablet, effective up to 72 hours—and with reduced efficacy up to 120 hours—after unprotected intercourse. It is safe for breastfeeding women and can be used multiple times in a cycle. Ulipristal acetate (UPA), a 30 mg selective progesterone receptor modulator, is more effective than LNG and remains effective up to 120 hours, even after the LH surge; however, breastfeeding women should discard breastmilk for 1 week postuse, and those on progestogen-based contraception should seek medical guidance due to potential interactions. The copper IUD, if inserted within 5 days, offers the most effective emergency and ongoing contraception, but timely access may be challenging.

Table 24.6 Age considerations and method-specific guidance for contraceptives

Age group	Nonhormonal	Combined hormonal contraception (CHC)	Depot medroxyprogesterone acetate (DMPA)	Implant/POP/ LNG-IUS
< 50 years	Stop after 2 years of amenorrhea	Continue until age 50[a]	Continue until age 50[a] (or beyond after individual risk–benefit discussion)	Continue to age 50 or longer[a]
≥ 50 years	Stop after 1 year of amenorrhea	Discontinue at 50 → switch to nonhormonal or POP	Discontinue at 50 → then: Switch to nonhormonal (stop after 2 y amenorrhea) Switch to POP/implant/ LNG-IUS (see right column) Continue DMPA with individualized risk discussion	If amenorrhoeic: Measure FSH twice (≥ 30 IU/L, 6 weeks apart) → stop Or stop at age 55 If still bleeding: Investigate abnormal bleeding Continue contraception until 1 year amenorrhea

[a]A woman wishing to stop before age 50 may switch off hormonal methods and cease once she's amenorrhoeic for 2 years (3 years if switching from DMPA)

24.9 When to Stop Contraception

Contraceptive use should continue until menopause is confirmed, typically after 12 months of amenorrhea in women not using hormonal contraception. Nonhormonal methods like copper IUDs are safe until menopause is assured. However, amenorrhea caused by progestin-only methods or continuous combined hormonal contraceptives (CHCs) may mask menopausal onset, making clinical confirmation challenging (NHS).

Women without contraindications may continue progestin-only methods or CHCs until age 50 yrs. For CHC users, cyclic regimens may not reliably indicate menopause due to scheduled bleeding, and continuous regimens often induce amenorrhea. As cardiovascular risk increases with age, CHC safety should be reassessed near menopause, and alternative methods considered if risks outweigh benefits (NHS) (Table 24.6).

24.10 Transition to Hormone Therapy (HT)

When stopping contraception, some women may choose to start menopausal hormone therapy (MHT). It is essential to counsel women that MHT does not prevent pregnancy, so additional contraception is needed for sexually active women who are not yet menopausal. It also affects FSH levels, so testing during MHT is not reliable. For those using combined hormonal contraception (CHC), menopause can be confirmed by checking FSH levels 14 days after stopping. For depot medroxyprogesterone acetate (DMPA) users, two FSH readings over 30 IU/L taken at least 90 days apart can confirm menopause.

The Mirena IUS gives endometrial protection for a maximum of 5 years and must be replaced after 5 years. Other progestogen-only methods like POP, implants, and DMPA don't have endometrial protection when used with estrogen-only MHT, but are safe for contraception alongside a sequential regime. CHC can be used in suitable women under 50 to manage menopause symptoms and help maintain bone strength.

24.11 Conclusion

In perimenopausal women, all contraceptive methods remain potentially viable, though age-related risks such as arterial vascular disease, venous thromboembolism, and hormonally sensitive cancers necessitate careful individual assessment, especially when considering estrogen-containing options. Estrogen-containing contraceptives are generally unsuitable for women over 50. Progestogen-only methods, excluding DMPA, which is second-line after age 45, can typically be used until menopause unless contraindicated by breast cancer or severe liver disease. Long-acting reversible contraceptives (LARCs), including the LNG-IUD and Cu-IUD, implants, offer extended use and are particularly beneficial for managing heavy menstrual bleeding or providing durable contraception with minimal contraindications. FSH testing can guide discontinuation in amenorrhoeic women over 50, though continuing contraception until age 55 is often appropriate. Understanding method-specific risks and benefits, alongside acquiring procedural skills for LARC insertion and removal, is essential for optimizing contraceptive care in this population.

Key Points

1. Perimenopausal women have diverse contraceptive needs influenced by hormonal fluctuations, comorbidities, and shifting fertility potential. Tailored, evidence-based counseling ensures safe and effective choices.
2. Use of structured assessment tools to evaluate cardiovascular, thromboembolic, and metabolic risks before initiating hormonal contraception, especially combined methods, is indispensable.
3. Although fertility declines, contraceptive need persists in perimenopause, due to erratic ovulation and the possibility of pregnancy.
4. Contraception should be continued until menopause is confirmed clinically or biochemically.
5. Contraceptives, especially hormonal methods, provide significant non-contraceptive health benefits, including regulation of menstrual cycles, reduction of heavy bleeding and dysmenorrhea, prevention of certain ovarian and endometrial cancers, relief of vasomotor symptoms, and promotion of bone health. These effects greatly enhance quality of life and reduce morbidity in midlife women.
6. Hormonal methods (e.g., LNG-IUS, progestin pills) also cater to important clinical issues in perimenopause, like heavy menstrual bleeding and perimenopausal symptoms, and provide endometrial protection, supporting a dual therapeutic role.

Long Answer Questions (LAQs)

1. Give role of contraception in managing perimenopausal symptoms.
2. A 47-year-old woman presents with irregular menstrual cycles, vasomotor symptoms, and concerns about contraception. She is a nonsmoker and normotensive, and has a BMI of 28. She has no significant medical history and is sexually active with a male partner. Discuss the contraceptive options available to her.

Short Answer Questions (SAQs)

1. What are the contraindications for combined hormonal contraception in perimenopausal women?

2. How does the levonorgestrel-releasing intrauterine system (LNG-IUS) benefit perimenopausal women beyond contraception?
3. At what point can contraception be safely discontinued in a healthy woman over 50 using a progestin-only method?
4. What are the advantages of using DMPA in perimenopausal women, and what are the concerns regarding bone health?

Multiple Choice Questions (MCQs)

1. Which of the following is a noncontraceptive benefit of the levonorgestrel-releasing intrauterine system (LNG-IUS) in perimenopausal women?
   A. Improves fertility
   B. Prevents vasomotor symptoms
   C. Reduces heavy menstrual bleeding
   D. Increases bone density
2. At what age can contraception be discontinued in a healthy woman using a progestin-only method, assuming she is amenorrhoeic?
   A. 45 years
   B. 50 years
   C. 55 years
   D. After age 50 with 1 years of amenorrhea
3. Which long-acting reversible contraceptive (LARC) provides both contraception and endometrial protection during hormone replacement therapy (HRT)?
   A. Copper IUD
   B. LNG-IUS
   C. DMPA
   D. Etonogestrel implant
4. Which of the following is a concern with long-term use of depot medroxyprogesterone acetate (DMPA) in perimenopausal women?
   A. Increased risk of ovarian cancer
   B. Decreased bone mineral density
   C. Increased risk of thromboembolism
   D. Endometrial hyperplasia
5. Which method is most suitable for a perimenopausal woman with hypertension and a BMI of 32?
   A. Combined oral contraceptive pill
   B. Progestin-only pill
   C. Transdermal patch
   D. Vaginal ring
6. Which of the following is true regarding combined oral contraceptives in perimenopausal women?
   A. They are contraindicated after age 40

   B. They can help manage vasomotor symptoms
   C. They increase bone loss
   D. They are preferred in smokers
7. What is the minimum duration of contraception recommended after the last menstrual period in women overs 50 not using hormonal contraception?
   A. 6 months
   B. 1 year
   C. 2 years
   D. Until age 55
8. Which of the following contraceptive methods is most appropriate for a perimenopausal woman with a history of deep vein thrombosis (DVT)?
   A. Combined oral contraceptive pill
   B. Vaginal ring
   C. Progestin-only pill
   D. Transdermal patch
9. Which contraceptive method may mask the onset of menopause due to its effect on bleeding patterns?
   A. Copper IUD
   B. LNG-IUS
   C. Barrier methods
   D. Fertility awareness methods
10. What is the primary contraceptive mechanism of the etonogestrel implant?
    A. Inhibition of ovulation
    B. Endometrial thinning
    C. Sperm immobilization
    D. Tubal blockage

Answers

1. C
2. D
3. C
4. B
5. B
6. B
7. B
8. C
9. B
10. A

References

1. Van Heertum K, Liu J. Contraception and conception in mid-life: a review of the current literature. Women's Midlife Health. 2017;3(3):3.
2. Fritz MA, Speroff L. Clinical gynecologic endocrinology and infertility. 8th ed. Philadelphia: Lippincott Williams & Wilkins; 2012.
3. Allshouse AA, Pavlovic J, Santoro N. Menstrual cycle hormone changes associated with reproductive aging and how they may relate to symptoms. Obstet Gynecol Clin N Am. 2018;45(4):613–28. https://doi.org/10.1016/j.ogc.2018.07.004.
4. Shaaban MM. The perimenopause and contraception. Maturitas. 1996;23(2):181–92. https://doi.org/10.1016/0378-5122(96)83915-6.
5. Faculty of Sexual and Reproductive Healthcare. Clinical guideline: contraception for women aged over 40 years. London: FSRH; 2018. [updated 2019; cited 2022 Jul 7].
6. Grandi G, Facchinetti F, Bitzer J. Contraception during perimenopause: practical guidance. Int J Women's Health. 2022;14:667–77. https://doi.org/10.2147/IJWH.S361217.
7. Australian Menopause Society. Contraception in perimenopause: practice points for GPs [internet]. Melbourne: AMS; 2023. [cited 2025 Jul 4].
8. Schunmann C. NHS Clinical guideline for perimenopausal contraception. NHS; 2022.
9. Antinori S, Gholami GH, Versaci C, Cerusico F, Dani L, Antinori M, et al. Obstetric and prenatal outcome in menopausal women: a 12-year clinical study. Reprod Biomed Online. 2003;6(2):257–61.
10. Hatcher RA, Trussell J, Nelson AL, Cates W, Kowal D, Policar M. Contraceptive technology. 20th rev ed. Valley Stream, NY: Ardent Media; 2011. p. 421–2.
11. Di Bella ZIK, Bianchi AMHJ, Araujo FFM, Sartori MGF, Girão MJBC. Contraception and family planning at the extreme of reproductive life—climacteric. Rev Assoc Med Bras. 2016;62(5):454–7.
12. Gambacciani M, Monteleone P, Ciaponi M, Sacco A, Genazzani AR. Effects of oral contraceptives on bone mineral density. Treat Endocrinol. 2004;3(3):191–6.
13. Cibula D, Gompel A, Mueck AO, et al. Hormonal contraception and risk of cancer. Hum Reprod Update. 2010;16(6):631–50.
14. Kamani M, Akgor U, Gültekin M. Review of the literature on combined oral contraceptives and cancer. Ecancermedicalscience. 2022;16:1416. https://doi.org/10.3332/ecancer.2022.1416.
15. Mueck AO, Rabe T. Hormonal contraception and risk of endometrial cancer: a systematic review. Endocr Relat Cancer. 2010;17(4):R263–71.
16. Westhoff C, Britton JA, Gammon MD, Wright T, Kelsey JL. Oral contraceptive use and benign ovarian tumors. Am J Epidemiol. 2000;152(3):242–6.
17. Schrijver LH, Vasen HF, Vos JR, van Engelen K, van Sandick JW, Kets CM, et al. Oral contraceptive use in BRCA1 and BRCA2 mutation carriers: absolute cancer risks and benefits. J Natl Cancer Inst. 2022;114(4):540–52.
18. Khan F, Creinin MD. Contemporary understanding of breast cancer risk with combined oral contraceptives. Contemp OB/GYN [Internet]. 2024; [cited 2025 Jul 1].
19. Nelson AL. Contraception: transdermal contraceptive patches. In: Post TW, editor. UpToDate [Internet]. Waltham (MA): UpToDate; 2022.
20. Bitzer J, Merki-Feld GS. The contraceptive patch: a review of current evidence. Eur J Contracept Reprod Health Care. 2020;25(4):279–85.
21. Bahamondes L, Ali M. Recent advances in long-acting reversible contraceptive methods. Best Pract Res Clin Obstet Gynaecol. 2020;66:28–40.

Nutrition and Lifestyle Management in Menopause

25

Vandana Parti

Abstract

Menopause is a significant physiological phase in a woman's life, marked by the decline of ovarian function. With the average age of menopause in Indian women occurring earlier than in the West, timely nutrition and lifestyle interventions are critical for improving quality of life and preventing long-term complications. This is an area which needs more attention.

This chapter explores evidence-based strategies for dietary and lifestyle modification during the menopausal phase and the peri- and post-menopausal years. Key dietary recommendations include adequate protein intake, complex carbohydrates with low glycaemic load, healthy fats, and micronutrients essential for bone and cardiovascular health, such as calcium, vitamin D, magnesium, and phytoestrogens. Hydration and weight loss by portion control and anti-inflammatory food further support metabolic balance. Lifestyle approaches, including structured physical activity (aerobic, resistance, and flexibility training), stress management, mindfulness practices, sleep hygiene, and social connectedness are emphasised for holistic well-being.

By integrating nutrition science, physical health strategies, and mental-emotional wellness, this chapter highlights a preventive, patient-centric approach to managing menopause by holistic mind body reset. Practical frameworks, sample dietary patterns, and lifestyle modifications are provided to empower women and healthcare professionals in transforming menopause into an opportunity for health optimisation and long-term health.

V. Parti (✉)
Department of Men's Health, Women's Health & Gerontology, Baba Farid University, Faridkot, Punjab, India

Children & Adolescent Health, Scottish High International School, Gurgaon, India

R. Malik et al. (eds.), *Menopause Essentials*,
https://doi.org/10.1007/978-981-95-7498-8_25

Keywords

Menopause · Nutrition · Lifestyle Modification · Women's health · Bone health · Cardiovascular risk

25.1 Introduction

Menopause is the point in a women's life which marks the end of her reproductive period, between 45 and 55 years, or sometimes even earlier with cessation of her menstrual cycle. This is also called 'change of life'. It is just a part of the biological aging process. It could be caused by surgery, chemotherapy, or certain medication.

The common symptoms are hot flashes, night sweats, mood swings, vaginal dryness, trouble in concentrating, headache, and joint and muscle pain. The peri-menopausal period too can be as troublesome as the post-menopausal period where the ovarian hormones oestrogen and progesterone are on the decline. The lifestyle modifications and right nutrition are very crucial during this period of menopause as they can significantly help to manage symptoms like hot flashes and night sweats, while also mitigating the increased risk of long-term health concerns like osteoporosis, cardiovascular diseases, cancer colon, and breast cancer by promoting healthy blood sugar levels, bone density, weight loss, mental well-being, and overall well-being during this life stage.

The quality of life can be improved, and women can lead a better, more productive healthier life with lifestyle changes. Not only physical but also the mental and emotional well-being are areas of major concern. The menopausal symptoms can hamper the performance and affect the routine of a normal woman. It was seen in a study that 1 out of 10 women leaves their jobs early due to these menopausal symptoms.

The role of each nutrient and each aspect of lifestyle will be covered in later sections of this chapter along with an ideal routine and a diet plan for a menopausal woman.

25.2 Physiological Changes During Menopause

It is very crucial to understand the hormonal and physiological changes during the peri-menopausal and menopausal period to manage the symptoms effectively through lifestyle and dietary changes. By doing that, you can empathise with the patient and handle not only the physical but mental and emotional challenges as well.

During this period, as you know the oestrogen, progesterone, and the testosterone fall, whereas FSH and LH rise. The level of oestrogen during child-bearing age falls from 15–350 pg/ml to <10 pg/ml. The decline in number of oocytes to a critical level and cessation of ovarian follicular activity leads to the changes in feedback mechanism between ovary, pituitary, and hypothalamus. Almost 80% of women have the menopausal symptoms, of which one-third are severe.

The decline in hormonal levels affects the fat, glucose metabolism, bones, heart, moods, etc. The ability to switch from fat utilisation during fasting to carbohydrate utilisation during hyperinsulinemia is defined as metabolic flexibility. Gonadal hormones might regulate metabolic flexibility at the level of the mitochondria, determining how nutrients are converted into energy. In post-menopausal women, metabolic flexibility diminishes due to oestrogen reduction, and more fat accumulates in the central depots.

Estrogen has a protective effect on cardiovascular health. It leads to the production of nitric oxide and prostacyclins which cause vasodilation. Estrogen also shifts the renin-angiotensin axis leading to increased production of angiotensin, thereby enhancing cardiovascular protection.

There are many changes affecting carbohydrate metabolism during menopause. In the absence of oestrogen, the insulin secretion of the pancreatic beta cells decreases. Decrease in insulin sensitivity in the muscles, causes increased gluconeogenesis as well as lipogenesis. It ultimately leads to accumulation of triglycerides and VLDL.

As a result of the reduced insulin effect on adipose tissue, lipolysis increases, the size of fat cells increases, and inflammatory mediators accumulate. The resulting metabolic changes lead to development of metabolic syndrome. Therefore, the risk of developing a carbohydrate metabolism disorder is related to the presence or absence of gonadal hormones [1].

25.3 Common Symptoms

Hot flashes and night sweats: Hot flashes are due to neuroendocrinal process. The hypothalamus, which regulates the body temperature, becomes sensitive to fluctuations in body temperature. Elevated central sympathetic activation, mediated through alpha 2 adrenergic receptors, is one of the factors responsible for narrowing of the thermoneutral zone. That is why paced respiration meliorates hot flashes and causes peripheral cooling. Night sweats too occur due to change in the night temperature. The factors like genetic, body weight, smoking, and stress can trigger or worsen these symptoms.

Anxiety and panic, mood swings, and irritability: Fluctuating hormones, particularly oestrogen decline, significantly impact the neurotransmitters serotonin and GABA leading to anxiety, mood swings, and irritability. This is especially prominent during the peri-menopausal when the hormones fluctuate more dramatically.

Sleep disturbance: The sleep disturbance is primarily due to hot flashes, night sweats, and anxiety, and managing these symptoms will help in better sleep. Progesterone has a sedative effect, and its reduction can lead to sleep fragmentation. Oestrogen regulates serotonin and melatonin and disrupts sleep; vasomotor symptoms cause nocturnal awakening.

Altered serotonin, dopamine, and GABA levels affect the process: Other factors like increased urinary frequency, restless legs syndrome, and obstructive sleep apnoea (OSA) in post-menopausal women alter the sleep pattern.

Palpitations: Although the symptom of palpitation has not been explained well, stress, anxiety, and lifestyle factors like coffee, alcohol, and nicotine use could worsen the symptom.

Vaginal dryness, loss of libido, and frequent vaginitis: The declining hormone causes thinning of vaginal epithelium, decreased glycogen content, and reduced vaginal secretions. There is also reduced vaginal blood circulation. The loss of lactobacilli increases vaginal PH, leading to irritation and itching and infection (atrophic vaginitis), resulting in painful intercourse. The loss of libido is also attributed to the fall in testosterone level.

Urinary incontinence: Loss of elasticity and thinning of urethral lining and weakening of pelvic floor muscles.

Weight gain: The fall in oestrogen level results in increases in fat storage. The hormones strongly influence the body fat distribution and adipocyte differentiation as well. There is increase in visceral fat. The BMR falls. As oestrogen plays a role in fat distribution around the hips and thighs, there is increased insulin resistance. The average weight gain in a year is 15 pounds or 0.68 g even if the diet and lifestyle remain same.

Skin changes in menopause: Dryness, thinning, wrinkles, sagging, hyperpigmentation, and facial hair are commonly seen.

Others: Joint stiffness, muscle pain and loss of muscle mass and decreased bone mass. Increased risk of cardiovascular disease, dyslipidaemia, and hypertension.

25.4 The Role of Nutrition in Menopause

There has been a growing interest in non-pharmacological approaches which have highlighted the crucial role of nutrition. Proper dietary choices can help manage symptoms, reduce long-term health risks, and improve overall well-being. This section explores the impact of nutrition on menopause and provides evidence-based recommendations for optimal dietary intake. Mediterranean style diet is recommended in menopause [1].

25.4.1 Macronutrients and Energy Balance

Protein

Protein is essential for maintaining muscle mass, bone health, and overall metabolic function during menopause. Menopausal women have muscle loss (sarcopenia) due to declining oestrogen levels, which play a role in muscle protein synthesis. The fall in testosterone level also contributes to the loss of muscle mass. Adequate protein intake helps maintain muscle strength, support metabolic health, and promote satiety. Ensuring adequate protein intake is crucial for preserving lean muscle mass and supporting bone health and overall strength and energy levels. In the menopausal transition, lowering oestrogen levels have been associated with loss of lean body mass (LBM) and increase in fat mass (FM). In the longitudinal study of women's health across the nation, LBM loss during the menopausal transition averaged 0.5% (a mean annual absolute decrease of 0.2 kg), and FM increased by 1.5% per year (mean annual absolute increase of 0.45 kg).

Aging increases dietary protein requirement because skeletal muscles reduce their capacity of activating protein synthesis in response to anabolic stimuli, possibly due to insulin resistance. In the women's health initiative study, higher protein intake of 1.5 g/kg body weight was associated with 32% lower quality and better physical function.

It prevents muscle loss and supports bone health. Protein is key component of bone structure, and when combined with calcium and vitamin D, it aids in preventing osteoporosis. Protein contributes to higher thermal effect, helping in maintaining a healthy weight by supporting metabolism and reducing fat accumulation. It enhances recovery and immunity by aiding in tissue repair.

Recommended intake: 1.0–1.2 g/kg body weight per day.

Sources: Lean meat, fish, eggs, dairy, legumes, soy, nuts, and seeds.

Healthy Fats

Dietary fat composition influences inflammation, cardiovascular health, and cognitive function. Omega-3 fatty acids are particularly beneficial in reducing inflammation and supporting brain function. Cholesterol is restricted to less than 300 mg [2, 3].

Sources: Fatty fish, flax seeds, walnuts, chia seeds, olive oil.

Avoid: Trans fats and excessive saturated fats, which can increase the cardiovascular risk.

Complex Carbohydrates

There are many changes during menopause that affect carbohydrate metabolism. Menopause is associated with an increased risk of insulin resistance and weight gain. Choosing complex carbohydrates with a low glycaemic index helps regulate blood sugar levels and support gut health. Complementing additional ways of characterising carbohydrate foods, such as fibre and whole green content, glycaemic index (GI) should also be considered particularly important in reducing total body FM and managing weight. Eating a meal with high GI elicits a quick pancreatic response to the rising blood glucose levels, with intense insulin secretion that rapidly lowers that glucose and causes hunger and over eating. Specifically in postmenopausal women, a clinical trial with low GI <55 dietary intervention aimed to balance energy needs has shown that despite similar energy intake and resting metabolic rate during 6 months of follow-up, all the participants have lost body and fat.

Sources: Whole grains (quinoa, brown rice, oats), legumes, fruits, and vegetables.

Fluid Intake in Menopause Adequate fluid intake is also extremely important during menopause, especially concerning cellular metabolism and maintaining the optimal function of a haemostasis. It has an important role in regulating heat balance, detoxification, maintaining the proper functioning of gastrointestinal tract and moisture of the membrane, as well as turgor of skin. Adequate daily fluid intake is important in the transport of nutrients and oxygen and contributes to the health of the skeletal system. Oestrogen and progesterone significantly affect not only the cardiovascular system but also fluid and electrolyte balance. During menopause, hormonal changes affect the third as well, which may result in a significant decrease in fluid intake. The individualised, appropriate amount of fluid to be taken is 33 ml/kg/day, which is recommended to be evenly distributed over the day.

25.4.2 Micronutrients in Menopause

Calcium and Vitamin D

Research indicates that up to 20% of bone loss can happen during menopause, and approximately 1 in 10 women over 60 is affected by osteoporosis worldwide. Women experience drop in bone density particularly in the first few years of menopause. Vitamin D and calcium play an important role in development of healthy bones. The National Osteoporosis Foundation recommends at least 1200 mg/day of calcium and 800–1000 IU per day of vitamin D. This should be ideally done by dietary intake but supplemented when if necessary. It is recommended for individuals at risk or with proven insufficiency. Early menopause, family history low calcium intake, vitamin D deficiency, and sedentary lifestyle are few factors that contribute to bone loss during menopause. Research found that adequate calcium intake in presence of adequate Vitamin D intake prevents bone loss and reduces fracture risk in peri- and post-menopausal women.

Although calcium is not an effective anti-resorptive agent (e.g. oestrogen, selective oestrogen-receptor modulators, or biphosphates), it is an essential component of anti-resorptive therapy for osteoporosis. Calcium has also been associated with beneficial effect in several non-skeletal disorders, primarily hypertension, colorectal cancer, and obesity, although not fully explored. Some studies suggest that vitamin D may also help in other menopausal symptoms like mood swings and dry vagina. [3]

Calcium sources: Dairy products, fortified plant-based milk, leafy vegetables like cabbage, broccoli not spinach, almonds, sesame seed, tofu, mushrooms.

Vitamin D sources: Fatty fish, fortified dairy products, egg yolk, sun exposure.

Magnesium

Magnesium plays a role in bone health, muscle relaxation, and nerve system function. It also improves sleep quality and reduces anxiety.

Sources: Nuts, seeds, whole grain, leafy vegetables, dark chocolate.

Recommended Intake: 320 mg/day.

Vitamin K2

Vitamin K2 helps direct calcium to bones and away from the arteries, reducing the risk of osteoporosis and cardiovascular disease.

Sources: Fermented foods, egg yolks, organ meat.

Recommended Intake: 90 mcg/day.

Vitamin B (B6, B12, Folate)

These vitamins support cognitive function, nerve health, and glucose metabolism. Vitamin B6 may also help in mood swings and irritability [3, 4].

Sources: Whole grains, eggs, dairy, leafy vegetables, legumes.

Recommended Intake: B6: 1.5 mg/day, B12: 2.4 mg/day, Folate: 400 mcg/day.

Phytoestrogens

Phytoestrogens are plant-derived compounds that mimic oestrogen in the body, potentially alleviating menopausal symptoms such as hot flashes and bone loss [5].

Sources: Soy products (tofu, tempeh, edamame), flaxseeds, chickpeas, lentils.

Clinical evidence: Studies suggest that soy isoflavones can reduce hot flashes frequency by 20–50%.

Antioxidants (Vitamin C, Vitamin E, Selenium, and Zinc)

Oxidative stress increases with aging, and oestrogen declines, contributing to inflammation and chronic disease. Antioxidants help neutralise free radicals.

Sources: Vitamin C: citrus fruits, bell peppers, berries. Vitamin E: Nuts, seeds, spinach, sunflower oil. Selenium: Brazil nuts, sea food. Zinc: shellfish, legumes, nuts.

25.5 Nutritional Supplements in Menopause

Supplements can play a crucial role in supporting women's health during menopause. However, they need to be prescribed based on individual needs, dietary intake, and the detailed personal history of the patient. A combination of proper nutrition, lifestyle modification, and targeted supplementation can significantly improve the menstrual health and well-being.

Although not much scientific proof and evidence is available about herbal and dietary supplement's role, some vitamins and minerals may help in these menopausal symptoms.

Protein Supplementation

Protein supplements can be given after taking the dietary history and medically assessment.

Sources of protein supplements:

- Whey protein: A complete protein with all essential amino acids, ideal for muscle preservation and recovery.
- Plant-based protein (soy, pea, hemp)—Suitable for those with lactose intolerance or a vegetarian diet.
- Collagen peptides—Supports skin elasticity, joint health, and bone strength.
- Casein protein—A slow digesting protein beneficial for prolonged muscle support, especially at night.

Post-menopausal women should take 1–1.2 g of protein per kg body weight per day.

The consumption should be evenly distributed throughout the day, with supplements taken post workout or between meals to support muscle synthesis and satiety. Protein works best when paired with strength training, calcium, vitamin D, and healthy fats to optimise muscle and bone health.

Magnesium: As magnesium supports bone health, reduces muscle cramps, improves sleep quality, and alleviates mood swings, daily dose of 320–400 mg preferably in the evening can promote relaxation and improve the sleep patterns.

Vitamin D & Calcium: Vitamin D has positive effect in hot flashes, mood swings, cognitive function, and vaginal dryness. If the dietary intake seems insufficient, calcium 1200 mg and vitamin 600–800 IU can be prescribed with meals for better absorption.

Vitamin B (B6, B12 and folate): These vitamins support energy production, nerve function, and cardiovascular health. Vitamin B12 is particularly important as absorption decreases with age. A daily dose can be prescribed in the morning to boost energy levels.

Vitamin E: Vitamin E has been used for symptoms of hot flashes. A daily dose of 200–400 IU with meals can be prescribed for optimal absorption.

Omega-3 Fatty Acids: 1000–2000 mg Omega-3 fatty acids daily with meals can help reduce cardiovascular risks, improve cognitive function, and reduce inflammation.

Phytoestrogens: Although there is no scientific proof, certain herbal preparations have been used in allaying menopausal symptoms. Black cohosh extract, red clover, and flax seeds have been used time and again.

These plant compounds mimic oestrogen and may help in hot flashes.

Isoflavones might have beneficial effect by its anti-inflammatory and anti-oxidant properties through the production of equal, an active metabolic formed from daidzein by gut microbiota.

25.6 Nutritional Strategies for Symptom Management

Hot Flashes and Night Sweats

- Increase phytoestrogens from soy and flaxseeds.
- Maintain hydration to offset fluid loss.
- Avoid triggers such as caffeine, alcohol, and spicy food.

Bone Health

- Ensure adequate calcium, Vitamin D, magnesium, and Vitamin K2 intake.
- Engage in weight-bearing exercises along with proper nutrition.

Cardiovascular Health

- Increase omega-3 fatty acids and fibre to lower cholesterol and improve lipid profiles.
- Reduce saturated fats, trans fats, and refined carbohydrates to prevent metabolic syndrome.

Mental Health and Cognitive Function

- Support brain health with omega-3 fatty acids, B vitamins, and antioxidants.
- Maintain stable sugar levels to prevent mood swings and brain fog.

Sleep and Stress Management

- Consume magnesium-rich foods (nuts, seeds, whole grains) to aid relaxation.
- Incorporate herbal teas (chamomile, valerian root) for better sleep quality.

25.7 Role of Lifestyle Modification in Menopausal Management

25.7.1 Role of Physical Activity

- Habitual participation in physical exercise results in many health benefits including longevity, cardiovascular disease, metabolic diseases, maintenance of energy balance, and improving musculoskeletal system and mental health.
- Research has shown that physical activity has a range of neuroendocrinal response on single bout and regular exercise as well. The increase in brain epinephrine and its metabolites distracts women from hot flashes [6].
- Bone density increases, and risk of osteoporosis and fractures associated with low bone density also reduce. Other symptoms like joint stiffness, fatigue, difficulty in concentrating, poor sleep, irritability, and depression are also improved by physical activity.
- Regular aerobic exercises can help lower blood pressure, improve cholesterol, and decrease the risk of cardiovascular disease. Exercise also improves anxiety, mood swings, and irritability by increasing the release of dopamine, serotonin, and endorphins.
- Sleep quality can improve which is a common menopausal symptom. Weight management by burning calories and preserving muscle mass by strength training is helpful. Studies have shown that exercise reduces the inflammation. In case of obesity or overweight, losing just 5 kg of weight improves the tolerability of hot flashes by 30%, and regular exercise ensures metabolic health and reduces the number and intensity of hot flashes.

Types of Exercise

- *Strength training:* Lifting weights strengthens and builds muscles using free weights, resistance bands, and machines at the gym [7].
- *High-intensity interval training (HIIT):* This also helps in reducing visceral abdominal fat and reducing the incidence of diabetes and heart disease.
- *Cardiovascular exercises:* Aerobic activities like jogging, brisk walking, swimming, dancing, and biking are equally important.
- *Flexibility exercises:* Stretching, yoga, and Pilates balancing acts like standing on one leg or tai chi improve stability.

25.7.2 Role of Stress Management

Hormonal decline leads to anxiety, stress, and sleep disturbances. Effective stress management is essential for maintaining overall well-being during this period. Below are the key strategies to help manage stress during menopause.

25.7.3 Lifestyle Modification

Regular exercise: Engaging in aerobic exercises and strength training helps reduce stress, improve mood, and enhance sleep.

Balanced diet: Eating a nutrient dense diet rich in whole grain, lean proteins, healthy fats, and fibre supports hormonal balance.

Adequate sleep: Poor sleep exacerbates stress. Establishing a regular sleep schedule, limiting screen time before bed, and practicing relaxation techniques improve sleep quality.

Mind and Body Practices

Yoga and meditation: These practices promote relaxation, reduce cortisol levels, and improve emotional resilience.

Breathing techniques: Diaphragmatic breathing (4–7–8 technique) helps control stress response [8].

Progressive muscle relaxation: It is a process of tensing and relaxing muscle groups systematically, thereby reducing tension and producing calmness [9].

GUT Health and Microbiome balance

The gut microbiome plays a role in oestrogen metabolism. A diet rich in probiotics and prebiotics can support hormonal balance.

- *Probiotic source:* Yogurt, fermented vegetables, kombucha.
- *Prebiotic source:* garlic, onions, bananas, asparagus, whole grains.
- *Hydration*

Hormonal changes can lead to increased water loss and dry skin with a higher incidence of urinary tract infections. Oestrogen decline also affects the body's ability to retain moisture, contributing to joint pain, fatigue, and headaches.

Staying well hydrated helps in temperature regulation and the proper metabolism. It promotes energy levels, cognitive functions, and overall well-being during menopause.

Smoking and Alcohol

Smoking and alcohol consumption can worsen menopausal symptoms and increase the health risks. Smoking further lowers the oestrogen levels leading to more severe hot flashes, osteoporosis, and cardiovascular diseases. It also accelerates skin aging and raises the risk of lung cancer. Alcohol triggers hot flashes, disrupts sleep, and contributes to weight gain. Women during menopause should quit smoking and limit alcohol intake.

Alcohol and caffeine limitation help reduce hot flashes and improve sleep.

Sleep Hygiene

Menopause often disrupts sleep due to hormonal changes, night sweats, and mood swings. Good sleep hygiene can improve the rest quality. The patient needs to be advised to maintain a consistent sleep schedule, create a cool and dark bedroom environment, and avoid screens before bed. Regular exercises, stress management techniques like meditation, and reducing caffeine and alcohol intake can help.

Wearing breathable sleep wear and using cooling bedding can minimise night sweats. If sleep disturbances persist, cognitive behaviour therapy for insomnia (CBT-I) may be considered. Prioritising sleep hygiene supports overall health, mood stability and daily functioning during menopause.

25.8 Managing Menopausal Symptoms with Diet and Lifestyle Modification

Holistic Care

The clinician needs to have a holistic approach while managing women. The physical, emotional, and psychological well-being needs to be addressed through an integrated approach. It combines lifestyle modifications, nutrition, exercise, stress management, and complementary therapies to manage the symptoms effectively. Mind-body practices such as yoga and meditation can alleviate anxiety, insomnia, and hot flashes.

A balanced diet rich in phytoestrogens, calcium, and omega-3 fatty acids supports hormonal balance and bone health. Emotional well-being is enhanced through counselling, social support, and cognitive behavioural therapy. By focusing on the whole person rather than just symptoms, holistic care promotes the quality life during menopause.

Personalised Care
Although the tips given in this chapter are relevant to all menopausal women, the personalised care role cannot be underplayed. Personalised care in menopause tailors treatment to an individual's symptoms, lifestyle, medical history, and ensuring effective and patient-centric management. Since menopause affects women differently, a one-size-fits-all approach is inadequate. Personalised care may include hormonal and non-hormonal therapy, lifestyle modifications, and integrative therapies based on individual needs.

Genetic, metabolic, and psychological factors are also considered to optimize treatment outcomes. Regular assessments help adjust interventions as symptoms evolve. By addressing unique concerns and preferences, personalised care enhances symptom relief, improves quality of life, and supports long-term health, empowering women to navigate menopause with confidence and well-being.

Hot Flashes and Night Sweats
Hot flashes are the commonest vasomotor symptoms, result from hypothalamic dysfunction due to oestrogen withdrawal, and are experienced by women during menopause.

- *Cooling strategies:* Wearing light clothes, maintaining a cool temperature in the room using cold packs if required.
- *Regular Exercise:* Yoga, aerobic exercises, and deep breathing techniques help in thermoregulation [10].
- *Stress Management:* Meditation, mindfulness, and adequate sleep will improve overall well-being.
- *Phytoestrogens intake:* Soy, flaxseeds, and legumes may alleviate symptoms.
- *Hydration and Balanced diet:* Whole grain, fruits and vegetables and avoiding caffeine and limiting alcohol.

Mood Swings and Anxiety
Regular exercises to boost endorphins and reduce stress can be advised. Yoga and tai chi can improve relaxation and emotional balance. Social support and counselling can be done for emotional well-being. A good sleep hygiene is advised. Mindfulness, deep breathing exercises, and CBT are advised to reduce stress.

Vaginal Dryness
Reduced oestrogen levels lead to thinning of vaginal epithelium, decreased glycogen content, and reduced vaginal secretions.

- Hydration: Intake of 2–3 litres of water is important for mucosal hydration, with reduction in caffeine and alcohol intake.
- Intake of omega-3 fatty acids from fish, flax seeds, and chia seeds will help maintain cell membrane integrity.
- Intake of Vitamin E and A from nuts, seeds spinach for mucosal integrity and carrots, eggs for epithelial healing.

- Intake of zinc (pumpkinseeds, fish) will support tissue healing, and magnesium will help in reducing inflammation (nuts and leafy vegetables).
- Regular physical exercises and stress management have a role too.
- Avoiding vaginal irritants like harsh soaps, douches, and scented products can prevent itching and dryness.
- Wearing cotton underwear and avoiding tight synthetic fabrics should be recommended.

Sleep Disturbances

Prevalence of sleep disturbances is common in menopausal women. Taking a good clinical history and assessing play significant role in management.

Sleep schedule is to be maintained. The patient is advised to avoid screen time before bed and to keep the room environment comfortable and cool. The patient is advised to limit caffeine, alcohol, and heavy meals before bedtime. Incorporate magnesium and tryptophan-rich food like nuts, berries, banana, and dairy. Regular physical exercise, yoga, meditation, and deep breathing are advisable for better sleep.

25.9 An Ideal Day in Life of a Menopausal Woman: Lifestyle and Diet

Morning routine

- Wake up and hydrate
- Drink a glass of lukewarm lemon water
- Avoid caffeine immediately upon waking to prevent cortisol spikes
- Gentle morning movements

  A walk or yoga and stretching

- Nutritious breakfast
- A balanced healthy meal with protein, healthy fat, and fibre
- For example, eggs with whole grain toast and herbal tea, or green tea

Mid-morning

- Work or activities that stimulate the brain or social engagement
- A healthy snack like handful of almonds or pumpkin seeds and avoid processed sugars

Afternoon

- A balanced lunch of protein, vegetables, and whole grain, or can take soy or flax seeds.
- A post-meal walk is advisable to help with digestion and blood sugar regulation.
- A short power nap or relaxation for 15–20 minutes is optional to avoid fatigue without disrupting night-time sleep.

Evening

- Physical activities like strength training 2–3 times a week and aerobic exercises like brisk walk, cycling, or dancing can be done. Even mind-body exercises like yoga or Pilates can be done in evening for stress and flexibility.
- Early light dinner with focus on lean protein, fibre-rich vegetables, and healthy fats. The need to limit heavy and spicy or sugar-rich foods should be emphasised.

Night-time

- It is better to engage in light relaxing activities like reading, journaling, or light stretching to unwind. A warm herbal tea can be taken to promote relaxation. Advise to avoid screen time 2 hours before bed to support melatonin production.
- Good quality sleep: Keeping the environment cool and having a consistent sleep schedule with mindfulness or deep breathing exercises ensures good sleep.

Key Points

- *Diet:* To take high protein, high fibre, low fat, and low carbohydrate meals with adequate calcium, vitamin D, and water intake
- *Exercise:* Regular physical activity with 3 times a week strength training is advisable.
- *Rest:* To take good 7–9 hours' sleep
- *Mind-set:* To manage stress by practicing mindfulness, meditation, and deep breathing exercises
- *Avoid* excess tea, coffee, alcohol, and highly processed foods.

Long Answer Questions (LAQs)

1. Discuss the physiological and hormonal changes that occur during menopause. How do these changes influence nutritional and lifestyle needs in menopausal women?
2. Describe the role of nutrition in managing menopausal symptoms. Highlight dietary modifications for common issues such as hot flashes, bone health, cardiovascular risk, and weight gain.
3. Explain the importance of physical activity, sleep hygiene, and stress management in menopause. How can lifestyle interventions be integrated into clinical care for midlife women?
4. Outline a comprehensive lifestyle management plan for a menopausal woman. Include key components of diet, exercise, mental health support, and preventive health screenings.

Short Answer Questions (SAQs)

1. List four common symptoms experienced by women during menopause.
2. Mention any two dietary sources of phytoestrogens and explain their role in menopause.

3. What are the recommended lifestyle modifications for improving sleep quality in menopausal women?
4. State two reasons why calcium and vitamin D are important during menopause.
5. Name two forms of physical activity beneficial during menopause and justify their inclusion.

Multiple-Choice Questions (MCQs)

1. Which of the following is a common vasomotor symptom of menopause?
   A. Insomnia
   B. Hot flashes
   C. Osteoporosis
   D. Mood swings
2. Which nutrient is most crucial for maintaining bone health during menopause?
   A. Vitamin A
   B. Vitamin C
   C. Calcium
   D. Iron

3. Phytoestrogens are plant-based compounds that mimic:
   A. Testosterone
   B. Cortisol
   C. Oestrogen
   D. Progesterone
4. Which of the following is a good dietary source of phytoestrogens?
   A. Cheese
   B. Soybeans
   C. Chicken
   D. Egg yolk
5. Which of the following lifestyle changes is recommended to manage menopausal weight gain?
   A. Intermittent fasting without exercise
   B. High-protein, balanced diet with regular physical activity
   C. Low-fat, high-sugar diet
   D. Complete elimination of carbohydrates
6. The risk of which of the following conditions increases after menopause due to oestrogen decline?
   A. Appendicitis
   B. Asthma
   C. Cardiovascular disease
   D. Cataracts
7. Which vitamin enhances calcium absorption and is especially important post-menopause?
   A. Vitamin E
   B. Vitamin D

   C. Vitamin B12
   D. Vitamin K
8. Which of the following is NOT a recommended practice for menopausal women?
   A. Regular strength training
   B. Smoking cessation
   C. Alcohol excess for stress relief
   D. Maintaining good sleep hygiene
9. What is the role of omega-3 fatty acids in menopause management?
   A. Increases bone demineralisation
   B. Reduces cholesterol and inflammation
   C. Induces weight gain
   D. Enhances oestrogen production
10. Which of the following is a mindfulness-based intervention beneficial for menopausal symptom management?
   A. Weightlifting
   B. Power yoga
   C. Mindful meditation
   D. HIIT workouts

Answers

1. B
2. C
3. C
4. B
5. B
6. C
7. B
8. C
9. B
10. C

References

1. Contributors WE. Menopause and good nutrition . WebMD. 2022. Available from: https://www.webmd.com/menopause/staying-healthy-through-good-nuitritio.
2. The evidence-based diet solutions to managing menopause. British Nutrition Foundation. 2025. Available from: https://www.nutrition.org.uk/news/revealing-the-evidence-based-diet-solutions-to-managing-your-menopause-symptom.
3. Erdélyi A, Pálfi E, Tűű L, et al. The importance of nutrition in menopause and perimenopause-a review. Nutrients. 2023;16(1):27. Published 2023 Dec 21.
4. Menopause Diet: what to eat to help manage symptoms. Cleveland Clinic. Available from: https://health.clevelandclinic.org/menopause-diet.

5. Silva TR, Oppermann K, Reis FM, Spritzer PM. Nutrition in menopausal women: a narrative review. Nutrients. 2021;13(7):2149. Published 2021 Jun 23.
6. Huber-Disla N. Lifestyle modifications to help you navigate menopause. Center for Nutrition Studies. 2024. Available from: https://nutritionstudies.org/lifestyle-modifications-to-help-you-navigate-menopause/.
7. Exercise, nutrition and lifestyle in menopause, Manchester University, NHS; 2024.
8. Managing menopausal symptoms without medication. Healthdirect.gov.au. Health direct Australia; 2024. Available from: https://www.healthdirect.gov.au/managing-menopausal-symptoms-without-medication.
9. Nilsson S, Henriksson M, Hammar M, Berin E, Sofia Sederholm Lawesson, Ward LJ, et al. A 2-year follow-up to a randomized controlled trial on resistance training in postmenopausal women: vasomotor symptoms, quality of life and cardiovascular risk markers. BMC Womens Health. 2024;24(1):511.
10. Balzer D. Mayo Clinic Minute: lifestyle changes to manage menopause symptoms. Mayo Clinic News Network. 2021. Available from: https://newsnetwork.mayoclinic.org/discussion/mayo-clinic-minute-lifestyle-changes-to-manage-menopause-symptoms/.

Setting Up Menopause Clinic

26

Ragini Agrawal and Kavita Kumari

Abstract

The global population of postmenopausal women is growing. Despite affecting half the population, menopause has long remained underdiscussed, underresearched, and underserved in routine healthcare. Today, establishing dedicated menopause clinics is not only timely, but it is essential. There are many public health challenges related to menopause such as discussing menopause is often a taboo within society, families, workplaces, or healthcare settings. Women get adequate care from adolescence to the reproductive-age group. But we have no existing policies for care of postmenopausal women.

Setting up a menopause clinic is a valuable initiative that can provide much-needed support for women experiencing menopause as well-managed menopause transition sets the stage for active and healthy aging. A comprehensive systemic medical record with regular checkups and symptom management is the need of the hour to provide appropriate care to midlife women for the rest of life which should be offered to her around 45 years of age. The menopause card is the most important tool to give comprehensive, appropriate, preventive care and management of menopausal symptoms. A menopause clinic offers specialized, comprehensive, and empathetic care tailored to the unique needs of midlife women. They serve as vital hubs for preventive health.

R. Agrawal (✉)
A.A. Dermascience, Complete Clinic for Women Health, Gurugram, Haryana, India

K. Kumari
Department of Obstetrics & Gynecology, Atal Bihari Vajpayee Institute of Medical Sciences & Dr. Ram Manohar Lohia Hospital, New Delhi, India

R. Malik et al. (eds.), *Menopause Essentials*,
https://doi.org/10.1007/978-981-95-7498-8_26

Keywords

Menopause · Menopausal clinic · Menopausal card

The global population of postmenopausal women is growing. Women at and above 50 years of age accounted for 26% of all women and girls globally as per 2021 data. Women are living longer. In 2019, a 60-year-old woman could expect to live an additional 21 years on an average worldwide [1]. Given that women are expected to live for around one-third of their lives beyond menopause, this demographic and epidemiological trend would make noncommunicable illnesses the leading cause of morbidity and mortality in middle-aged and older women [2].

The purpose of menopausal hormonal therapy is to reduce or eliminate menopausal symptoms and thus improve women's quality of life [3]. Postmenopausal symptoms are sometimes so troublesome affects personal and professional lives. Menopause brings about some changes that will impact a woman's health as she gets older. With increasing life expectancy, there are enhanced chances for women to suffer from somatic and psychological symptoms due to aging and hormonal deficiency. It is important to understand menopausal problems. The factors affecting perimenopausal women's health will largely be depending upon prior health, reproductive history, lifestyle, and environmental factors.

The common age for menopause is between the ages of 45 and 55. During this period, women need to reassess her physical well-being, opportunities, and goals.

26.1 Necessity of Menopause Clinic

Despite affecting half the population, menopause has long remained underdiscussed, underresearched, and underserved in routine healthcare. Today, establishing dedicated menopause clinics is not only timely but it is essential. The symptoms of menopause—ranging from hot flashes, mood swings, and sleep disturbances to osteoporosis and cardiovascular risk—are multifactorial and can significantly impair quality of life. Yet, many women suffer in silence, often dismissed or misdiagnosed in general practice settings. A dedicated clinic ensures that these symptoms are addressed holistically and with evidence-based interventions. It is needed to fill a lacuna in the services of senior women.

There are public health challenges related to menopause such as discussing menopause is often a taboo within families, society, workplaces and healthcare settings. Menopausal women have limited access to quality health services, communities, and support systems. Healthcare awareness and access to menopause-related scientific information and services remain a significant challenge. Women may not know about menopausal and treatment options available that can alleviate discomfort.

Healthcare professionals might not have the necessary training to identify postmenopausal symptoms and offer therapeutic alternatives. Menopause does not receive its due importance in the training curriculum. The sexual well-being of menopausal women is overlooked. GSM is often ignored. It is a chronic progressive condition for which timely intervention is necessary. But considering it, a normal part of aging women suffers silently. It's possible that older women do not think they are at risk for STIs, including HIV, or that their healthcare practitioners do not advise them to get tested or engage in safer sexual behavior.

In low-resource settings, where there are frequently other pressing and conflicting priorities for health funding, menopause-related therapies present a problem. Women get adequate care from adolescence to the reproductive-age group. However, there are currently no policies in place for the treatment of postmenopausal women. It is an obvious gap in managing the health issues of midlife women (45–60 years).

26.2 Aim of the Menopause Clinic

- Increasing awareness about menopause and how it affects women both personally and socially, as well as the health and socioeconomic advancement of nations.
- Stressing the importance of a life course approach to health and well-being, including sexual health and well-being, by making sure women have access to the right health information and services to support healthy aging and a high standard of living prior to, during, and following menopause.
- Promoting the inclusion of menopausal symptom management diagnosis, treatment, and counseling in universal health coverage.
- Promoting the inclusion of training on menopause and treatment options in preservice curricula for health workers.

Setting up a menopause clinic is a valuable initiative that can provide much-needed support for women experiencing menopause as well-managed menopause transition sets the stage for active and healthy aging.

Defining Menopause Clinic's Vision and Scope
- *Mission Statement:* Clarify purpose (e.g., improving women's quality of life during menopause)
- *Scope of Services:* Possible areas include medical hormone therapy (MHT), nutritional counseling, psychological support, pelvic floor therapy, bone health and osteoporosis prevention, physical rehabilitation, and support groups.

Understand Legal and Regulatory Requirements
- Like MHT requires counseling documentation and consent.

Secure Funding and Resources
- *Budget Planning*: Includes costs for location, equipment, staff, marketing, and initial operating expenses
- *Funding Sources:* Explore private investors, grants, or partnerships with healthcare institutions

- *Space and Equipment Needs:* A welcoming clinic space and equipment for consultations and diagnostics (e.g., bone density scanners) are crucial.

Assembling a Qualified Team

- *Medical Staff:* Include gynecologists, endocrinologists, or general practitioners with expertise in menopause care
- *Support Staff:* Consider psychologists, nutritionists, and physiotherapists for a holistic approach
- *Administrative Team:* Ensure efficient appointment scheduling and patient communication

Develop Clinical Protocols

Establish evidence-based protocols for diagnosis (e.g., evaluating symptoms, hormone level tests, treatment (e.g., HRT, lifestyle advice), monitoring, and follow-up care). Partnership with local labs for tests like hormone panels, bone density scans, etc. may be done.

Educate and Engage the Community

- *Awareness Campaigns*: Host seminars, workshops, or webinars about menopause
- *Patient Education Materials:* Provide resources on symptoms, treatment options, and lifestyle management
- *Community Partnerships:* Collaborate with local health organizations or fitness centers for outreach programs

26.3 Menopausal Card

In menopausal women due to deficiency of estrogen, there are many symptoms (like hot flushes, night sweats, mood swings etc.) and there is an increased risk of many chronic diseases. The health services should be planned according to the needs of menopausal women because they are different from reproductive age. Even the International Classification of Diseases lists this natural phenomenon as a disease to provide coverage to medical care of older women for menopausal problems.

A proper medical record of midlife management is very necessary as it can span for more than two decades of a woman's life. This is the time when she requires preventive care as well as management of her menopausal issues.

A comprehensive systemic medical record with regular checkups and symptom management is the need of the hour to provide appropriate care to midlife women for the rest of life which should be offered to her around 45 years of age.

The menopause card is the most important tool to give comprehensive, appropriate, preventive care and management of menopausal symptoms and long-term issues (Table 26.1).

Table 26.1 Component of menopause card

History	**General examination**	**Breast and vulvovaginal examination**
Lab tests	**Imaging**	**Special tests**

26.4 History

General Questions—Illicit why she is visiting the clinic. Is she complaining or she has just come to discuss preventive care. Her awareness regarding menopause should be judged and entered.

Menstrual History—Details like whether she has attained menopause, years post menopause, type of menopause (Premature/ Natural/Early/ Surgical) should be asked. If surgical menopause then only hysterectomy or ovaries were also removed, indication of hysterectomy, any change in the menstrual cycle before attaining menopause. Any issues during transition, some directed questions like any changes in her mood, any treatment taken for any symptom during transition phase etc. should be asked.

Obstetrical History—Parity, any abortion, self-conception/ any infertility treatment/ IVF, any obstetrical complications like GDM, PIH, history of anticoagulant during pregnancy, and contraception history should be asked.

Medical History—Any known comorbidity, duration, and treatment.

Personal History—Use of tobacco, alcohol, recreational drugs, etc.

Family History—Diabetes/BP/thyroid, cancer (type of cancer, relation with person).

Sexual History—Heterosexual /LGBTQ+, active/ not active. If active- frequency, use of condom, any issues in intimacy should be discussed. Use of some questionnaires is very important. FSFI is a good questionnaire. One can modify for their own use (https://www.apta.org/contentassets/a10dbafd45234c7a98ae3dd98385cdab/fsfi_test.pdf).

Few directed questions about libido, dyspareunia, and vaginal discomfort should be included.

Immunization History—Menopause is a crucial time in life when preventative medical care can make a big difference. However, vaccination recommendations are frequently disregarded, which causes needless illness and mortality in older women. Healthcare professionals have a duty to offer vaccinations and educate patients about vaccination protocols and related risks, given the significance of immunization and the need to reduce vaccine-preventable diseases (Table 26.2) [4].

Psychological Evaluation

Psychological issues are a major part of menopausal transition. Women who have a history of depression, often face more problems due to hormonal fluctuation. Circumstances such as retirement from job, empty nest syndrome, loss of spouse/ apathy of spouse, financial setback, and onset of disabilities, worsen the situation.

Table 26.2 Immunization schedule especially for older females

Name of vaccine	Schedule
Influenza inactivated (IIV3, CCIIV3)Influenza recombinant (RIV3)	1 Dose annually
Zoster recombinant	2 Doses
Pneumococcal vaccination (after 50 years)	1 Dose repeat after 5 years
RSV	Age 75 years or older Unvaccinated: 1 dose (Arexvy or Abrysvo or mResvia). Additional doses not recommended.

Rest routine vaccination should also be checked

26.5 Examination

Detailed general and systematic examination: Age, height/weight/BMI, hip–waist ratio, any facial hairs/sign of acanthosis nigricans, pulse/BP/temperature, CVS/chest/abdomen.

Focused breast and external genital organ examination: Bilateral clinical breast examination. This is the time to teach her to do by herself monthly.

Clinicians play a crucial role in recognizing the signs of GSM because majority of women are reluctant to report these symptoms.

Examination of vulva in detail (any sign of atrophy, any lesion and examination of vagina. Use of tools to document examination at time of booking and further changes or response to treatment is a must.

Few tools for vaginal examination are as follow:

Vaginal Maturation Index (VMI)

By calculating the proportion of superficial, intermediate, and parabasal cells, the VMI shows the level of tissue maturation. The following formula is used to get the maturation value (MV): MV = % surface cells + (0.5 × % intermediate cells) [5].

Genitourinary Syndrome of Menopause and Vaginal Health Index

A method for assessing the level of genitourinary tract atrophy is the Vaginal Health Index Score. By assigning a single score to each of the five parameters—vaginal elasticity, vaginal secretion, pH, epithelial mucous membrane, and vaginal hydration—this method enables us to determine a final score (Table 26.3). Each element is rated from 1 (worst) to 5 (best). More severe atrophy is indicated by lower scores.

Table 26.3 Vaginal Health Index

Score	Overall elasticity	Type of fluid secretion and consistency	Vaginal pH	Vaginal epithelial mucosa	Moisture
1.	None	None	6.1	Petechiae observed prior to contact	None, mucosal inflammation present
2.	Poor (scanty)	Thin-yellow	5.6–6.0	Bleeds with light touch	None, no inflammation of mucosa
3.	Fair (superficial)	Thin-white	5.1–5.5	Bleeds with scraping	Minimal
4.	Good (moderate)	Thin-white	4.7–5.0	Not friable, thin mucosa	Moderate
5.	Excellent	Normal white flocculent	<=4.6	Not friable, normal mucosa	Normal

26.6 Investigations

Laboratory tests—FSH if considering premature ovarian insufficiency.

Annually—CBC, Vitamin D3, B12, TSH, HbAIC, LFT, KFT, urine routine and microscopy, urine culture sensitivity. Pap smear—LBC with HPV done 5 yearly till 65 years.

Imaging—Breast USG and mammography, whole abdomen USG with TVS, central dual X-ray absorptiometry (DXA). Additional tests can be added in special circumstances with type of comorbidities.

Salient features of menopause clinic are:

- Customized treatments
- Room for yoga, acupressure, massage, and exercise
- Focus on a holistic approach toward menopause management
- Multidisciplinary team
- Fall prevention measures equipped building

The term "perimenopause" refers to a time when monthly irregularities, such as amenorrhea, might persist for years. The time of *menopausal transition*, which is linked to the loss of fertility in women over 40, is when hormonal changes that result in both bodily and psychological changes start even earlier.

The severity of menopause can be assessed by following scoring system:

Table 26.4 Modified Greene Scale

	Score before MHT	3 months after starting MHT	6 months after starting MHT
Hot flushes			
Light headed feelings			
Headaches			
Brain fog			
Irritability			
Depression			
Unloved feelings			
Anxiety			
Changes in mood			
Lack of sleep			
Unusual tiredness			
Backache			
Pain in the joints			
Pain in the muscle			
New facial hair			
Dry skin			
A crawling sensation beneath the skin			
Less sexual feelings			
Vaginal dryness			
Uncomfortable sexual intercourse			
Urinary frequency			
TOTAL			

Severity of problem is scored as: None = 0; Mild = 1; Moderate = 2; Severe = 3
(not all of the symptoms listed are necessarily estrogen deficiency symptoms)

Symptom Score (Modified Greene Scale) [6]—It is used to document symptoms and monitor response to treatment. It should NOT be used to diagnose perimenopause or menopause. Perimenopause commences when menstrual cycle changes occur, with differences in length of consecutive cycles. Menstrual cycle changes cannot be used to diagnose perimenopause or menopause for people on hormonal contraception, or who have undergone endometrial ablation or hysterectomy (Table 26.4).

26.7 Osteoporosis

Osteoporosis Screening Tool for Asians (OSTA) [7] is recommended to identify the individual's risk for osteoporosis in clinics as first step and high-risk cases are referred for dual x-ray absorptiometry (DEXA).

26.8 Cardiac Assessment Tool

10-year risk for cardiovascular diseases according to the WHO prediction chart:

Using the best available mortality and risk factor data of these populations in low- and middle-income countries, WHO/ISH risk prediction charts forecast the 10-year risk of combined myocardial infarction and stroke risk, both fatal and non-fatal. Although these charts are necessarily crude but they are straightforward, secure, and helpful resources for directing individual management and treatment choices. The charts may help avoid heart attacks and strokes, especially if primary healthcare providers are able to utilize them [8].

Sarcopenia assessment—SARC-F score:

- The total score range is from 0 to 10 (0–2 points for each component; 0 = best to 10 = worst).
- Assess for signs of sarcopenia; the European Working Group on Sarcopenia in Older People 2 (EWGSOP2) suggests using a chair stand test or grip strength with particular cut-off values for each test.
- EWGSOP2 sarcopenia cut-off points for low strength by chair stand and grip strength: Grip strength <16 kg, Chair stand >15 s for five rise (Table 26.5).

Table 26.5 SARC-F questionnaire

Component	Question	Scoring
Strength	How hard is it for you to lift and carry ten pounds?	None—0 Some—1 A lot or unable—2
Assistance in walking	How hard is it for you to walk across a room?	None—0 Some—1 A lot, use aids, or unable—2
Rise from a chair	How hard is it for you to get out of bed or a chair?	None—0 Some—1 A lot or incapable without assistance—2
Climb stairs	How hard is it for you to climb ten steps?	None—0 Some—1 A lot or unable—2
Falls	In the last year, how many times have you fallen?	None—0 1–3 falls—1 ≥3 falls—2

26.9 Menopause Hormone Therapy

Before starting MHT, certain objectives should be fulfilled like proper counseling, discussion with the patient, all pros and cons, and documentation of whole discussion and information about alternative treatments. For hormone replacement therapy to be effective, the menopausal symptoms must be accurately identified. Adequate knowledge of the several kinds of progesterone and estrogen treatments available for hormone replacement therapy is crucial. Menopausal symptoms can be effectively treated with hormone replacement therapy by following clinical guidelines. Apply interprofessional team strategies to improve care coordination and outcomes in patients using hormonal replacement treatment [9].

To address female sexual dysfunction in midlife women, sometime testosterone therapy is used:

Testosterone therapy indications

After conventional HRT has been tried and other explanations have been ruled out, women with female sexual interest and arousal dysfunction may benefit from the addition of testosterone medication. Currently, no FDA-approved testosterone product is available for women. However, transdermal testosterone therapy at a dose suitable for postmenopausal women may be used to increase sexual desire, arousal, and orgasm.

Testosterone (gel/cream) should be applied to clean, dry skin on the upper thighs or lower abdomen. Hands should be washed immediately after application, and contact with others should be avoided until it is completely dry. After application, the area shouldn't be washed for two to three hours. In 2019, a global consensus statement regarding testosterone treatment was made after a collaboration between several international confederations to provide clearer guidelines for clinicians who prescribe testosterone to postmenopausal women.

As per some recommendations, total testosterone and sex hormone binding globulin should be measured prior to starting testosterone therapy and consent for Hormone Replacement Therapy should be taken. To ensure that testosterone levels are not greater than usual for premenopausal women, ACOG advises measuring testosterone levels at baseline, three months, and six months after treatment begins [10].

Tailor-made MHT prescription and informed consent [11]

With customized treatment programs that take into account each woman's risk factors, a patient-centered approach is essential. The patient's values and preferences are crucial to the treatment process when the patient and the medical team collaborate to make decisions. Frequent monitoring and follow-up enable therapy modifications, maximizing efficacy and safety. Informed consent, in which patients are given impartial, explicit information regarding the advantages and disadvantages of hormone replacement therapy, is one of the most important ethical factors.

Consent for Hormone Replacement Therapy for Women

The "Informed Consent Form" is intended to educate women about Menopause Hormone Therapy (MHT). Before deciding whether to consent to this therapy, the woman is advised to carefully read this form and ask any questions. As with any treatment, there may be advantages and disadvantages to both alternative therapy and treatment. All treatment options have the potential risk complications and poor outcomes.

The woman is asked if she has an absolute or relative lack of any hormones, such as progesterone, testosterone, estrogen, or a mix of these. Hormonal supplements may be beneficial for her. The main goal is to provide the woman with the most up-to-date treatment options. She should be aware of the rationale for the prescription of this therapy as well as the possible hazards associated with it and the possibility of treatment refusal.

It is vital to let her know that there are significant controversies about the best ways to diagnose and treat menopausal and perimenopausal symptoms, as well as the best ways to monitor therapy. She should be provided with comprehensive information so that she may comprehend the rationale for the diagnosis, the course of therapy, and the possible risks and advantages. She should thoroughly understand the potential risks and benefits of therapy, and then only give consent for treatment.

Expected benefits of hormone replacement therapy may include control of the symptoms brought on by declining hormone levels. It may help prevent, reduce, or control physical ailments and dysfunction associated with decreasing estrogen levels. The long-term effects of these hormones have not been established, especially in relation to thrombosis, cardiovascular disease, and breast cancer.

Estrogen (estradiol and/or estriol)

This hormone can be administered via troche, cream, patch, oral tablet, or subdermal pellet. When taken during the first ten years of menopause, this hormone reduces hot flashes, nocturnal sweats, and vaginal dryness, lowers the risk of osteoporosis and cardiovascular disease, and boosts energy and well-being. Additionally, this hormone improves memory and cognition, lowers the risk of dementia, and helps with sleep and urinary incontinence.

Testosterone

There are various ways to administer this hormone. These methods include injection, troche, subdermal pellet, and transdermal cream. The FDA has not authorized the use of testosterone in postmenopausal women. Reduced hot flashes, increased libido, energy, and well-being, less frequent and severe headaches, increased energy, increased muscle mass and decreased visceral fat, increased insulin sensitivity, prevention of osteoporosis, decreased risk of dementia, improved cognition and memory, assistance with sleep problems, lower risk of reproductive cancers, and lower risk of cardiovascular disease are some benefits of using this hormone.

Risks of testosterone replacement are erythrocytosis, decreased insulin requirements in insulin-dependent diabetics, elevated estradiol levels, edema (fluid retention), reproductive malignancies, and cardiovascular disease.

Side effects of testosterone: enlarged clitoris, hair loss, temporary water retention, acne, irritability, and voice changes. Most of the side effects are resolved after reducing the dose. Premenopausal women must use some form of contraception to prevent accidental pregnancy and embryopathy.

Alternative to Hormone Replacement Therapy

The patient should be aware of the following alternatives to hormone replacement therapy which simply lessen the symptoms of hormone insufficiency; and do not replace hormones. This alternative can necessitate treating illnesses or dysfunctions linked to declining hormone levels.

These complementary therapies include sleeping medications, herbal remedies, essential oils, selective serotonin uptake inhibitors (antidepressants), and lifestyle changes including yoga, stress reduction, and weight loss.

Some of these hormones are used "off-label," meaning the FDA has not approved them, consulting a different healthcare professional who supports the use of FDA-approved menopausal treatments and/or nonbioidentical synthetic hormones like Premarin.

Signed by a patient with name and date ....

26.10 Marketing of Menopausal Clinic

- Digital Presence: Create a professional website and use social media to share information and success stories.
- Referral Networks: Connect with local GPs and gynecologists to establish referral relationships.
- Patient Testimonials: Encourage satisfied patients to share their experiences.

Evaluate and improve: Regularly collect feedback through surveys or interviews. Stay updated on the latest menopause research and integrate innovations into your practice. Measure success through patient outcomes and satisfaction.

In a nut shell, menopausal clinic should have: old age friendly architecture, compassionate staff, dedicated trained menopause specialists, and multidisciplinary clinics. Educational materials and support groups should be formed.

Key Points

- A menopause clinic offers specialized, comprehensive, and empathetic care tailored to the unique needs of midlife women.
- They serve as vital hubs for preventive health. Menopause is a critical window for screening and managing long-term health risks such as heart disease, metabolic syndrome, and cognitive decline.

- Equally important is the role of these clinics in education and empowerment. They provide women with accurate information, dispel myths, and foster informed decision-making about their bodies and treatment options.
- In an era advocating gender-equitable, life-stage-appropriate care, menopause clinics are no longer a luxury but a necessity. They represent a shift from reactive to proactive care, ensuring that women in midlife receive the attention, respect, and medical support they deserve.

- By working as a cohesive team and involving the patient in every step of the decision-making process, results are better, care is safer, and the patient experience is enhanced.

Long Answer Questions (LAQs)

1. What is the rationale behind setting up a menopausal clinic?
2. What are the aims of menopausal clinic?
3. What is menopausal card? What are its components?
4. What are the prerequisites of setting up a menopausal clinic?

Short Answer Questions (SAQs)

1. What are the questionnaires that can be used in a menopausal clinic?
2. What do you understand by "Tailor-made MHT prescription"?
3. Write short notes on "Informed consent" regarding MHT.
4. How should the functioning of menopausal clinic be evaluated and improved?

Multiple Choice Questions (MCQs)

1. What is the dose schedule of pneumococcal vaccine after 50 years?
   A. One dose only
   B. 2 Doses
   C. 3 Doses
   D. None of the above
2. Which is the most common hormone whose deficiency leads to menopausal symptoms?
   A. Estrogen
   B. Progesterone
   C. Androgen
   D. All of the above.
3. Which tool is used for detecting genitourinary atrophy?
   A. OSTA
   B. DEXA

   C. VMI
   D. None of the above
4. What is the recommendation of ACOG for testing testosterone level before starting testosterone therapy?
   A. Testing baseline testosterone level at 3 months and at 6 months
   B. No need for testing testosterone level
   C. Testing at 3 months
   D. Testing at 3 months and 6 months
5. Which test is commonly done for detection of osteoporosis?
   A. DEXA scan
   B. X ray
   C. USG
   D. None of the above
6. Pap smear is recommended till what age?
   A. 50 years
   B. 55 years
   C. 60 years
   D. 65 years

Answers

1. B
2. D
3. C
4. A
5. A
6. D

References

1. World Health Organization. Menopause. World Health Organization; 2024. Available from: https://www.who.int/news-room/fact-sheets/detail/menopause.
2. Meeta M, Aggarwal N, Chawla N. Menopause management: a manual for primary care practitioners and nurse practitioners. J Mid-Life Health. 2022;13(5):2.
3. Paszkowski T, Bińkowska M, Dębski R, Krzyczkowska-Sendrakowska M, Skrzypulec-Plinta V, Zgliczyński W. Menopausal hormone therapy in questions and answers—a manual for physicians of various specialties. Menopausal Rev. 2019;18(1):1–8.
4. Brown V. Immunization for midlife women. Menopause. 2022;29(10):1204–9.
5. Domenici L, Musella A, Bracchi C, Lecce F, Schiavi MC, Colagiovanni V, et al. Comparison of anogenital distance and correlation with vulvo-vaginal atrophy: a pilot study on premenopausal and postmenopausal women. J Menopausal Med. 2018;24(2):108.
6. Greene JG. Constructing a standard climacteric standard. Maturitas. 1998;29:25–31.
7. Latt TS, Aye TT, Ko K, Myint T, Thaung M, Chit TT. Myanmar clinical practice guideline for osteoporosis. J ASEAN Fed Endocr Soc. 2012;27(2):151–5.

8. World Health Organization. Cardiovascular diseases (CVDs) [internet]. World Health Organisation; 2021. Available from: https://www.who.int/news-room/fact-sheets/detail/cardiovascular-diseases-(cvds).
9. Harper-Harrison G, Shanahan MM, Carlson K. Hormone replacement therapy [internet]. National Library of Medicine: StatPearls Publishing; 2023. Available from: https://www.ncbi.nlm.nih.gov/books/NBK493191/.
10. Levy B, Simon JA. A contemporary view of menopausal hormone therapy. Obstetrics and gynecology (New York 1953 Online)/Obstetrics and Gynecology. 2024.
11. Consent for Hormone Replacement Therapy for Women. Available from: https://www.rhett-womenscenter.com/wp-content/uploads/2018/09/Hormone-Consent-Women.pdf.

Artificial Intelligence in Menopause

27

Meenakshi Ahuja, Aarshika Singh, and Yukti Wadhawan

Abstract

Artificial intelligence (AI) is emerging as a transformative tool in menopausal healthcare, offering solutions that move beyond traditional, generalized approaches. Menopause, a universal yet highly individualized transition, is often associated with vasomotor symptoms, mood disturbances, cognitive changes, and increased risks of osteoporosis and cardiovascular disease. Conventional management strategies rely on subjective assessment and broad treatment protocols, leaving gaps in personalized care. AI technologies—including machine learning, natural language processing, and digital therapeutics—are bridging these gaps by enabling individualized symptom tracking, predicting menopausal onset, stratifying long-term health risks, and optimizing hormone therapy. AI-powered wearables, apps, and chatbots are expanding accessibility, providing real-time support, and empowering women with tailored guidance. These innovations hold potential to improve quality of life while enhancing clinical decision-making and research. However, significant challenges remain, including algorithmic bias, data privacy concerns, limited validation, and ethical considerations. Realizing the promise of AI in menopause care will require robust clinical trials, regulatory oversight, and inclusive datasets. This article reviews current applications, highlights opportunities, and underscores the need for responsible integration of AI into routine menopause management.

Keywords

Artificial intelligence · Menopausal healthcare · Osteoporosis · Cardiovascular · AI

M. Ahuja (✉) · A. Singh
Fortis la femme, New Delhi, India

Y. Wadhawan
Yukti IVF & Gynaecology, New Delhi, India

R. Malik et al. (eds.), *Menopause Essentials*,
https://doi.org/10.1007/978-981-95-7498-8_27

27.1 Introduction

Artificial intelligence (AI) is rapidly transforming the landscape of healthcare, and its integration into menopausal care represents a promising frontier. Menopause, a natural biological transition affecting millions globally, presents a variety of symptoms ranging from vasomotor disturbances and mood changes to long-term risks such as osteoporosis and cardiovascular disease. Traditional approaches to diagnosis and treatment often rely on subjective assessment and generalized protocols, failing to account for individual variability in symptom presentation and progression.

AI, particularly through machine learning (ML) and natural language processing (NLP), offers the potential for personalized, data-driven management of menopause. Applications include symptom tracking through wearable technology, prediction of menopausal onset using genomic and clinical data, cognitive decline risk stratification, and digital therapeutics for hormone replacement therapy (HRT) optimization. Moreover, chatbots and telemedicine platforms powered by AI have enhanced patient engagement and access to care, particularly during the COVID-19 pandemic.

Despite these advances, the use of AI in menopause care is still nascent. Concerns about algorithmic bias, data privacy, lack of clinical validation, and ethical issues remain significant. Integrating AI into routine practice will require rigorous clinical trials, regulatory oversight, and inclusive datasets that reflect the diversity of menopausal experiences. This chapter explores the role of AI in menopause—from technological innovations to clinical applications and prospects—highlighting both its transformative potential and the challenges that must be addressed to harness it effectively.

Menopause, defined as the cessation of menstruation for twelve consecutive months, marks a significant phase in a woman's life and is associated with multifaceted physiological and psychological changes. While it is a natural biological transition, the associated symptoms can significantly affect quality of life. Common symptoms include hot flashes, mood disturbances, sleep difficulties, and cognitive impairments, in addition to long-term risks such as osteoporosis and cardiovascular disease [1]. Traditional approaches to menopause management rely heavily on clinical judgment, symptom diaries, and general treatment guidelines. These methods often lack personalization and fail to incorporate the multifactorial nature of the menopausal transition, which can vary widely across individuals based on genetics, environment, comorbidities, and cultural context [2].

The rise of artificial intelligence (AI) has brought transformative potential to healthcare, promising data-driven personalization of care. AI encompasses machine learning (ML), natural language processing (NLP), and deep learning (DL)—technologies capable of analyzing vast datasets to uncover patterns, predict outcomes, and assist clinical decision-making [3]. In women's health, AI applications have traditionally focused on areas such as breast cancer detection, fertility prediction, and obstetric monitoring. However, menopause care remains an underexplored but critical domain.

This chapters aims to bridge that gap by exploring how AI can revolutionize menopause management. From symptom tracking to risk prediction and therapeutic decision-making, AI offers the potential to personalize care, enhance accessibility, and improve outcomes. We also examine current limitations, ethical concerns, and the future direction of AI in this space.

27.2 Understanding Menopause

Menopause typically occurs between the ages of 45 and 55, with the average age around 51. The transition, known as perimenopause, can span several years and is marked by hormonal fluctuations, particularly a decline in estrogen levels [4]. This hormonal shift affects multiple organ systems and manifests as vasomotor symptoms (hot flashes, night sweats), sleep disturbances, anxiety, depression, and memory lapses. In the long term, reduced estrogen increases the risk of osteoporosis, cardiovascular disease, and cognitive decline [5].

Managing menopause requires a multidisciplinary approach, involving gynecologists, endocrinologists, psychiatrists, and sometimes neurologists. However, a lack of menopause-specific training among healthcare professionals, combined with underreporting of symptoms by patients, contributes to gaps in care [6]. These complexities present an opportunity for AI-driven tools to assist in early detection, symptom profiling, and individualized treatment plans.

27.3 The Rise of AI in Healthcare

AI in healthcare is primarily used for prediction, classification, image recognition, natural language processing, and decision support. AI models are trained on electronic health records (EHRs), wearable sensor data, medical imaging, genomics, and patient-reported outcomes. In recent years, FDA-approved AI applications include algorithms for diabetic retinopathy detection, breast cancer risk prediction, and cardiac event forecasting [7].

Key AI techniques used in healthcare include:

- Supervised learning: Trains models using labeled datasets (e.g., hot flash severity scores) to predict future outcomes.
- Unsupervised learning: Identifies hidden patterns (e.g., clustering menopausal profiles based on symptoms).
- Reinforcement learning: Useful in optimizing treatment strategies over time.
- Natural Language Processing (NLP): Extracts insights from clinical notes and patient feedback.

Given the growing interest in personalized medicine, AI offers promising opportunities to tailor menopause management to individual needs, accounting for lifestyle, symptoms, and biomarkers [8].

27.4 AI Applications in Menopausal Symptom Management

27.4.1 Vasomotor Symptoms and Wearable Tech

Vasomotor symptoms (VMS) such as hot flashes and night sweats affect up to 80% of menopausal women and significantly impair sleep and daily functioning. Traditional symptom tracking relies on self-reported diaries, which are subjective and intermittent. AI-enhanced wearables bring objectivity and continuity to this domain.

For example, the Embr Wave device combines a wrist-worn cooling mechanism with an onboard ML algorithm that monitors skin temperature, heart rate, sweat, and activity levels to detect imminent hot flashes. Once early physiological signs are recognized, the device activates cooling, potentially interrupting or softening the flash within seconds.

Similarly, identifyHer (Peri) is a torso-adhering biosensor platform optimized for detecting hot flashes, night sweats, sleep changes, and anxiety during perimenopause. Its ML-based "digital fingerprints" were developed to isolate symptomatic signals from confounders such as ambient temperature and exercise.

Wearables like Oura rings, in collaboration with Clue and academic researchers, are being studied to capture heart rate variability, skin temperature, and sleep patterns in relation to menopausal phases. These data streams, when analyzed by AI, could illuminate early perimenopause markers and improve symptom anticipation.

A pilot study applying AI to sternal skin conductance achieved 81% sensitivity and 97% specificity in VMS detection. Through adaptive feedback loops, these systems may personalize behavioral or cooling interventions in real time.

27.4.2 Mood and Sleep Tracking

AI-powered mobile apps and chatbots are emerging to monitor and support emotional and behavioral health during menopause.

The Caria digital therapeutic app uses ML to assess self-reported mood and sleep metrics, offering personalized cognitive-behavioral therapy techniques and lifestyle recommendations. A randomized evaluation found Caria significantly reduced hot flashes and improved behavioral health scores in menopausal women [9].

NLP-enabled chatbots like Vira Health's "Stella" provide context-aware counseling on symptom management, including mood swings and insomnia. These bots typically score above 4 out of 5 in clinical faithfulness and relevance.

Apps also use mood prediction models incorporating voice analysis, typing behaviors, and wearable data. By providing just-in-time mental health support, these tools may alleviate menopause-related distress without requiring clinician access.